ATLAS OF FOOT AND ANKLE SURGERY

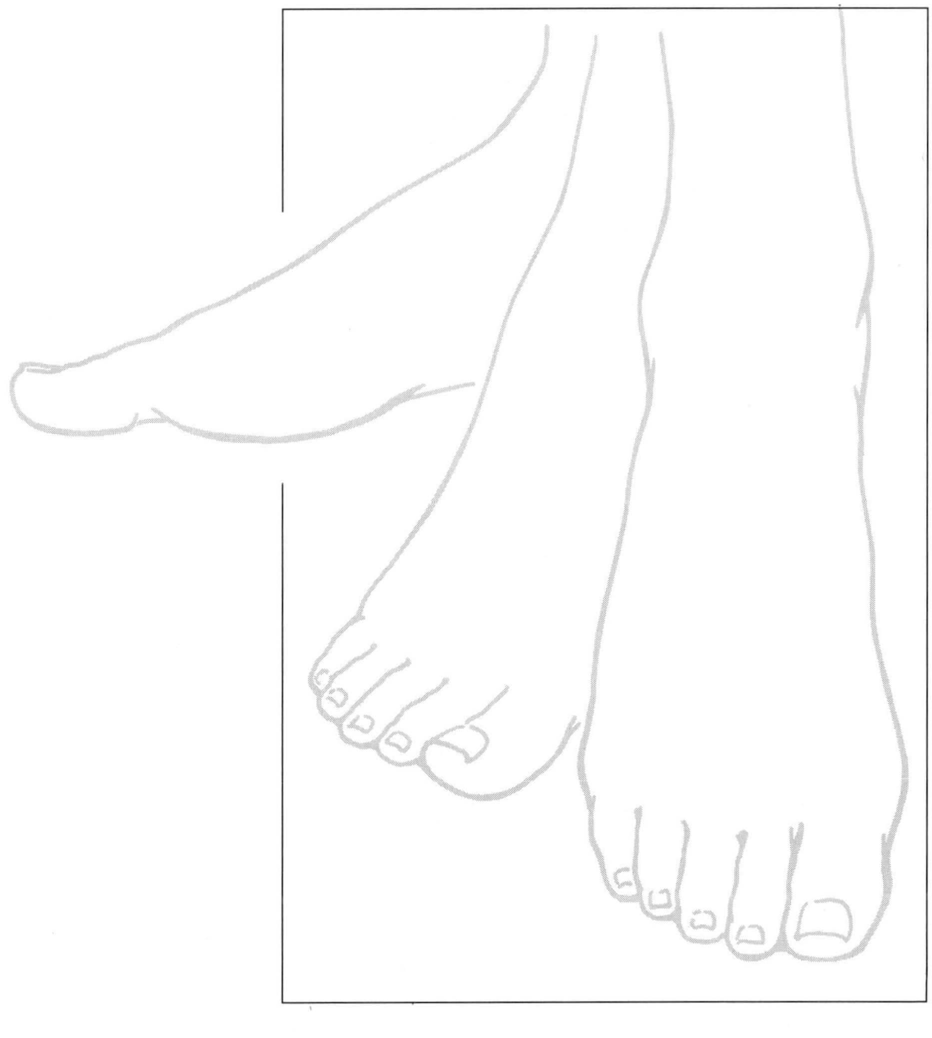

Illustrated by

PAT THOMAS

Certified Medical Illustrator, AMI

W.B. SAUNDERS COMPANY

A Division of Harcourt Brace & Company

Philadelphia London Toronto Montreal Sydney Tokyo

MICHAEL J. SHEREFF, M.D.
Director, Division of Foot and Ankle Surgery
Associate Professor, Department of Orthopaedic Surgery
Medical College of Wisconsin
Milwaukee, Wisconsin

ATLAS OF FOOT AND ANKLE SURGERY

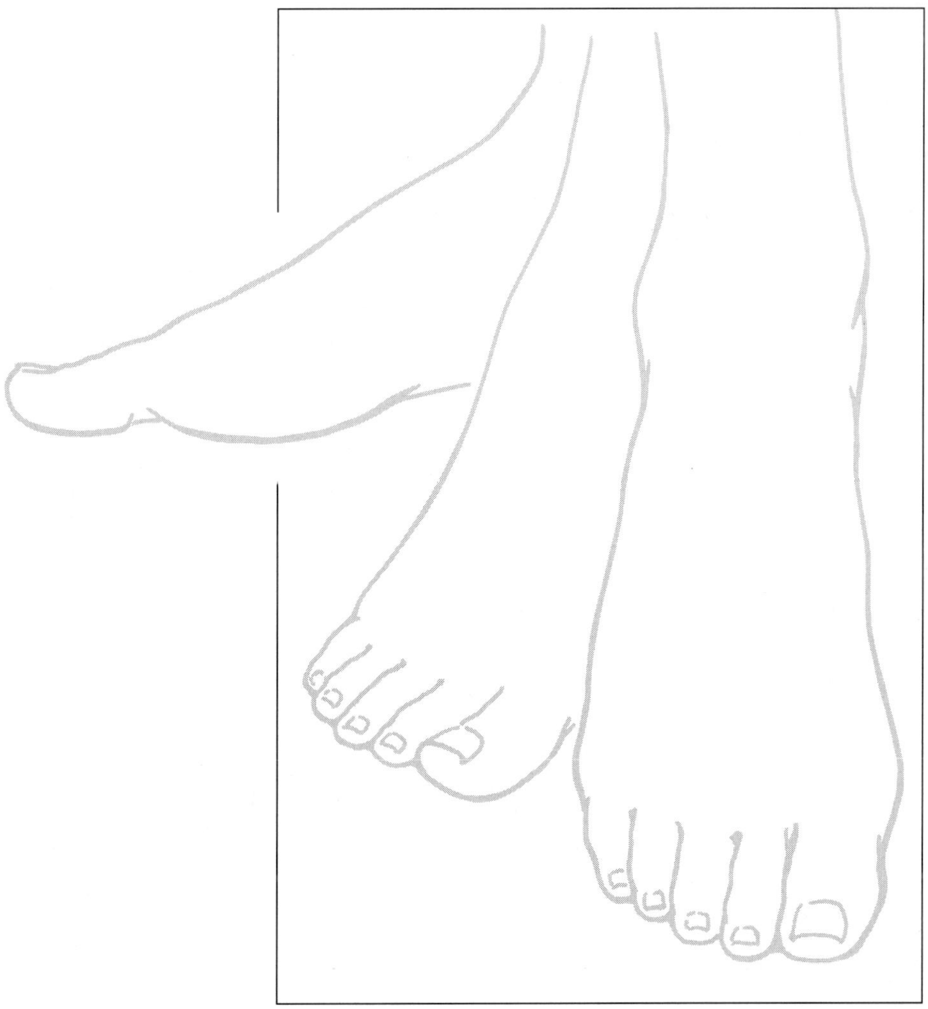

W. B. SAUNDERS COMPANY
A Division of
Harcourt Brace & Company

The Curtis Center
Independence Square West
Philadelphia, Pennsylvania 19106

Library of Congress Cataloging-in-Publication Data

Shereff, Michael J.
Atlas of foot and ankle surgery / Michael J. Shereff; illustrated by Pat Thomas.

p. cm.

ISBN 0–7216–3537–7

1. Foot—Abnormalities—Surgery—Atlases. 2. Ankle—Abnormalities—Surgery—Atlases. I. Title. [DNLM: 1. Ankle—surgery—atlases. 2. Foot—surgery—atlases. WE 17 S551a]

RD781.S53 1993

617.5′85059—dc20

DNLM/DLC 90-19403

Atlas of Foot and Ankle Surgery ISBN 0–7216–3537–7

Printed in the United States of America.

Last digit is the print number: 9 8 7 6 5 4 3 2 1

To my wife, Cobby, for her enthusiasm, support, and love.

To my children, Rebecca and Daniel, for their patience and understanding.

To my parents for providing me with the opportunities
with which to accomplish my goals.

Preface

The evaluation and treatment of disorders of the foot and ankle have been long neglected in the orthopaedic literature. Detailed descriptions of relevant surgical procedures and operative techniques can be found in few textbooks and only sporadically in journal articles. The subspecialty field of foot and ankle surgery has attracted more interest in recent times, as evidenced by the establishment and development of The American Orthopaedic Foot and Ankle Society, as well as the publication of the official journal of that organization, *Foot and Ankle.*

The purpose of this text is to provide a step-by-step description of some of the more common surgical procedures utilized for the correction of disorders of the foot and ankle. It is hoped that this atlas will serve as a guide to both residents in training and practicing orthopedists in clinical decision-making and preparation prior to surgery.

To present surgical techniques in a concise manner, each operative description has been structured to include the following:

- An introductory statement as to the purpose of the procedure
- Indications
- Contraindications
- Operative technique presented in a stepwise manner
- Postoperative care
- Technical pitfalls
- Potential complications

Each surgical procedure is illustrated by drawings to provide insight into technical details. It is anticipated that this atlas will be used in conjunction with a more traditional textbook of foot and ankle disorders to give the practitioner a complete understanding of the history, development, and expected outcome of the surgical procedures described.

Acknowledgments

I would like to express my heartfelt appreciation to all those individuals who have devoted their time and effort to the production of this textbook.

I would like to thank my devoted teachers and colleagues at The Hospital for Joint Diseases, Orthopaedic Institute; The Mayo Clinic and Graduate School of Medicine; and The Medical College of Wisconsin. These wonderful people provided me with their insight and expertise regarding the subspecialty field of orthopaedic foot and ankle surgery. In particular, I am indebted to Melvin H. Jahss, MD, Kenneth A. Johnson, MD, and John S. Gould, MD, for their wisdom and friendship.

I would like to thank my former fellows from whom I learned so much and who instilled in me their enthusiasm.

I would like to thank my colleagues in The American Orthopaedic Foot and Ankle Society who imparted their knowledge freely at various meetings and courses.

I would like to thank my secretary, Rani Eckenrod, who devoted extensive time and effort in the organization and preparation of this work.

I am indebted to the editors at W.B. Saunders for their guidance and support. I would like to thank Ed Wickland, Jennifer Mitchell, and Kathleen McCarthy for their personal attention, as well as their sage advice.

I am most grateful to Wendy Harrison Hashmall, whose enthusiasm and judicious counsel enabled me to bring this project to fruition.

Most importantly, I will always be indebted to Pat Thomas, the medical illustrator with whom I have been so fortunate to work on this project. Her creative talents and organizational abilities have made this arduous task a joyful one.

Introduction

This textbook is designed as a general guide outlining some of the more common surgical procedures utilized in orthopaedic foot and ankle surgery. The reader is advised to consult any of the fine textbooks listed in the bibliography section to review those operative techniques not included in this volume.

Each individual patient presents a unique clinical problem. The surgical technique used must be tailored to each specific case. Variations in technique are required for each patient depending on the specific clinical presentation, as well as the medical status, activity level, and temperament of the patient. In addition, the quality of the soft tissue and osseous structures encountered may dictate modifications of the operative procedure. Based on these and other factors, the surgeon will be required to alter his or her approach, including choice of instruments, suture material, and the nature of internal fixation implants. It will often be necessary for the surgeon to add, delete, or modify various steps of the operation.

This textbook should not be used as the sole source of information for the surgeon preparing for an operative case. The reader should review the procedure in one or more of the standard textbooks of orthopedic foot and ankle surgery prior to its performance. In particular, readers are referred to one or more of the following classic works:

Gould, J.S. Operative Foot Surgery. Philadelphia: W.B. Saunders, 1993.

Jahss, M.A. Disorders of the Foot and Ankle: Medical and Surgical Management. 2nd ed. Philadelphia: W.B. Saunders, 1991.

Johnson, K.A. Surgery of the Foot and Ankle. New York: Raven Press, 1989.

Mann, R.A. Surgery of the Foot. 5th ed. St. Louis: C.V. Mosby, 1986.

Contents

SECTION 3

Midfoot

SECTION 4

Hindfoot

SECTION 5

Ankle

SECTION 1

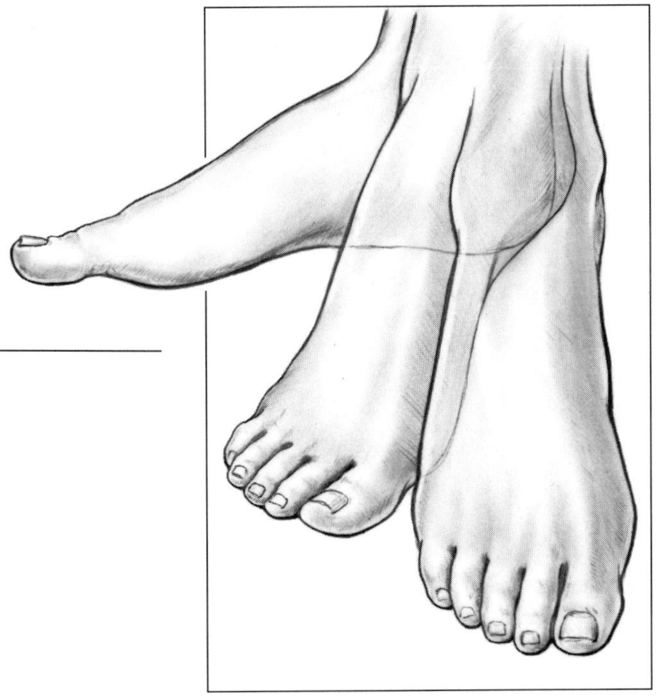

General Principles of Foot and Ankle Surgery

GENERAL CONSIDERATIONS

The foot serves as a platform that supports body weight during standing. It also functions as a lever that raises and propels the body forward during ambulation and other activities. The foot is truly the focal point to which all body weight is transmitted in weight-bearing activities. It is well designed for this function in part because of the thick heel and toe pads on the plantar surface of the foot that absorb the shock associated with standing and ambulation.

The foot consists of 33 joints that allow for adjustments required for effective balance on a variety of terrains. Despite this ability to adjust, however, the stresses applied to the foot during activities of daily living may lead to problems. Because of the magnitude of the forces applied to the distal peripheral extremity, the foot is particularly susceptible to the development of numerous acquired deformities that do not occur elsewhere in the musculoskeletal system. Common examples include hallux valgus, disorders of the lesser toes, interdigital neuromas, and metatarsalgia. In addition, these same stresses may be responsible for the fact that the foot is a common site of manifestation of various general systemic disorders, including diabetes, arthritis, and other metabolic and infectious arthropathies.

Disorders of the foot and ankle have been the source of much interest on the part of orthopedic surgeons and other clinicians. This is in part because of the fact that foot disorders are common in the general population. An epidemiologic study performed at the University of Vermont estimated that 40% of the American population have foot problems, with 74 million people affected each year. The vast majority of foot and ankle disorders are most appropriately treated with conservative modalities. Most of these clinical problems respond to nonoperative measures such as shoe modifications, pads, inserts, and medications. Surgery is the last resort and should be reserved for patients in whom conservative measures have failed to provide relief of symptoms. It is important that patients are educated with regard to the limitations of surgical intervention. In certain cases surgery may serve to alleviate pain and improve deformity in the lower extremity. It can also improve the structural configuration of the extremity and thus provide a more plantigrade foot that may allow the patient to wear relatively normal footwear and improve the patient's ability to ambulate. Unfortunately, surgery cannot re-create a normal foot. The patient should be provided with realistic expectations as to the results of surgical intervention for disorders of the foot and ankle.

PREOPERATIVE DISCUSSION

Part of the physician's responsibility is to instruct the patient regarding the nature of the disease process, as well as the treatment recommended. Clinical evaluation includes the initial patient history and physical examination. During both this initial interaction and subsequent visits, the physician should take the opportunity to develop a sense of cooperation with the patient. Only after failure of conservative modalities of treatment should surgical intervention be considered. Alternative forms of treatment, which usually consist of continued nonoperative measures, should be discussed in great detail. The nature of the surgery is explained, and the patient is encouraged to ask questions related to the operative technique as well as postoperative care. Possible problems and complications of the specific operation, in addition to those associated with foot and ankle surgery in general, are discussed. Problems that can occur in foot and ankle surgery include, among others, infection, permanent numbness, tender scar, joint stiffness, and loss of motion. A limp may be associated with decreased motion at the articulations of the distal peripheral extremity. A prolonged period of postoperative pain and swelling is typical following many surgical procedures in the foot and ankle. The fact that all the body weight is transmitted through the foot may be the reason for the slow resolution of postoperative symptoms. Recurrence of deformity and pain is possible, and unfortunately, further progression of symptoms may occur even after the surgical procedure.

Most importantly, the patient must be provided with realistic expectations regarding the results of surgical procedures in the foot and ankle. Surgery will not restore the foot and ankle to its preinjury or predisease state. Medicine is not a precise science, and there is great individual variation with respect to healing and ultimate recovery. There is no way to predict to what extent preoperative symptoms will be relieved, if at all, and there is no guarantee that surgery will be successful. The patient should understand that preoperative symptoms and deformity may persist or recur. The patient should also be informed that further surgery may be required in the future.

A patient who is well informed and well educated will have realistic expectations with regard to the outcome of the surgical intervention. The patient must be willing to accept the possible risks and complications of surgery in hopes of obtaining partial relief of symptoms. The preoperative discussion provides the physician with the opportunity to instill in the patient the desire to participate in the treatment plan and an understanding of the goals and limitations of foot and ankle surgery.

PREOPERATIVE EVALUATION

The preoperative visit provides the physician with the opportunity to plan the proposed surgical procedure. The physician correlates the physical examination of the patient with the preoperative radiographic evaluation. The laboratory results are also reviewed. Evaluation prior to surgery may include the review of the results of consultations with other physicians. The patient's primary care physician is often consulted with regard to medical clearance for surgery and anesthesia. Preoperative anesthesia evaluation may be helpful in acquainting the anesthesiologist with the patient's medical status. Consultation with a neurologist may be appropriate in those cases in which an underlying neuropathic disorder is suspected, and a vascular evaluation is commonly necessary to ascertain the status of the circulation to the distal peripheral extremity prior to surgery. Patients who have had previous surgeries may benefit from preoperative evaluation or even intraoperative assistance by a plastic surgeon, who may provide valuable insight into the placement of operative incisions, advisability of various surgical approaches, and techniques of wound closure. Patients who have other associated medical disorders should be reviewed by their primary care physicians or other medical specialists with regard to requirements for perioperative medication and other modalities. In particular, consideration is given to those patients requiring perioperative antibiotics, steroids, anticoagulants, or other medications for underlying systemic disorders.

Preoperative evaluation and instruction by a physiatrist or a physical therapist may be appropriate. Preoperative ambulation training with crutches may allow early discharge from the hospital and more rapid rehabilitation.

INSTRUMENTATION

Foot and ankle surgery requires the use of fine instruments for meticulous and precise handling of soft tissue and osseous structures. These instruments must be kept in good working order. Drill points, osteotomes, and other cutting instruments must be kept sharp. It is most helpful to review the required instrumentation with the surgical nursing staff prior to the procedure. In addition, the foot and ankle surgeon should establish a standardized instrument tray that includes instruments commonly used for soft tissue and bone surgery in the distal peripheral extremity.

Instruments required for handling of soft tissue include forceps, retractors, hemostats, and probes (Fig. 1). Incision and sharp dissection of soft tissue structures require scalpels and various types of scissors (Fig. 2).

Instruments required for exposure, cutting, and shaping of osseous structures include periosteal elevators, osteotomes, a mallet, an awl, rongeurs, bone cutters, curets, and rasps (Fig. 3).

Special instruments utilized for specific operative techniques reviewed in this textbook include the lamina spreader, Marin reamers, the Johnson neuroma retractor, and the Hewsen or other tendon passer (Fig. 4). Instruments frequently needed to determine linear and angular measurements include a ruler and a digital goniometer (Fig. 5).

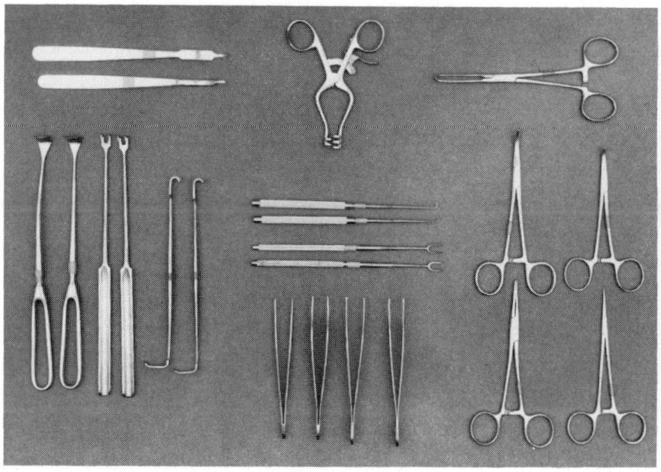
FIGURE 1

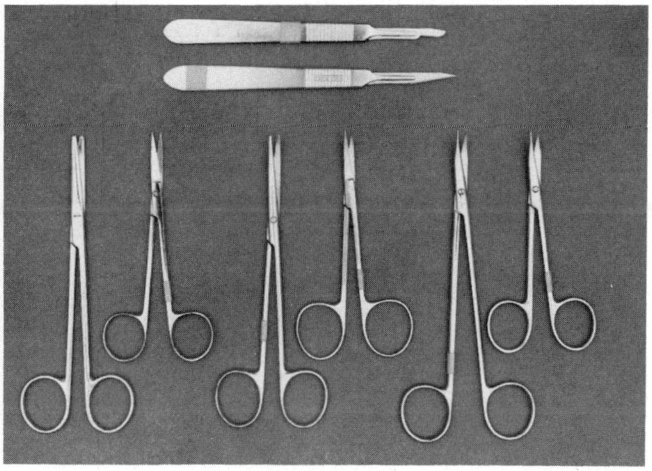
FIGURE 2

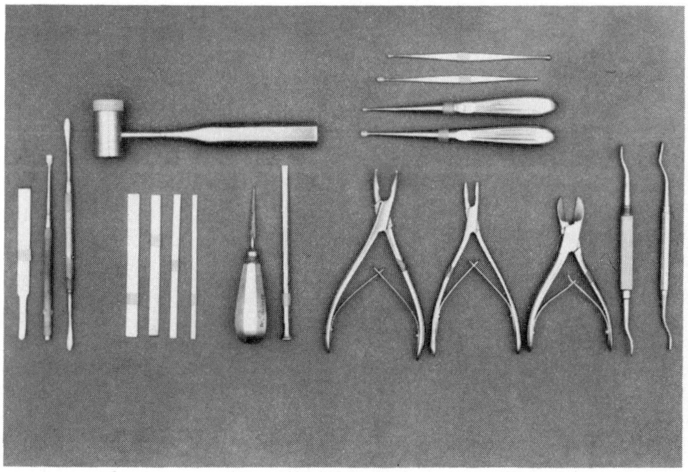
FIGURE 3

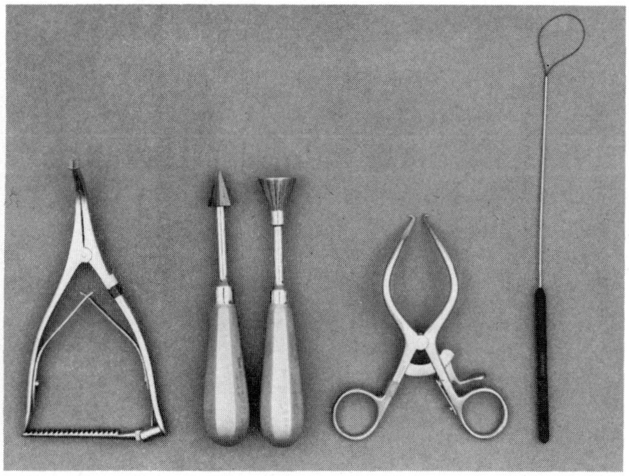
FIGURE 4

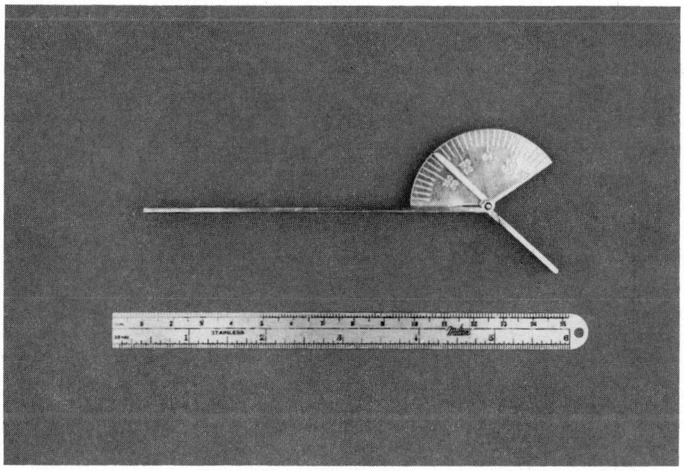
FIGURE 5

Power instruments commonly utilized include a small microsagittal saw (Fig. 6), a micro-oscillating saw (Fig. 7), a wire driver, and a small power drill (Fig. 8).

Internal fixation devices used for foot and ankle surgery include small fragment implants and instruments for osteosynthesis, including cancellous screws, cortical screws, various small plates; K wires; and smooth Steinmann pins (Fig. 9). Arthrodesis, osteotomy, and internal fixation may sometimes require a cortical or cancellous bone graft. A separate bone graft instrument tray is used for such procedures (Fig. 10).

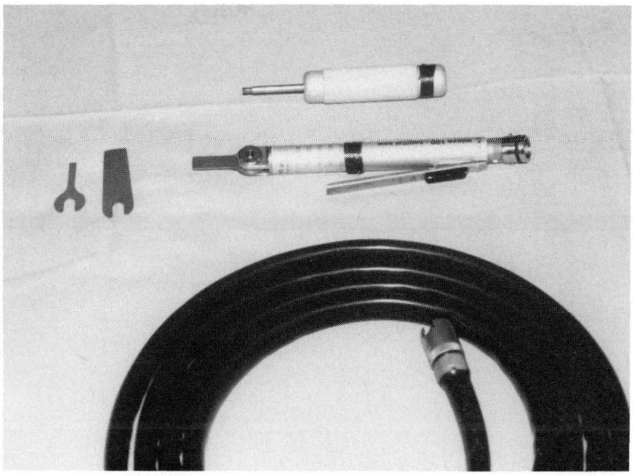

FIGURE 6

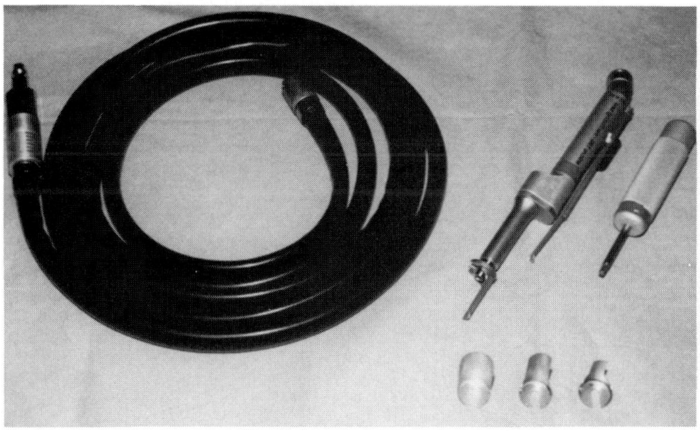

FIGURE 7

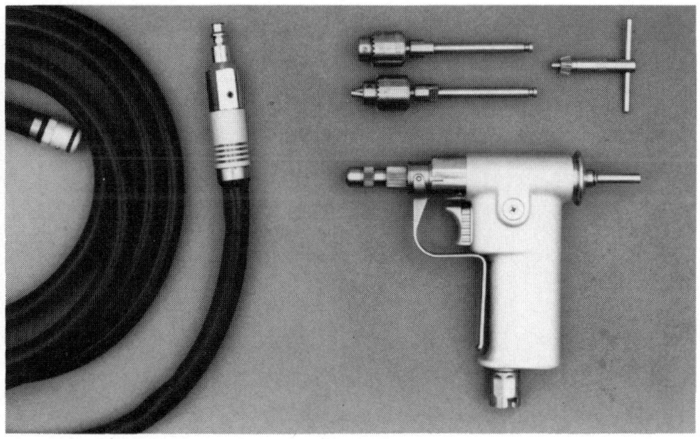

FIGURE 8

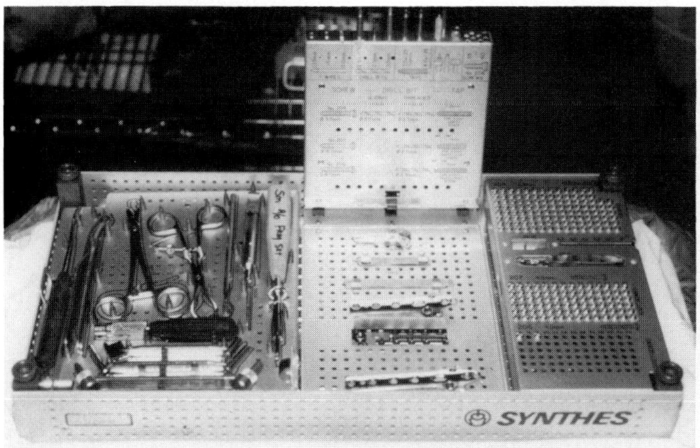

FIGURE 9

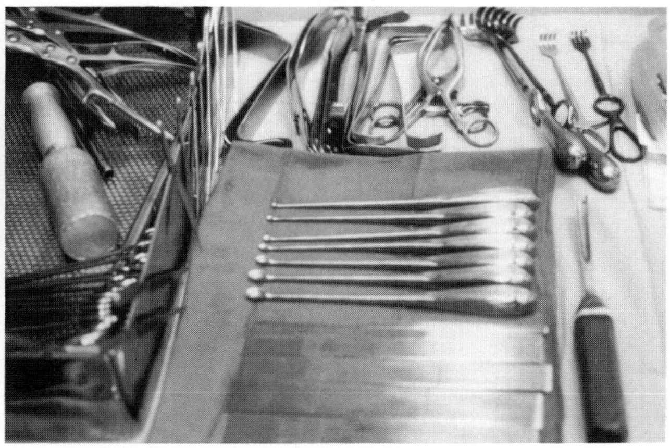

FIGURE 10

Arthroscopy of the ankle requires optical instrumentation, including a light source, light cable, and video camera (Fig. 11). Various instruments such as forceps, probes, rongeurs, burs, and articular shavers allow for arthroscopic surgery (Fig. 12).

Some orthopedic foot and ankle surgeons find that occasional use of magnification loops may be advantageous for fine surgery on soft tissues (Fig. 13).

Photographic equipment that can be utilized intraoperatively includes a camera body, macro lenses, and flash units (Fig. 14).

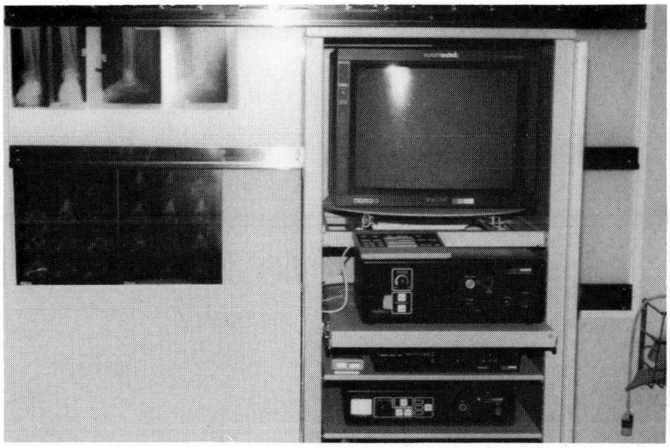

FIGURE 11

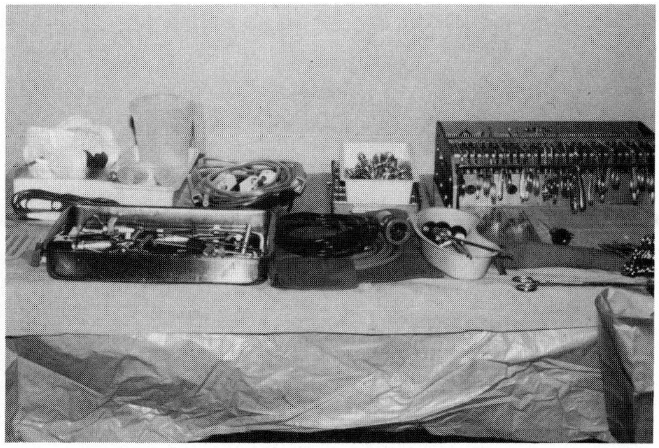

FIGURE 12

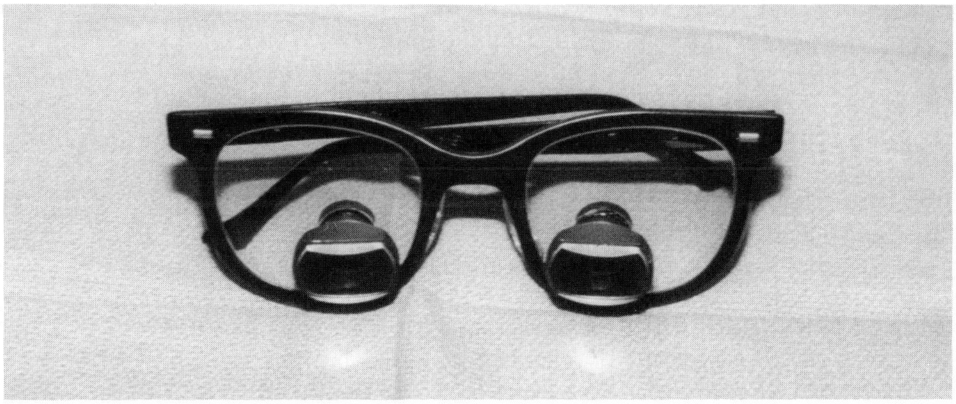

FIGURE 13

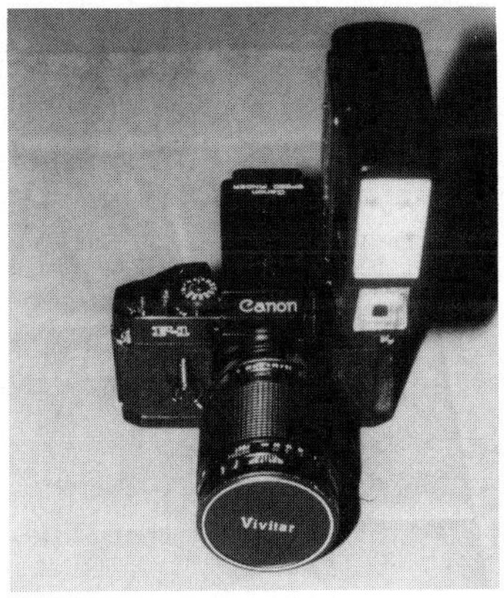

FIGURE 14

OPERATING ROOM SETTING

Surgical procedures are carried out in an operating room setting under strict aseptic conditions. The patient's medical records are kept in the operating room. Radiographs obtained preoperatively and intraoperatively are kept in the room during the surgery, and relevant radiographs are hung on view boxes for reference.

The patient is usually placed in the supine position for most foot and ankle procedures. For forefoot surgery it may be useful to have the heel positioned at the very end of the table so that the forefoot slightly overhangs the foot plate. This enables the physician to sit at the end of the table, allowing easy access to the forepart of the foot. Folded sheets or a sand bag placed under the hip can be used to internally rotate the extremity and thus provide access to the lateral aspect of the foot and ankle. This same technique may be useful in making the iliac crest more prominent under the skin, which may be helpful in obtaining iliac bone graft. The use of sterile bolsters consisting of folded towels may allow effective positioning of the distal peripheral extremity for a particular surgical technique.

Some procedures that require posterior approaches to the foot and ankle may be more easily performed in a prone position. This is particularly true for an Achilles tendon repair or when using a posterolateral approach to the ankle for excision of an os trigonum.

Preoperative preparation should include discussions with the nursing staff and the other operating room personnel. By reviewing the patient's medical status, surgical plan, and required instrumentation with the operating room team, all individuals involved in patient care will be prepared for the upcoming operation. The education of operating room personnel will inevitably enhance and expedite both perioperative patient management and the surgical procedure. The operating team will perform in an effective manner if instruction and guidance are provided by the operating surgeon.

Restriction of traffic and conversation in the operating room may provide a quiet and calm atmosphere for the patient and operating room personnel. In general, foot and ankle surgery must be carried out in a logical, systematic, and methodical manner. Complete preoperative evaluation and planning are necessary to provide an optimum clinical result. Meticulous soft tissue management and fine bone surgery with careful attention to procedural details are required. Intraoperative radiographs and clinical assessment ensure adequate achievement of the goals of surgery.

ANESTHESIA

Foot and ankle surgery may be carried out under various forms of anesthesia. General, regional, or local anesthesia may be appropriate depending on the age, medical condition, and temperament of the patient, as well as the preference and experience of the surgeon and anesthesiologist.

A general anesthetic may be preferable for more extensive foot and ankle surgery, especially those procedures that require concomitant iliac bone graft. General anesthesia may also be preferable for situations in which foot and ankle surgery will be carried out concurrently with surgery elsewhere on the body.

Regional anesthesia for foot and ankle surgery may include the use of a spinal or epidural anesthetic. Sciatic femoral blocks, as well as knee blocks, have been effective for surgery on the distal peripheral extremity. Regional ankle block is most appropriate for surgery in the midfoot and forefoot regions. Digital block may be very effective for surgery on isolated digits. This technique has proved to be quite useful for toenail surgery and other digital procedures. The local infiltration of anesthetic agents may be adequate for removal of pins and other hardware.

The actual choice of anesthesia may best be determined by the anesthesiologist and the patient, with input from the operating surgeon.

TOURNIQUETS

The use of a tourniquet in foot and ankle surgery may help provide a bloodless field, which enables adequate visualization of soft tissue and osseous structures encountered during the surgical procedure. Various techniques of tourniquet application for the purpose of obtaining hemostasis have been described in the literature. In general, the use of a pneumatic tourniquet at the level of the thigh has been most effective for reconstructive surgical procedures in the region of the ankle, hindfoot, and midfoot (Fig. 15). It is recommended that several layers of soft padding be applied about the skin under the tourniquet to avoid local skin irritation or injury. In general, the tourniquet is set to about 100 mm Hg higher than the systolic blood pressure and is inflated after exsanguination of the leg with an Esmarch bandage (Fig. 16). For long surgical procedures, the tourniquet is deflated after 90 minutes but may be reinflated, if necessary, after deflation for a 15-minute period.

For procedures in the forefoot and for some surgery in the midfoot, it may be preferable to use an Esmarch or Martin bandage as a tourniquet. Beginning at the tip of the toes and proceeding proximally, the bandage is applied in layers that do not overlap (Fig. 17). At the mid portion of the leg at the level of the muscular region of the calf, three layers are completely overlapped. The remainder of the roll is tucked under the last layer (Fig. 18A and B). Beginning distally, the bandage is then unwrapped up to the level of the midcalf, where the multiple layers are left undisturbed (Fig. 19A and B).

Toenail and digital surgery may be performed under more discrete hemostasis obtained by means of a Penrose drain used as a tourniquet (Fig. 20). A 1/2- or 5/8-inch Penrose drain may be rolled as a Martin or Esmarch bandage. The digit is exsanguinated by wrapping from the distal tip of the toe to the base of the web (Fig. 21). At that location, two layers are overlapped and held with a small curved hemostat. The bandage is unwrapped distally to the level of the clamp (Fig. 22).

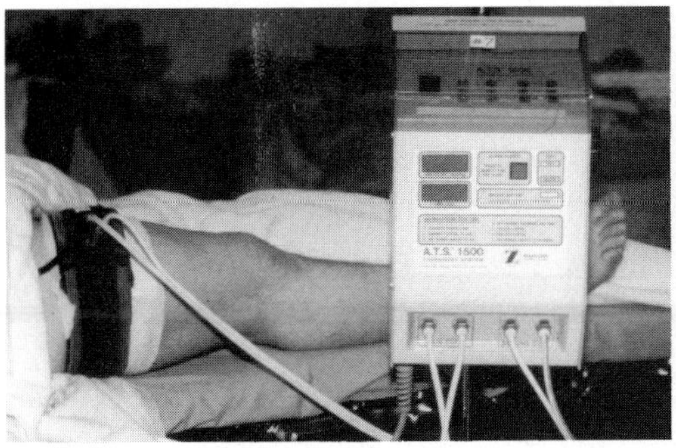

FIGURE 15

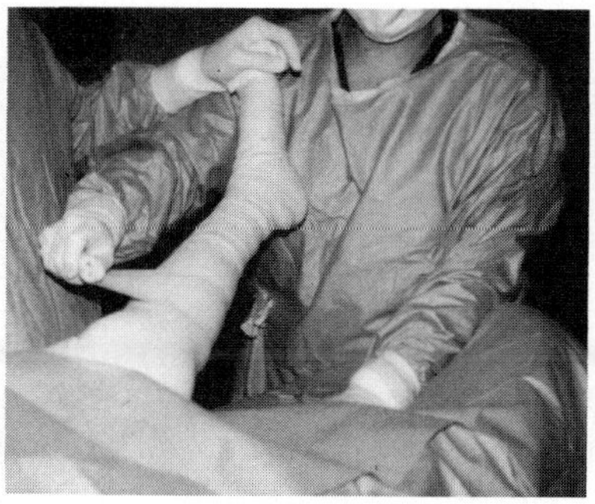

FIGURE 16

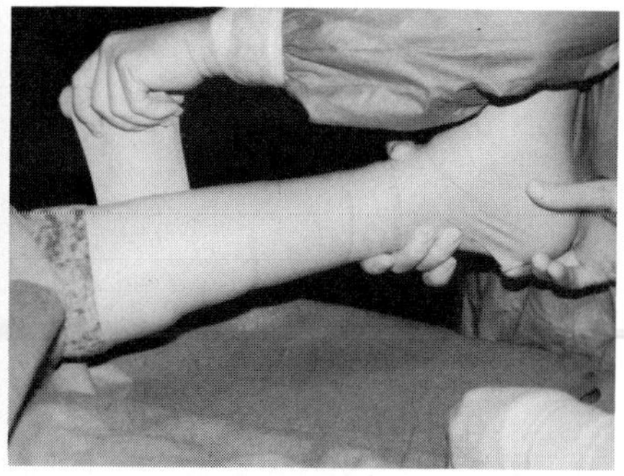

FIGURE 17

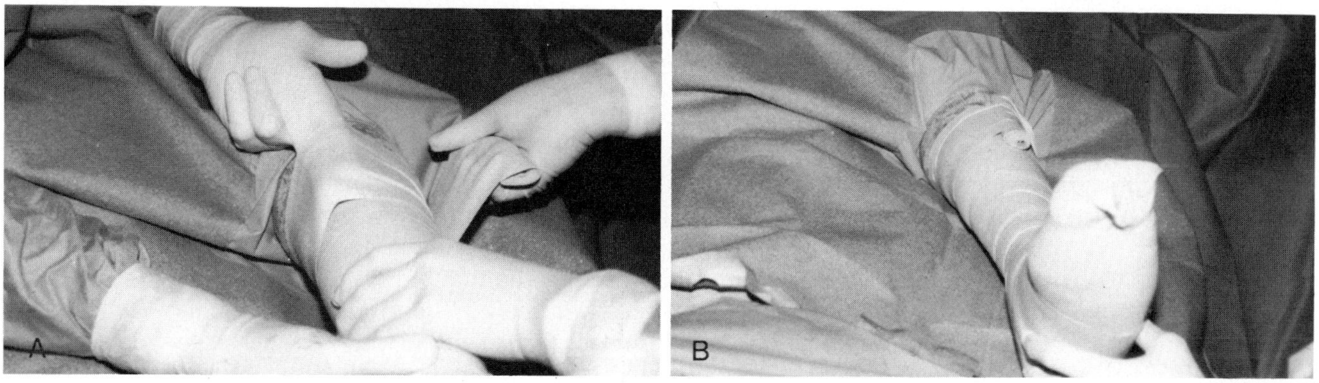

FIGURE 18

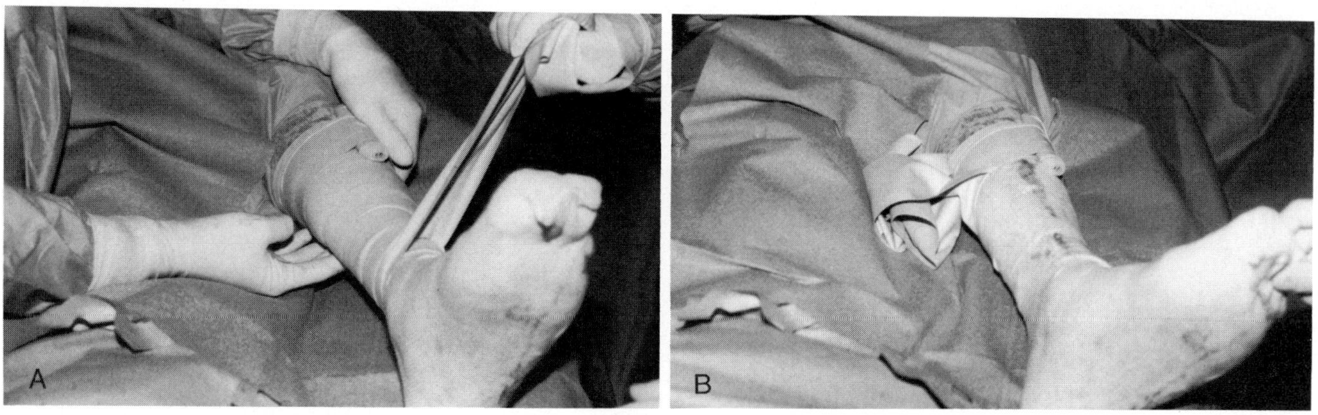

FIGURE 19

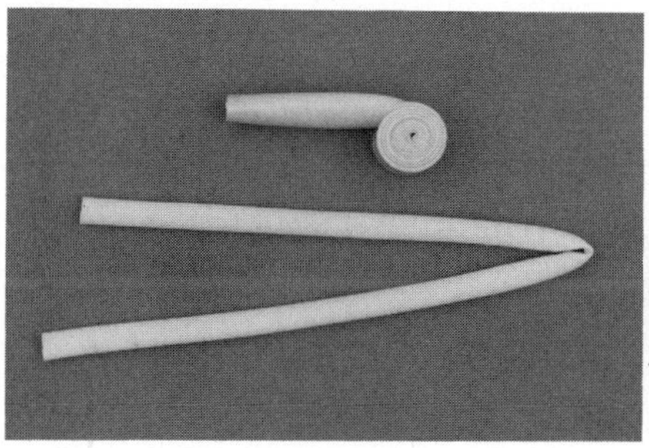

FIGURE 20

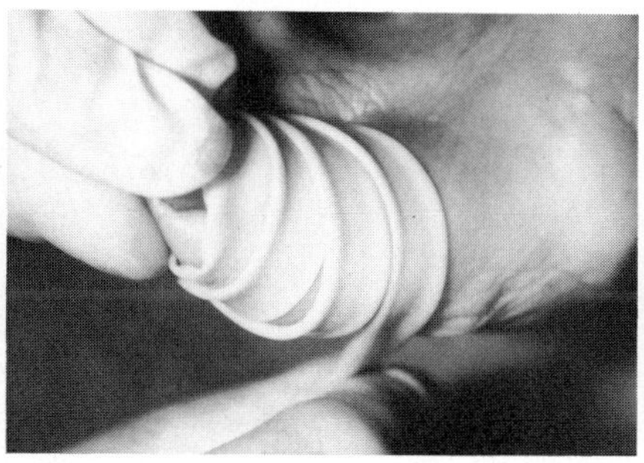

FIGURE 21

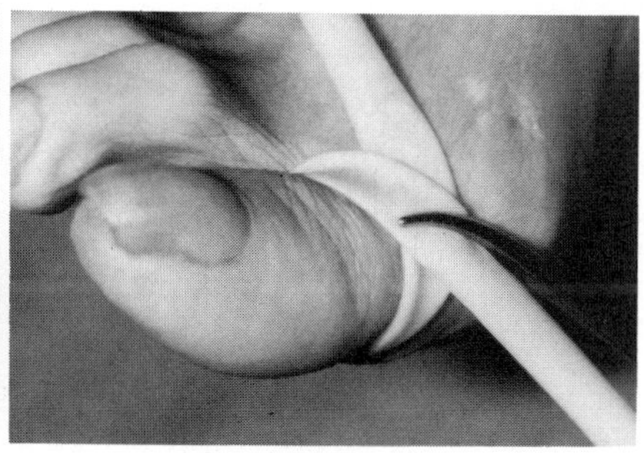

FIGURE 22

SKIN PREPARATION AND DRAPING

For all foot and ankle surgical procedures, the limb is prepped and draped in the usual sterile manner. For those cases in which a pneumatic tourniquet is used on the thigh, the limb is generally prepped and draped up to the level of the tourniquet. Many surgical procedures performed in the region of the forefoot and midfoot may require skin preparation and draping only to the level of the knee.

The patient is instructed to clip and clean the toenails and remove any nail polish before surgery. In the operating room or prep area the skin is shaved in the region of the incision. The skin is prepared by scrubbing with antiseptic solution for a 10-minute period (Fig. 23). Begin at the incision site and move in a centrifugal fashion until the region has been prepared. Excess solution is removed by blotting (Fig. 24), and the limb is painted or sprayed with an antiseptic solution such as povidone-iodine (Betadine) (Fig. 25).

If the entire extremity is to be draped free, a sterile towel is folded lengthwise and placed circumferentially around the tourniquet and held with a penetrating towel clamp (Fig. 26). This is applied while an assistant holds the limb elevated by means of a sterile towel placed under the heel. A large surgical glove is applied to the toes to isolate them from the rest of the surgical field (Fig. 27). A stockinette is then placed on the toes and unrolled proximally to the level of the towel that encircles the tourniquet (Fig. 28).

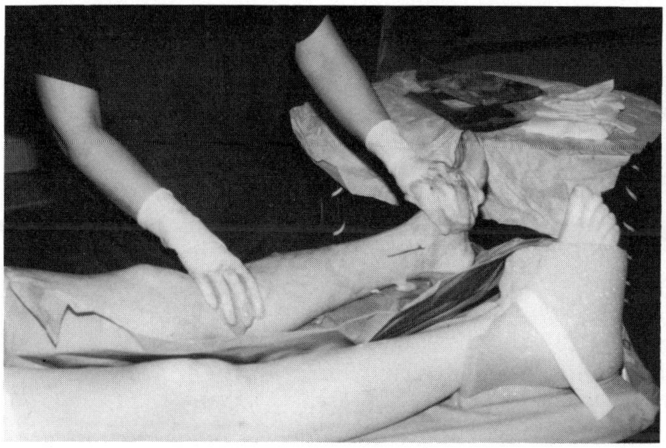

FIGURE 23

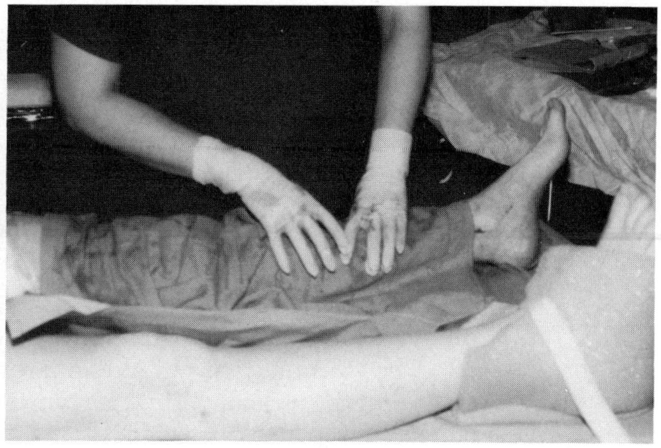

FIGURE 24

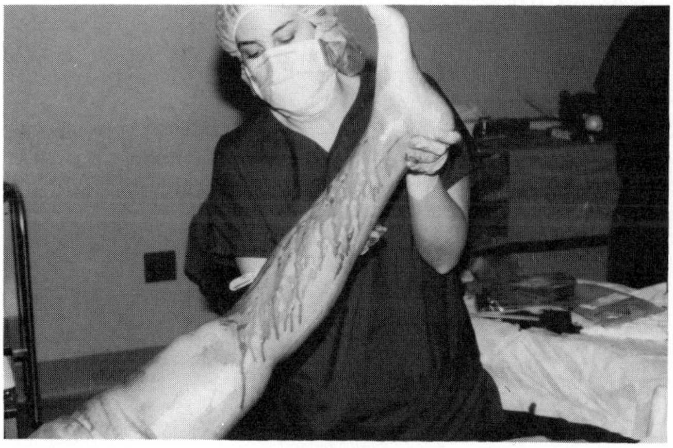

FIGURE 25

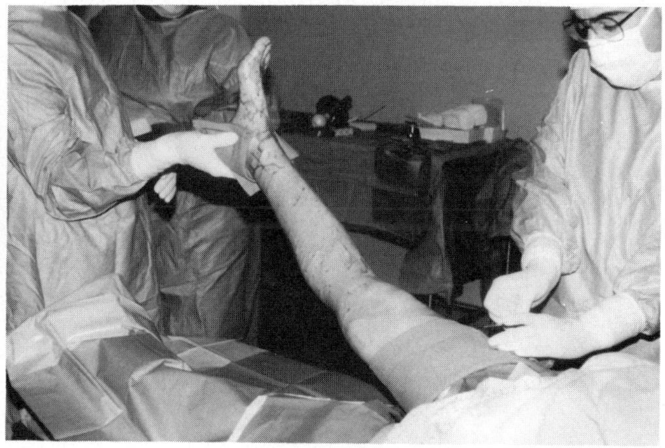

FIGURE 26

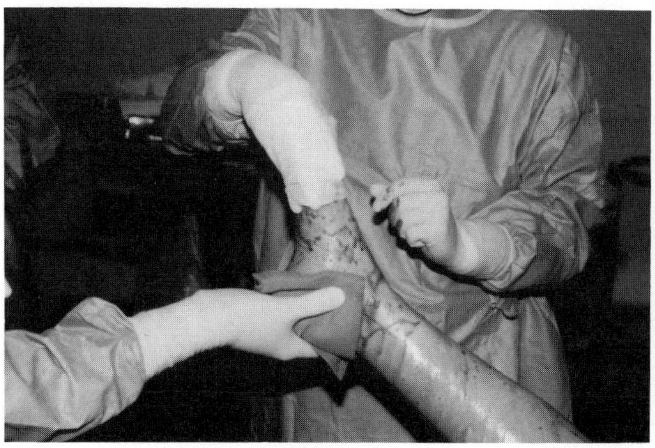

FIGURE 27

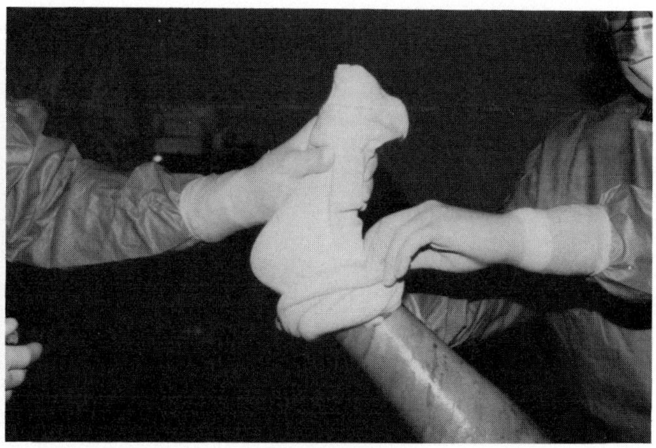

FIGURE 28

An impervious sheet is used to cover the table. Two sterile "bottom" sheets are placed over the table. A cuff is left at the level of the tourniquet (Fig. 29), and the limb is then lowered down to the table. A "top" sheet is applied, with a cuff left at the level of the tourniquet. The top sheet, "bottom" sheets, and unrolled portion of the stockinette are clipped together with nonpentrating towel clamps (Fig. 30). One clamp is applied to the lateral aspect of the limb, and a second towel clamp is applied to the medial aspect. An extremity drape with a hole is applied over the limb to ensure adequate sterile draping of the extremity (Fig. 31).

For exposure of an operative site in the region of the midfoot, hindfoot, or ankle, a collar-and-cuff configuration of the draped extremity is utilized (Fig. 32). The stockinette is cut circumferentially distal and proximal to the site of the surgical incision. This portion of the stockinette is removed, and the portion of the stockinette distal and proximal to the surgical incision is made to adhere to the skin by applying a circumferential 2- or 3-inch band of self-adhesive Vi-Drape. This technique effectively isolates the area of the surgical procedure.

The surgical incision is outlined with a marking pen. Other superficial landmarks, as well as structures to be avoided, are also marked. A lap pad is applied over the region of the surgical site. The Esmarch or Martin bandage is then applied from distal to proximal (Fig. 33). The knee is flexed, and the pneumatic tourniquet is inflated (Fig. 34).

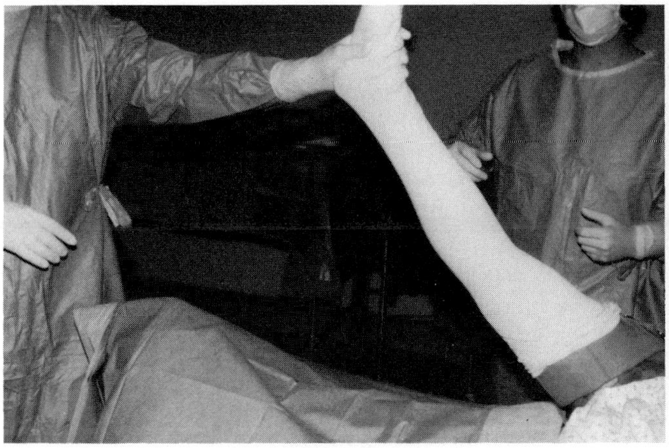

FIGURE 29

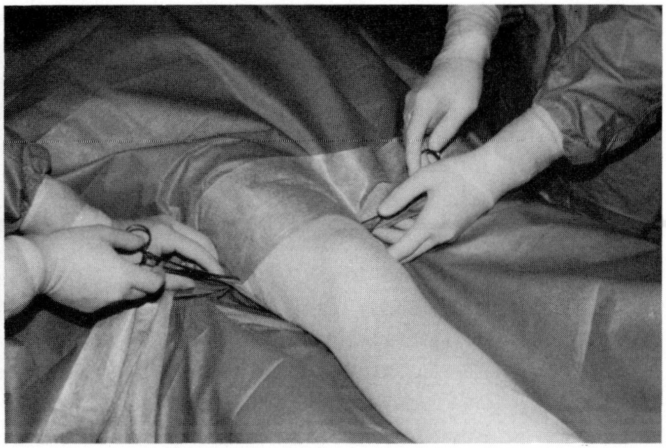

FIGURE 30

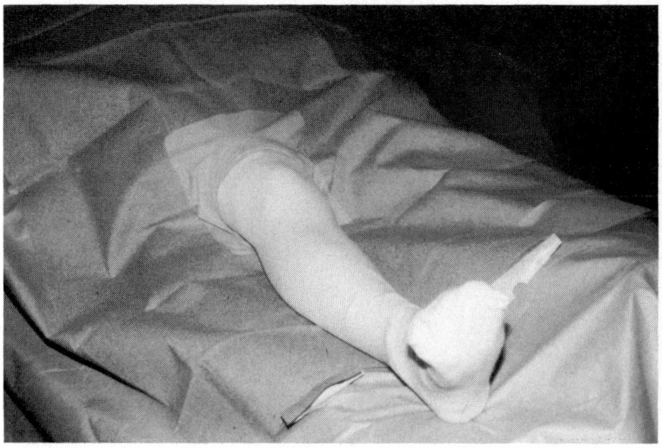

FIGURE 31

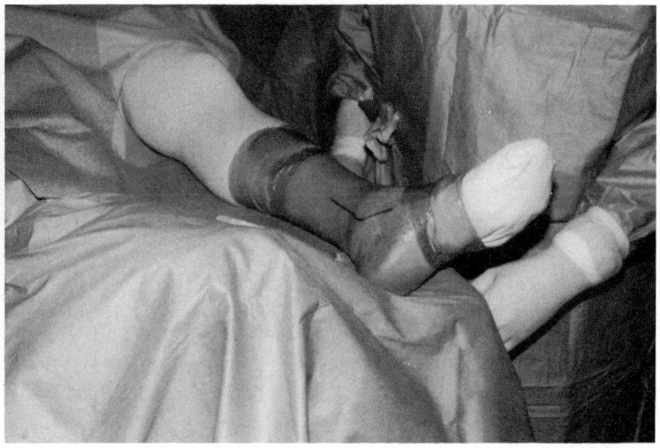

FIGURE 32

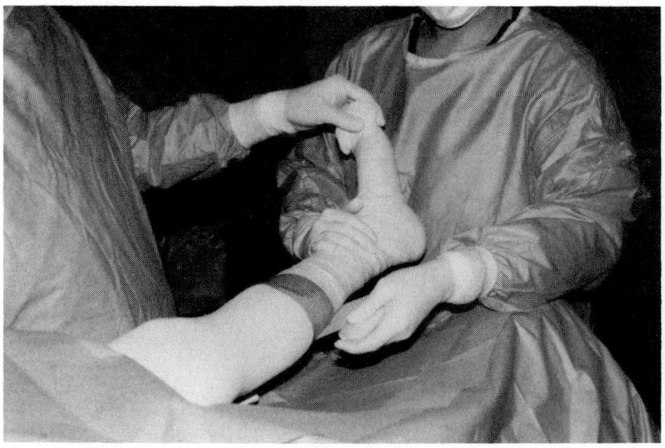

FIGURE 33

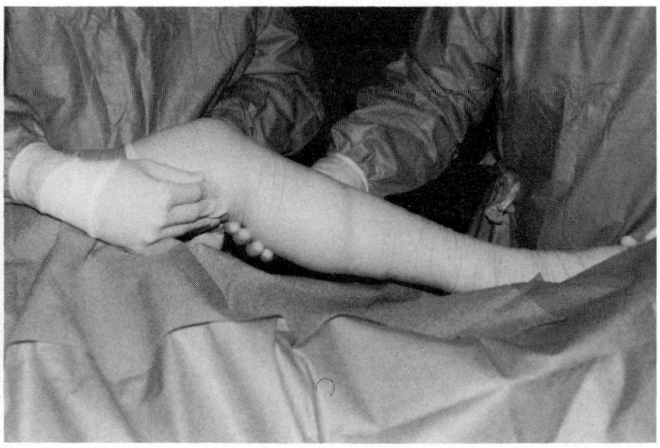

FIGURE 34

For surgical procedures involving the more distal aspects of the extremity, a less elaborate draping technique may be utilized. The skin is prepared up to the level of the knee (Fig. 35). A towel folded along its longitudinal axis is wrapped circumferentially about the leg at the most distal aspect of the skin preparation and clamped with a small penetrating towel clamp (Fig. 36). A stockinette is then applied distally and unrolled, proceeding proximally so that the unrolled portion at the proximal aspect of the stockinette lies over the sterile towel (Fig. 37). An impervious sheet is applied to cover the table while the limb is held elevated. Two "bottom" sheets are applied to the table, with the cuff of the uppermost sheet left unfolded at the level of the unrolled portion of the stockinette (Fig. 38). A "top" sheet is applied with a cuff at the level of the unrolled portion of the stockinette. The top sheet, bottom sheet, and unrolled portion of the stockinette are clipped with a nonpenetrating towel clamp on the medial side and another on the lateral side to effectively isolate the sterile portion of the limb (Fig. 39). An extremity drape with a hole is then passed over the limb, with its bottom portion unfolded to cover the table and its top portion unfolded to cover the remainder of the patient, and hung by two intravenous poles on either side of the operating room table. Thus a screen is formed at the level of the patient's upper body (Fig. 40). An Esmarch bandage is then wrapped at the level of the midcalf (Fig. 41). A hole is cut in the stockinette in the region of the forefoot and pulled over the foot proximally to expose the distal portion of the foot.

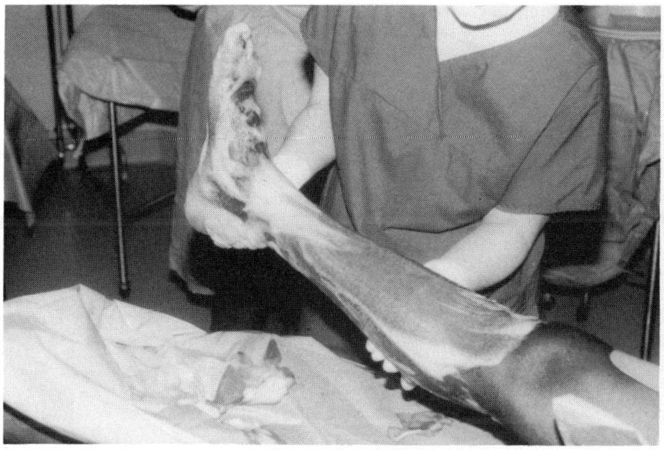

FIGURE 35

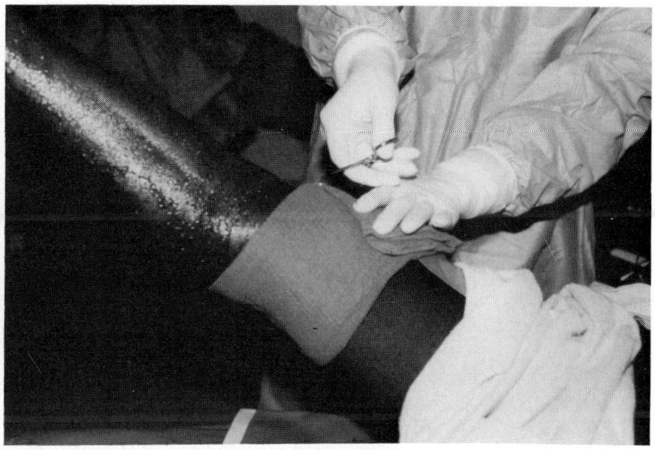

FIGURE 36

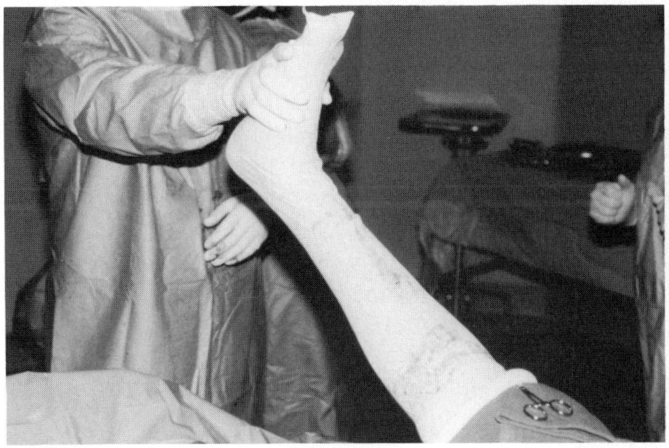

FIGURE 37

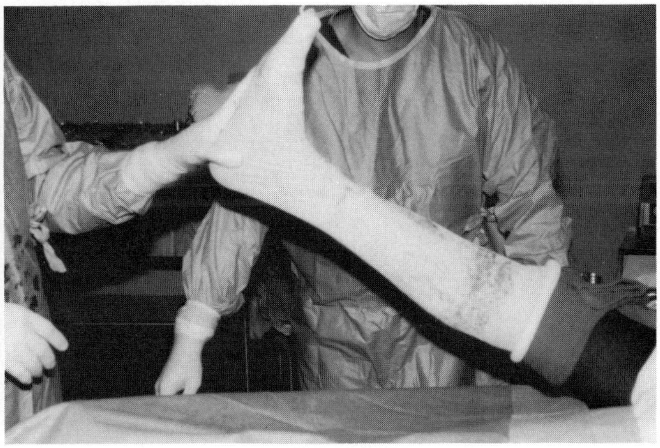

FIGURE 38

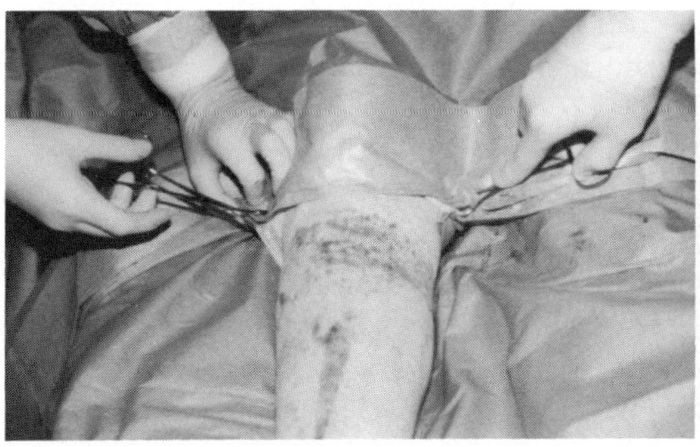

FIGURE 39

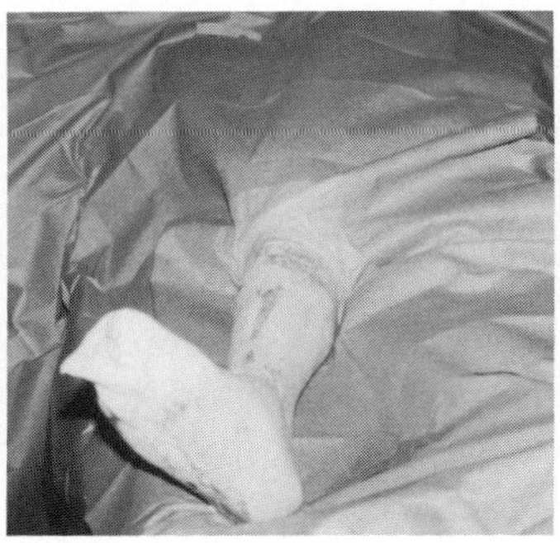

FIGURE 40

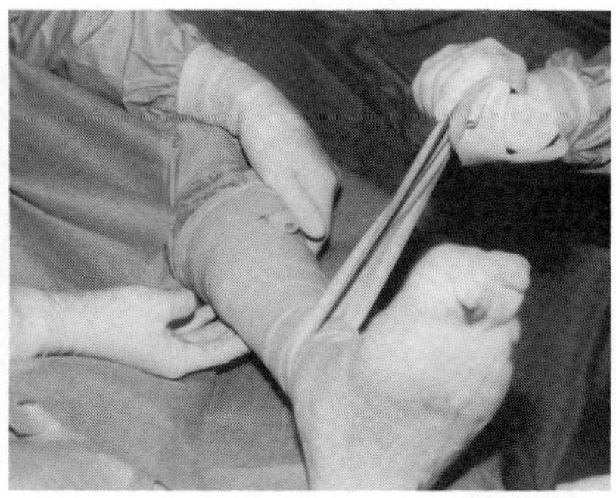

FIGURE 41

POSTOPERATIVE CARE

Initial postoperative orders include routine requirements for postsurgical monitoring in the recovery room as well as in the hospital and later at home. Vital signs are taken according to the usual postoperative routine, and input and output are monitored. Postoperative radiographs may be taken in the operating room, the recovery room, or subsequently during the postoperative period. Neurovascular observation is required to check circulatory status and sensation. The foot is elevated, and the patient is advised to maintain elevation while sitting or lying down. Initially, the operated foot is kept above the patient's heart. A foot cradle attached to the end of the bed for inpatients may prevent the sheets and blankets from touching the toes, which may be a source of discomfort for the patient postoperatively. Activity is generally restricted, ranging from complete bed rest to restricted ambulation with or without aids. Patients are often kept non–weight bearing on crutches or a walker during the early postoperative period. The physician must then determine at which point the patient may begin partial weight bearing. Generally a slow, gradual progression from non–weight bearing to partial weight bearing to full weight bearing provides adequate rest for the operated extremity. Immobilization devices may include a Robert Jones compression dressing, most often utilized with plaster U-shaped and/or posterior splints. The use of a well-padded short-leg cast may be appropriate in certain procedures. Some smaller soft tissue procedures may be amenable to postoperative mobilization in a stiff-soled shoe.

If surgery is performed on one foot, then a support stocking should be used on the contralateral limb. This device, combined with early mobilization of the patient, may help avoid complications such as phlebitis, thrombosis, and embolism. Incentive spirometry may avoid postoperative pulmonary problems. Physical therapy is often required for ambulation training and transfers.

Medications used during the early postoperative period typically include analgesics, sedatives, laxatives, antiemetic agents, and prophylactic antibiotics. Deep vein thrombosis prophylaxis may require the use of aspirin or other medications.

Once the patient is stable, discharge may be contemplated. Adequate postoperative instructions are required, particularly regarding the specific restrictions to ambulation. Elevation is maintained routinely during the postoperative period. Patients are discharged from the hospital with appropriate analgesic medications and guidelines regarding cast and bandage precautions. Patients are instructed to contact the operating surgeon regarding any problems that may arise during the recuperative period, including increasing discomfort, swelling, numbness and paresthesias, and fever or chills.

Guidelines and recommendations for the postoperative regimen for specific operative procedures are provided in the individual chapters describing these surgical techniques.

SECTION 2

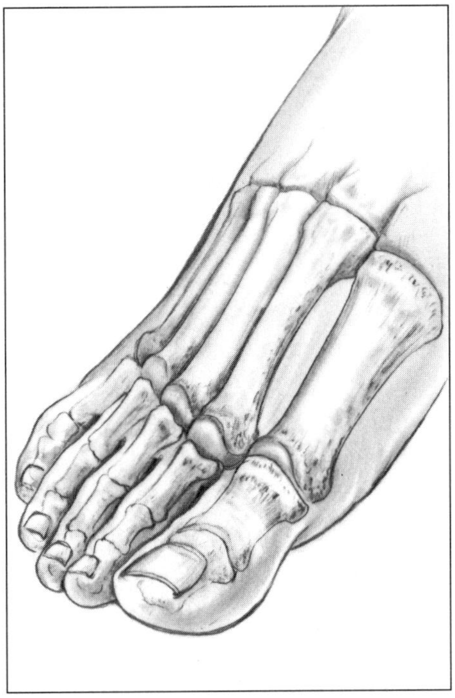

Forefoot

PART 1

Operations for Hallux Valgus

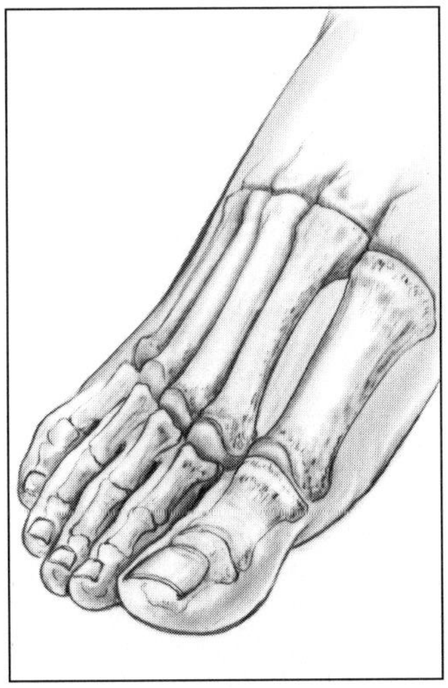

CHEVRON OSTEOTOMY

General Considerations

The chevron osteotomy is a transverse V-shaped distal osteotomy of the first metatarsal used to correct hallux valgus deformity. This procedure provides for reduction of the metatarsus primus varus, narrowing of the forefoot width, resection of the prominent medial eminence, and correction of the valgus deviation of the great toe.

Comparison of Chevron Osteotomy With Other Distal Osteotomies

Advantages. The advantages of chevron osteotomy are increased stability, rapid healing, and minimal shortening. This procedure can be performed with or without internal fixation.

Disadvantages. The primary disadvantage is that the procedure is technically demanding.

Patient Selection

Indications

1. Hallux valgus, metatarsus primus varus, and prominent medial eminence
2. Mild to moderate deformity
   a. Intermetatarsal angle up to 15 degrees
   b. Metatarsophalangeal angle up to 30 degrees
3. Middle-aged patient younger than 60 years

Contraindications

1. Arthrosis of the first metatarsophalangeal joint
2. Severe metatarsus primus varus
3. Older patient

Surgical Procedure

Operative Technique

1. A medial longitudinal incision 6 cm long is made slightly dorsal to the midline. The incision extends from the midpoint of the proximal phalanx to 2 cm proximal to the exostosis (Fig. 1). The skin and subcutaneous tissue are reflected to visualize the capsule. Care is taken to avoid injury to the dorsomedial cutaneous nerve.
2. Create a distally based Y-shaped capsular incision (Fig. 2). Reflect subperiosteally to expose the metatarsal head and neck.
3. Excise the exostosis parallel to the medial border of the foot (Fig. 3).
4. Make a transverse V-shaped osteotomy distally with the microsagittal saw (Fig. 4). (Angle of osteotomy, <60 degrees).

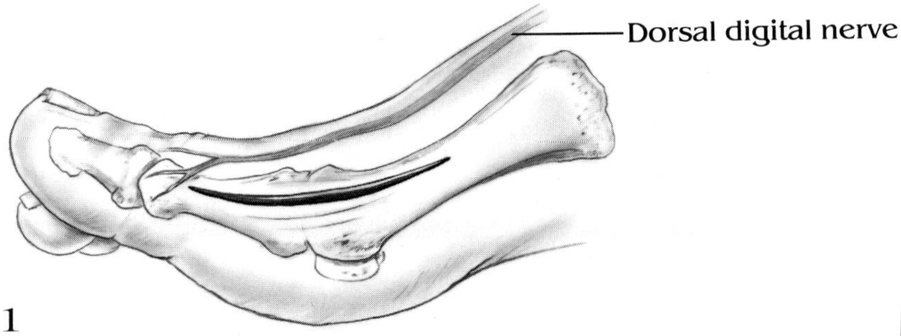

1

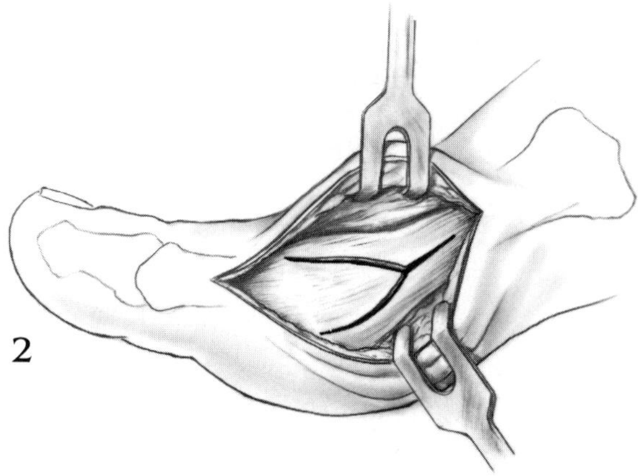

2

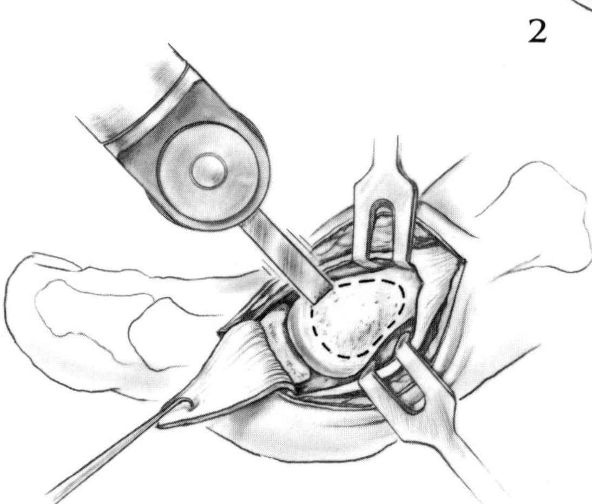

3

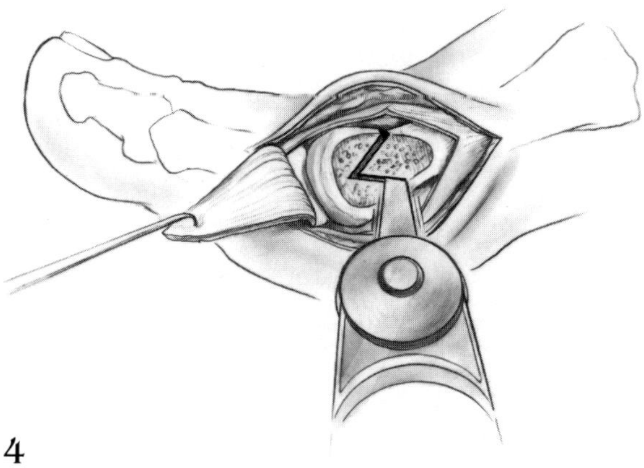

4

5. While holding the shaft with a towel clip or bone-holding forceps, push the metatarsal head laterally 2 to 4 mm (Fig. 5).
6. Fix the osteotomy with an oblique 0.045-inch Kirschner wire inserted from dorsodistal to plantar proximal through a separate stab incision. Cut off and bend the pin above the skin (Fig. 6).
7. Excise the prominent edge of bone remaining along the medial aspect of the metatarsal shaft with the power saw (Fig. 6).
8. While holding the hallux in slight overcorrection varus and plantarflexion, close the capsule with a horizontal mattress tension suture of 2-0 Vicryl (Fig. 7). Close the remainder of the capsule with interrupted simple 2-0 Vicryl sutures. Close the skin with a running subcuticular 3-0 Prolene suture (Fig. 8).

Postoperative Care

1. Soft compression dressing for 48 hours
2. Short-leg walking cast for 3 weeks
3. Sutures and pin removed at 3 weeks
4. Wooden-soled shoe for 3 weeks

Technical Pitfalls

1. Excessive soft tissue stripping
2. Excessive resection of prominent medial eminence
3. Improper osteotomy:
   a. Angle > 60 degrees
   b. Apex too far distal or proximal
   c. Not parallel in mediolateral plane
4. Instability of the distal fragment
5. Excessive removal of the bony projection of the metatarsal shaft

Potential Complications

1. Nonunion of the osteotomy
2. Avascular necrosis of the metatarsal head
3. Lateral transfer metatarsalgia
4. Recurrence of deformity

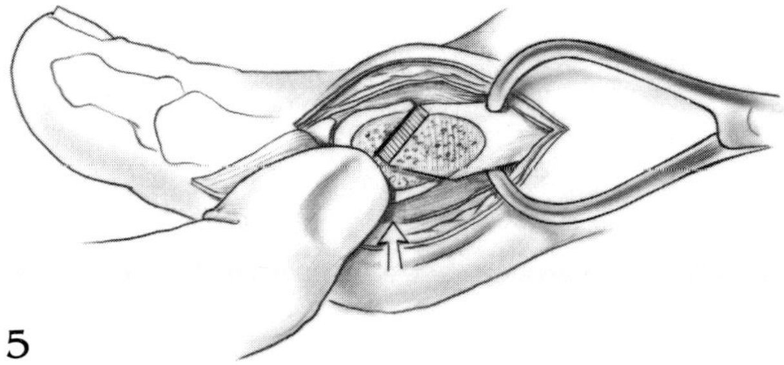

5

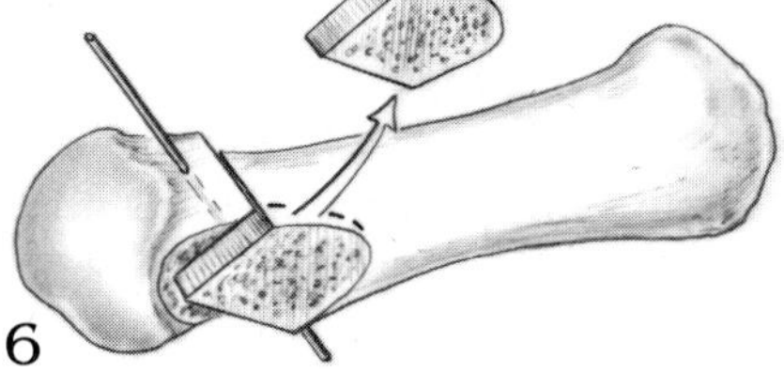

6

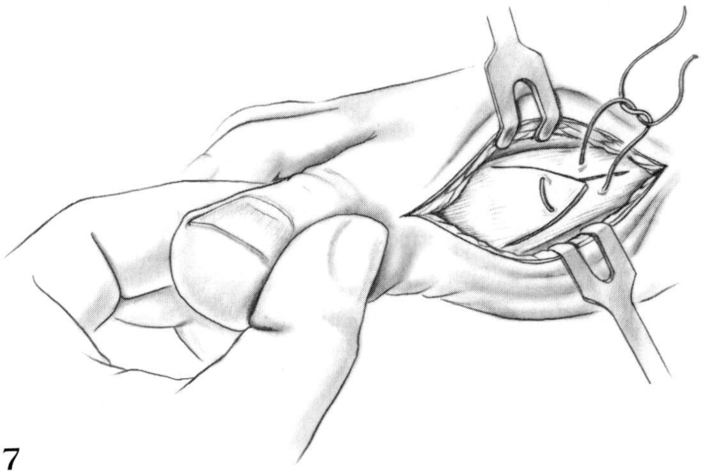

7

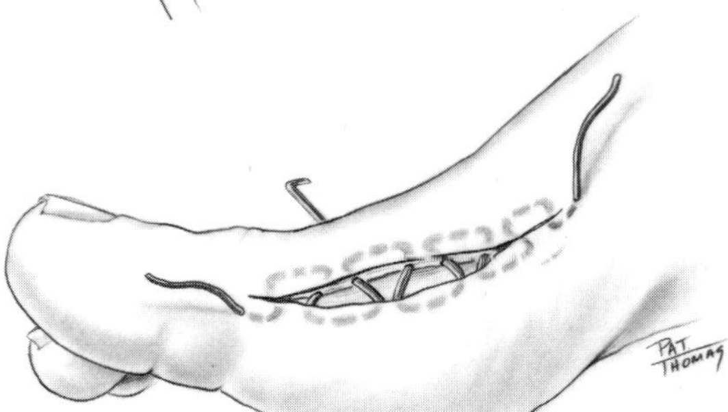

8

MODIFIED MITCHELL OSTEOTOMY

General Considerations

The modified Mitchell osteotomy, also used to correct hallux valgus, provides correction of the metatarsus primus varus, narrowing of the forefoot width, resection of the prominent medial eminence, and correction of the valgus deviation of the great toe. In this procedure, a transverse osteotomy is made perpendicular to the longitudinal axis of the first metatarsal at its neck, and the metatarsal head is shifted laterally and plantarward. Plantar displacement of the distal fragment allows for increased weight bearing at the first metatarsal head. This procedure is most effective in patients with hallux valgus and significant lateral metatarsalgia with hyperkeratotic lesions and tenderness at the plantar aspect of the lesser metatarsal heads. Fixation is best accomplished with two crossed Kirschner wires (K wires).

Comparison of Modified Mitchell Osteotomy With Other Osteotomies

Advantages. The modified Mitchell osteotomy is technically easier, plantar translocation of the distal fragment increases the weight-bearing capacity of the first metatarsal head, and shortening is minimal.

Disadvantages. The primary disadvantages of the procedure are that it requires fixation and a longer postoperative immobilization period.

Patient Selection

Indications

1. Hallux valgus, metatarsus primus varus, and a prominent medial eminence
2. Mild to moderate deformity
   a. Intermetatarsal angle < 18 degrees
   b. Metatarsophalangeal angle < 40 degrees
3. Middle-aged patient younger than 60 years
4. Especially suited for patients with a hyperkeratotic lesion or tenderness at the plantar aspect of the lesser metatarsal heads

Contraindications

1. Arthrosis of the first metatarsophalangeal joint
2. Severe metatarsus primus varus
3. Older patient

Surgical Procedure

Operative Technique

1. A dorsomedial incision is made from the midpoint of the proximal phalanx to 1 cm proximal to the exostosis (Fig. 1). The subcutaneous tissue is incised along the line of the skin incision to expose the capsule. Care is taken to avoid injury to the dorsal digital nerve.
2. A Y-shaped capsular incision based distally is made with the apex of the "V" arms meeting just proximal to the exostosis (Fig. 2). This V-flap is reflected from the bone by sharp dissection.
3. The exostosis is excised with a power saw (Figs. 3 and 4). The cut edge is then smoothed with a rasp.

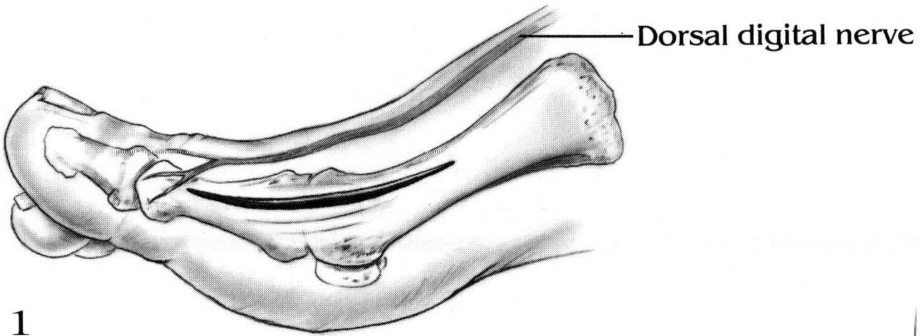

1

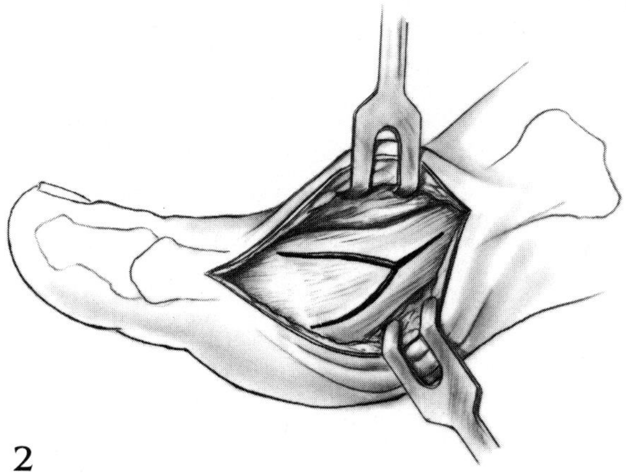

2

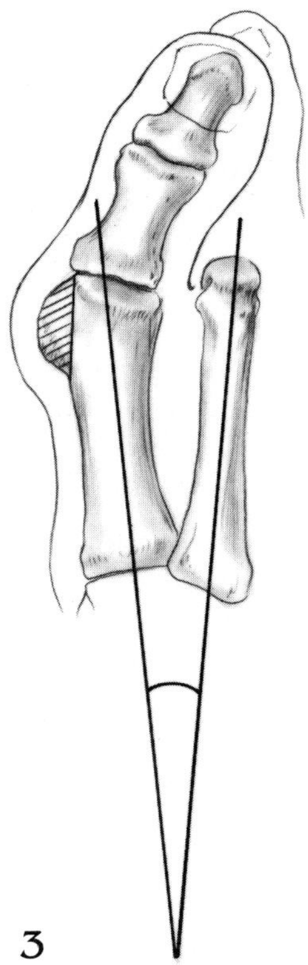

3

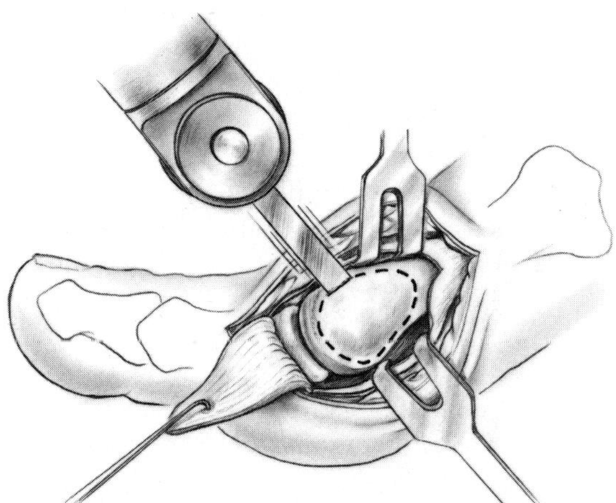

4

4. A transverse osteotomy is made at the level of the metatarsal neck with a microsagittal saw. This osteotomy is oriented perpendicular to the longitudinal axis of the first metatarsal (Fig. 5). The distal fragment is shifted laterally and plantarward (Fig. 6).
5. With the metatarsal head fragment held in its corrected position, two 0.045-inch Kirschner wires are inserted in a crosswise fashion to fix the osteotomy. These wires are bent and cut off under the skin.
6. The prominent edge of the remaining metatarsal shaft is then excised with a power saw and smoothed with a rasp (Fig. 6).
7. With the hallux held in slight overcorrection varus and plantarflexion, the capsule is sutured with a horizontal mattress tension suture of 2-0 Vicryl (Fig. 7). The remainder of the capsule is closed with interrupted simple 2-0 Vicryl sutures. The skin is closed with interrupted vertical mattress 4-0 nylon sutures (Fig. 8).

Postoperative Care

1. Soft compression dressing for 48 hours
2. Short-leg walking cast for 6 weeks
3. Suture removal at 3 weeks
4. Pin removal at 6 weeks

Technical Pitfalls

1. Injury to the dorsal digital nerve
2. Inadequate plantar displacement of the distal fragment, leading to decreased weight bearing under the first metatarsal head and lateral transfer metatarsalgia
3. Inadequate internal fixation, leading to dorsal displacement of the first metatarsal head with lateral metatarsalgia
4. Osteotomy performed too far distally
5. Excessive stripping of the surrounding soft tissue and capsule, which may lead to delayed union or avascular necrosis
6. Inadequate lateral transposition of the distal fragment, which may lead to incomplete correction

Complications

1. Nonunion of the osteotomy
2. Avascular necrosis of the metatarsal head
3. Lateral transfer metatarsalgia

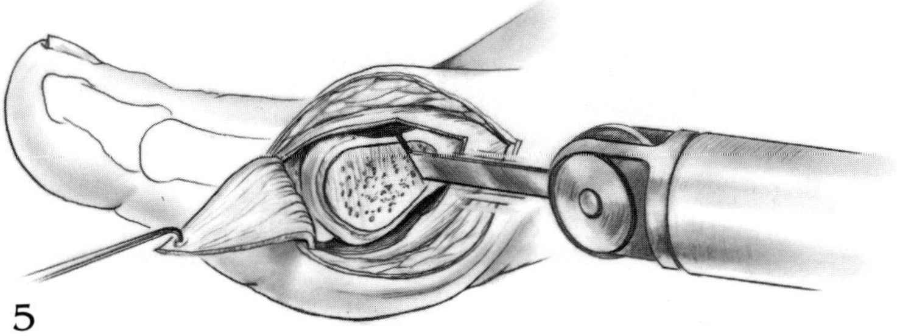

5

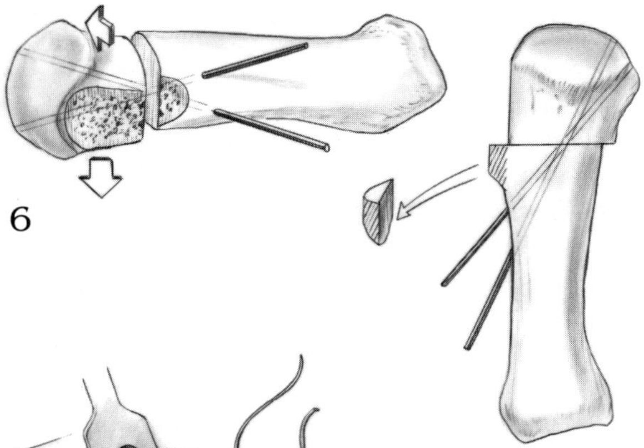

6

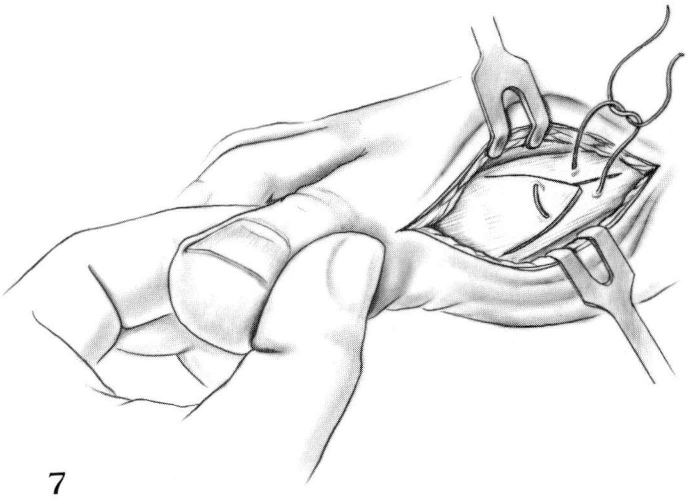

7

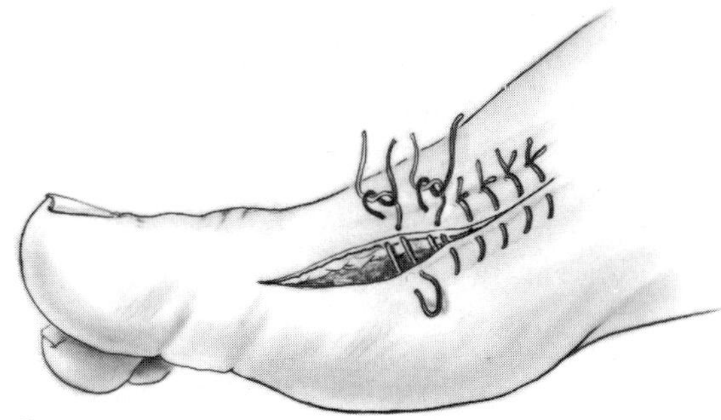

8

BASILAR CRESCENTIC OSTEOTOMY AND FIRST WEB SPACE RELEASE

General Considerations

Patients with moderate to severe hallux valgus deformity often require more extensive reconstructive procedures to gain correction of the various components of the deformity. The involved foot often displays significant metatarsus primus varus, marked hallux valgus, and a prominent medial eminence resulting from uncovering of the medial aspect of the first metatarsal head associated with subluxation of the first metatarsophalangeal joint. Patients frequently have associated abnormalities of the second toe because of mechanical abutment by the laterally deviated hallux; these include hammering or clawing of the second toe, which may come to underride or override the hallux. Because of the abnormal forces applied to the second metatarsophalangeal joint, these patients may display dorsal subluxation or even dislocation of that joint with synovitis. Lateral deviation of the great toe leads to attenuation of the medial capsule and contracture of the lateral capsule and the adductor hallucis muscle. The sesamoids and the extrinsic muscle tendon units subluxate laterally.

Reconstructive surgery in these patients often requires release of the contracted lateral soft tissue structures, medial capsulorrhaphy, excision of the prominent medial eminence, and osteotomy at the proximal aspect of the first metatarsal. Basilar osteotomy provides greater improvement of more severe medial deviation of the first metatarsal, as correction is obtained at the apex of the deformity. The basilar crescentic osteotomy described by R. A. Mann allows for good correction of the metatarsus primus varus with minimal shortening of the metatarsal. Excision of the prominent medial eminence allows for decompression at the medial aspect of the first metatarsal head. The web space release includes lateral capsulotomy of the first metatarsophalangeal joint, as well as tenotomy of the adductor hallucis tendon at its insertion on the base of the proximal phalanx. Web space release combined with medial capsulorrhaphy allows for realignment of the hallux and restoration of the anatomic alignment of the hallux sesamoids under the first metatarsal head. Pronation of the hallux, which is a common associated abnormality, may be improved by means of the medial capsulorrhaphy.

In general, this procedure is reserved for more severe forefoot deformities and is most appropriate for patients who display an intermetatarsal angle of greater than 15 degrees and a hallux valgus angle of greater than 25 degrees.

Patient Selection

Indications

1. Patients with moderate to severe hallux valgus, metatarsus primus varus, and a prominent medial eminence who fail to respond to conservative methods of treatment.
2. Patients whose preoperative anteroposterior standing radiographs reveal severe deformity with an intermetatarsal angle of greater than 15 degrees and a first metatarsophalangeal angle of greater than 25 degrees.
3. Patients in whom soft tissue procedures or distal metatarsal osteotomies are deemed inadequate for correction of the deformity.
4. Recurrent hallux valgus after prior isolated soft tissue procedures or distal metatarsal osteotomies.

Contraindications

1. Patients who have arthritis in the first metatarsophalangeal joint generally require either resection arthroplasty or arthrodesis of the joint depending on their age and activity level.
2. Patients with less severe deformities are better treated by distal metatarsal osteotomies.
3. Elderly patients with a limited ambulatory status may obtain satisfactory relief of symptoms with a Keller resection arthroplasty or isolated excision of the prominent medial eminence.
4. Patients with neuropathic disorders or vascular dysfunction may be at increased risk for infection and problematic wound healing.

Surgical Procedure

Operative Technique: Excision of the Prominent Medial Eminence

1. A medial longitudinal incision 6 cm long is made just dorsal to the midline. The incision extends from the midpoint to the proximal phalanx to 2 cm proximal to the exostosis (Fig. 1). The subcutaneous tissue is incised along the line of the skin incision. The skin and subcutaneous tissue are reflected to expose the capsule.
2. Create a distally based Y-shaped capsular incision with the apex of the "V" portion just proximal to the exostosis (Fig. 2). Reflect the "V" portion distally to expose the metatarsal head and neck, as well as the metatarsophalangeal joint.
3. Excise the prominent medial eminence flush with the metatarsal shaft using the microsagittal saw (Fig. 3). Smooth the cut surface with a rasp.

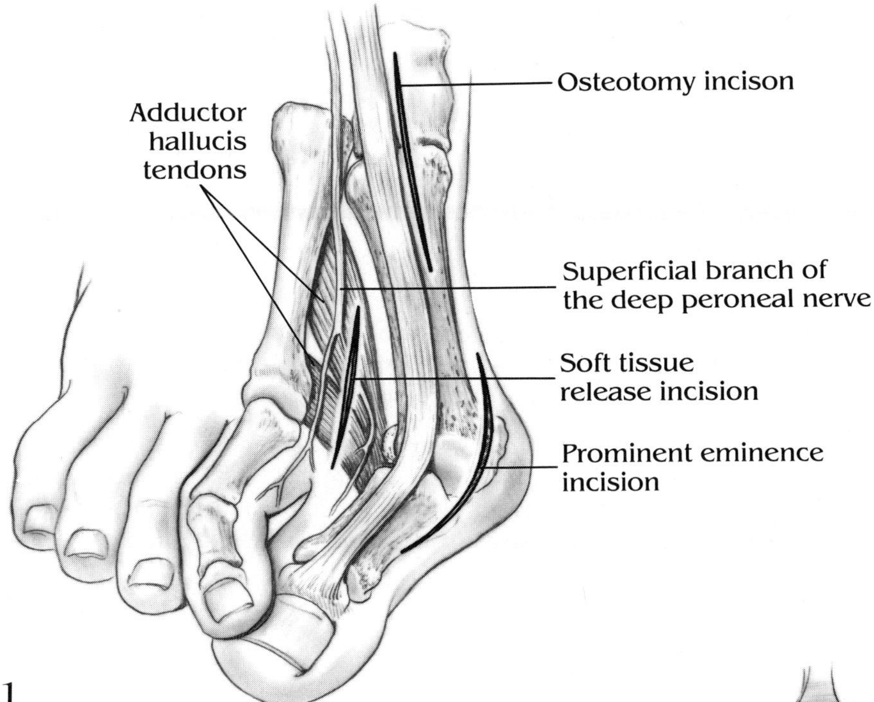
Osteotomy incison
Adductor
hallucis
tendons
Superficial branch of
the deep peroneal nerve
Soft tissue
release incision
Prominent eminence
incision

1

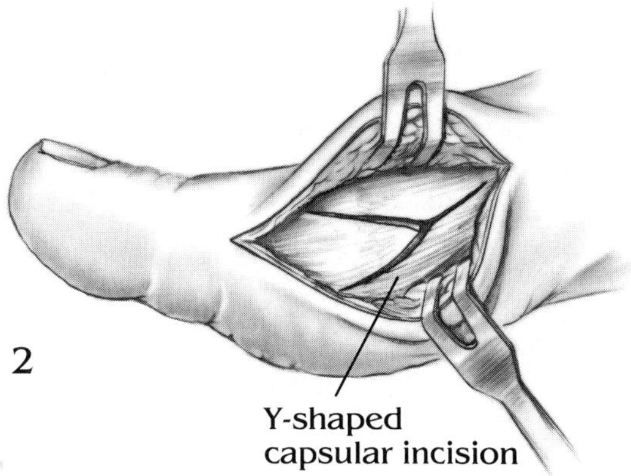
Y-shaped
capsular incision

2

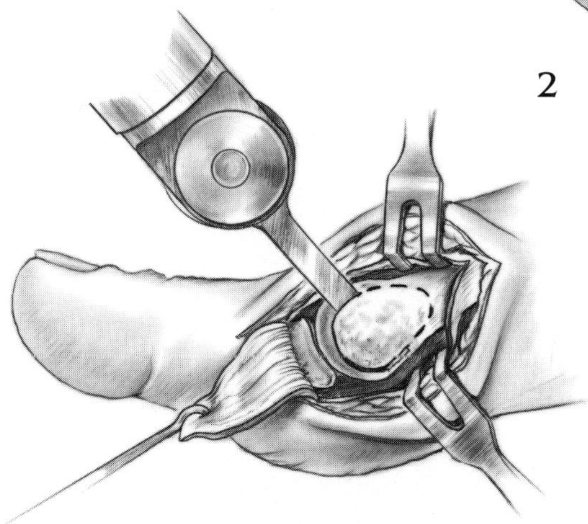

3

Operative Technique: Soft Tissue Release First Web Space

1. A dorsal longitudinal incision 4 cm long is made in the center of the first web space between the first and second metatarsals (see Fig. 1). Avoid injury to the superficial branches of the peroneal nerve. Incise subcutaneous tissue along the line of the skin incision. Insert a Weitlaner retractor to enhance exposure. Deepen the incision through subcutaneous tissue and fat to identify the adductor hallucis tendon (Fig. 4). Trace the adductor hallucis to its insertion at the base of the proximal phalanx. Identify the lateral joint capsule.
2. Detach the adductor hallucis insertion from the base of the proximal phalanx with a scalpel. Incise the attachments of the adductor hallucis to the lateral aspect of the lateral sesamoid (Fig. 4).
3. Reposition the Weitlaner retractor between the metatarsal heads and open it to apply tension to the intermetatarsal ligament (Fig. 5). Incise the intermetatarsal ligament, avoiding injury to the common digital nerve to the first web space, which lies in the fat pad beneath the ligament.
4. Incise the lateral capsule horizontally by making multiple perforations with a scalpel. Manipulate the hallux to 30 degrees of varus to ensure sufficient release of the contracted lateral capsule (Fig. 6).
5. Insert two or three simple sutures of 2-0 Vicryl in the first web space, incorporating the capsular tissue on the medial aspect of the second metatarsal head, the stump of the released adductor hallucis tendon, and the remaining capsular tissue on the lateral aspect of the first metatarsal head (Fig. 7). These sutures will be tied later.

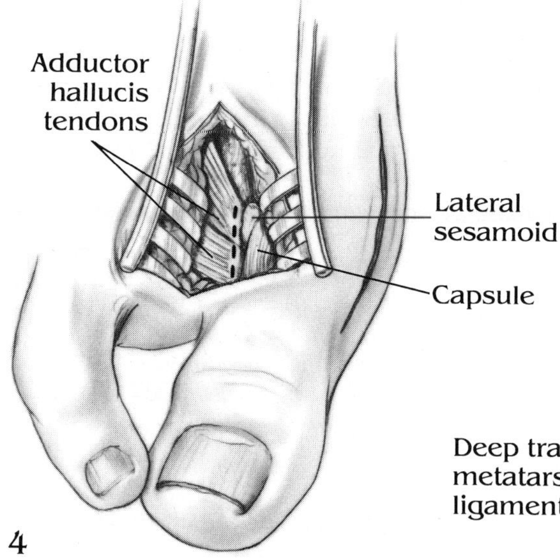
Adductor
hallucis
tendons
Lateral
sesamoid
Capsule

4

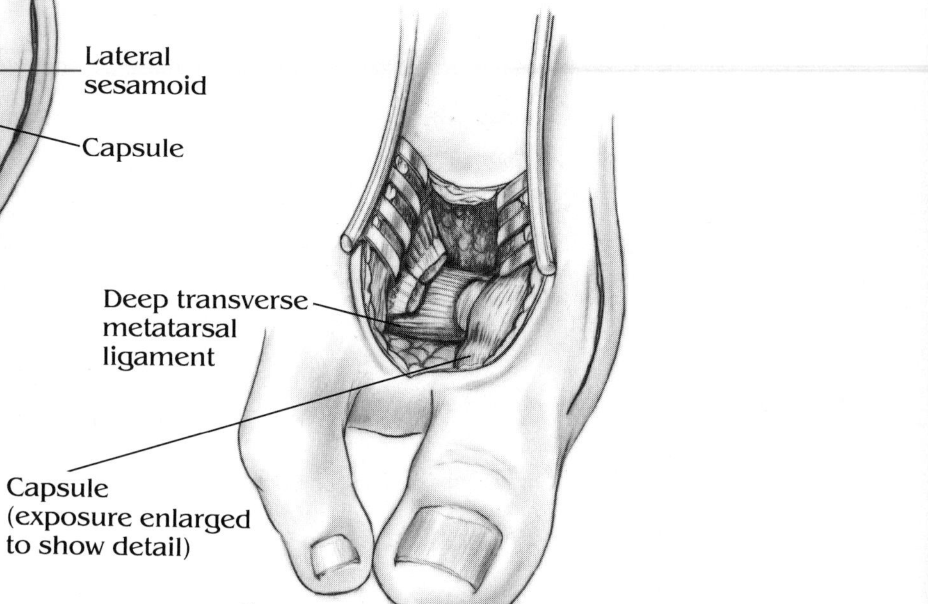
Deep transverse
metatarsal
ligament
Capsule
(exposure enlarged
to show detail)

5

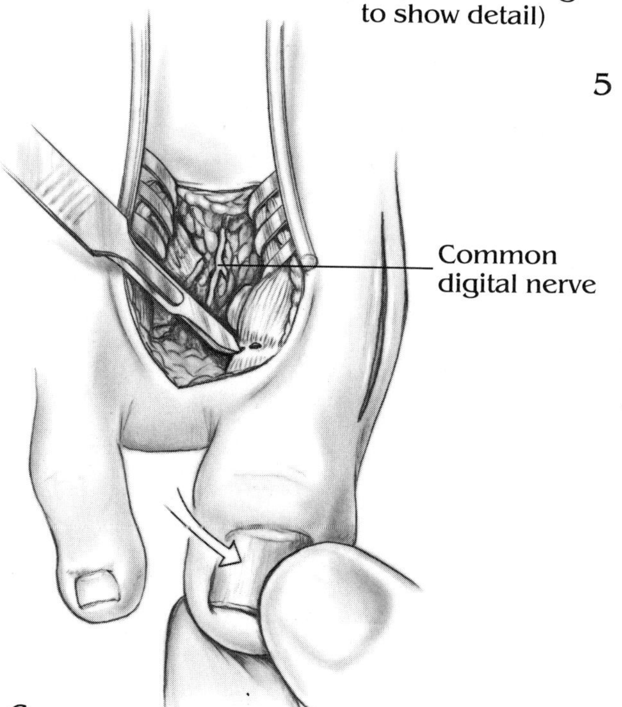
Common
digital nerve

6

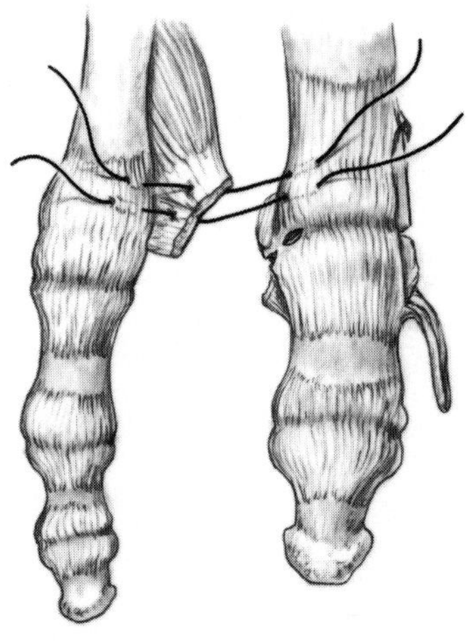

7

Operative Technique: Basilar Crescentic Osteotomy

1. A dorsal longitudinal incision 5 cm long is made medial to the extensor hallucis longus tendon and centered over the base of the first metatarsal (see Fig. 1). Incise the subcutaneous tissue along the line of the skin incision, and expose the base of the first metatarsal subperiosteally.
2. Create a crescentic osteotomy with a micro-oscillating saw. The osteotomy is made 1 cm distal to the base of the first metatarsal and is oriented perpendicular to the longitudinal axis of the metatarsal shaft (Fig. 8).
3. Rotate the distal fragment laterally while applying a medially directed force to the proximal fragment (Fig. 9).
4. Fix the osteotomy with two crossed 0.062-inch Kirschner wires (Fig. 10). Bend the wires to form a loop, and cut off the wires under the skin.
5. Tie the sutures in the first web space (Fig. 10).
6. While holding the hallux in a few degrees of varus, close the first metatarsophalangeal capsule with a horizontal box suture of 2-0 Vicryl. Close the remainder of the capsule with simple 2-0 Vicryl sutures.
7. Close all three incisions in layers. If necessary, reapproximate the subcutaneous tissue with interrupted simple 3-0 Vicryl sutures. Close the skin with interrupted vertical mattress 4-0 nylon sutures.

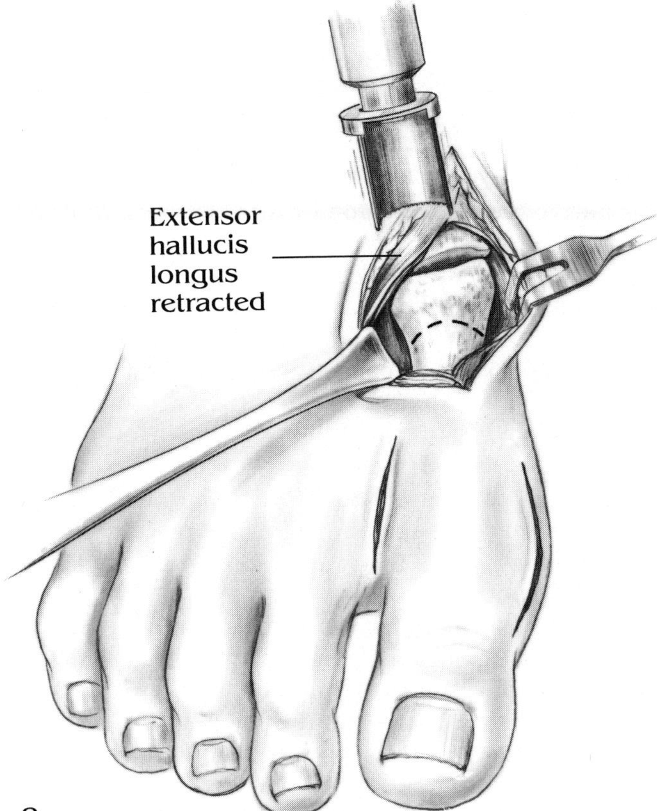

8

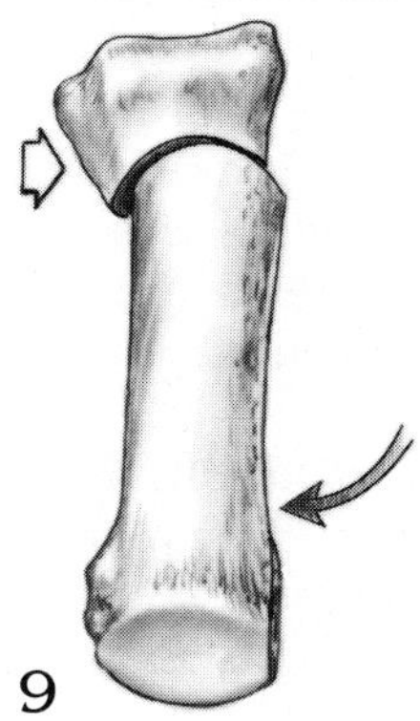

9

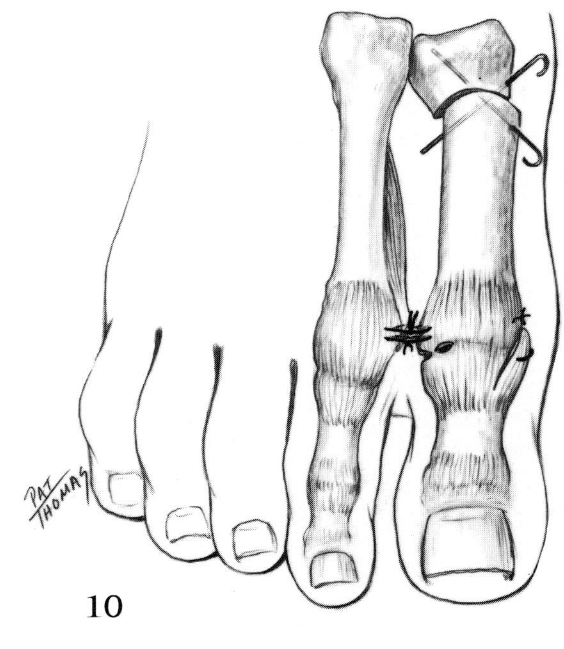

10

Postoperative Care

1. The patient may be placed in a short-leg cast. An alternative postoperative regimen includes the use of corrective strapping, which may be changed on a weekly basis.
2. The patient may be kept non–weight bearing on crutches until the osteotomy heals. An alternative treatment allows protected heel walking in a stiff-soled postoperative shoe.
3. Sutures are removed at 2 to 3 weeks after surgery.
4. Pins are removed at approximately 6 weeks after surgery once radiographs indicate osseous union.
5. Patients are then permitted a slow, gradual return to weight bearing within limits of discomfort.

Technical Pitfalls

1. The prominent medial eminence is excised flush with the shaft of the metatarsal. If excessive bone is excised, instability of the metatarsophalangeal joint may result. This may cause the hallux to deviate medially, resulting in a hallux varus deformity.
2. Excessive plication of the medial capsulorrhaphy of the metatarsophalangeal joint may also lead to medial deviation of the hallux.
3. Insufficient lateral transposition of the distal fragment at the osteotomy site may lead to insufficient correction of the metatarsus primus varus.
4. Inadequate soft tissue release in the first web space may lead to recurrent deformity.
5. Inadequate fixation of the osteotomy may lead to displacement at the osteotomy site. In particular, dorsal displacement of the distal fragment with plantar angulation at the osteotomy site has been reported.

Potential Complications

1. Hallux varus resulting from excessive bony resection of the prominent medial eminence or excessive lateral displacement of the metatarsal osteotomy
2. Recurrence of deformity related to inadequate release of contracted soft tissues in the first web space or inadequate correction of the metatarsus primus varus
3. Injury to the sensory nerves during the soft tissue dissection at the three operative incisions
4. Delayed union or nonunion of the metatarsal osteotomy
5. Malunion of the metatarsal osteotomy
6. Stiffness and loss of motion at the first metatarsophalangeal joint

PROXIMAL PHALANGEAL OSTEOTOMY (MODIFIED AKIN PROCEDURE)

General Considerations

Osteotomy of the proximal phalanx is an effective procedure for correction of hallux valgus deformity in those situations in which the apex of the deformity is located in the distal aspect of the first ray. It is particularly useful for the correction of hallux valgus interphalangeus, in which the lateral deviation of the great toe occurs at the interphalangeal joint, and it may also provide adequate correction for patients with hallux valgus with minimal metatarsus primus varus. The surgical technique described is a modification of the Akin procedure. This technique may be advantageous, because it avoids the shortening usually inherent in a medial-based closing wedge osteotomy. In addition, the arcuate configuration of the osteotomy allows for intraoperative correction of the alignment of the great toe if intraoperative radiographs reveal correction to be either inadequate or overzealous.

Patient Selection

Indications

1. Hallux valgus interphalangeus
2. Hallux valgus without metatarsus primus varus
3. Recurrent hallux valgus after other procedures
4. Second toe disorders associated with lateral deviation of the hallux
5. In combination with other procedures to correct severe hallux valgus

Contraindications as an Isolated Procedure

1. Osteoarthritis of the first metatarsophalangeal joint
2. Severe metatarsus primus varus
3. Significant incongruity of the first metatarsophalangeal joint

Surgical Procedure

Operative Technique

1. A dorsal longitudinal incision is made medial to the extensor hallucis longus tendon from the neck of the proximal phalanx to 1 cm proximal to the exostosis (Fig. 1).
2. Incise the subcutaneous tissue along the line of the skin incision to visualize the capsule. The capsule is incised longitudinally (Fig. 2).
3. Expose the proximal phalanx and exostosis subperiosteally.
4. Excise the exostosis parallel to the medial border of the foot (Fig. 3). Smooth the cut surface with a rasp.
5. Create a crescentic osteotomy with its convexity directed proximally at approximately 1 cm distal to the articular margin of the base of the proximal phalanx (Fig. 4).
6. Swing the distal fragment medially and fix the osteotomy with two crossed Kirschner wires inserted from medial to lateral (Fig. 5).
7. Close the capsule with interrupted simple 2-0 Vicryl sutures.
8. Close the skin with interrupted vertical mattress 4-0 nylon sutures.

Postoperative Care

1. Soft compression dressing for 48 hours
2. Short-leg walking cast for 4 to 6 weeks
3. Percutaneous pins removed at 4 to 6 weeks

Complications

1. Nonunion of the osteotomy
2. Malunion of the proximal phalanx
3. Avascular necrosis of the base of the proximal phalanx
4. Shortening of the great toe

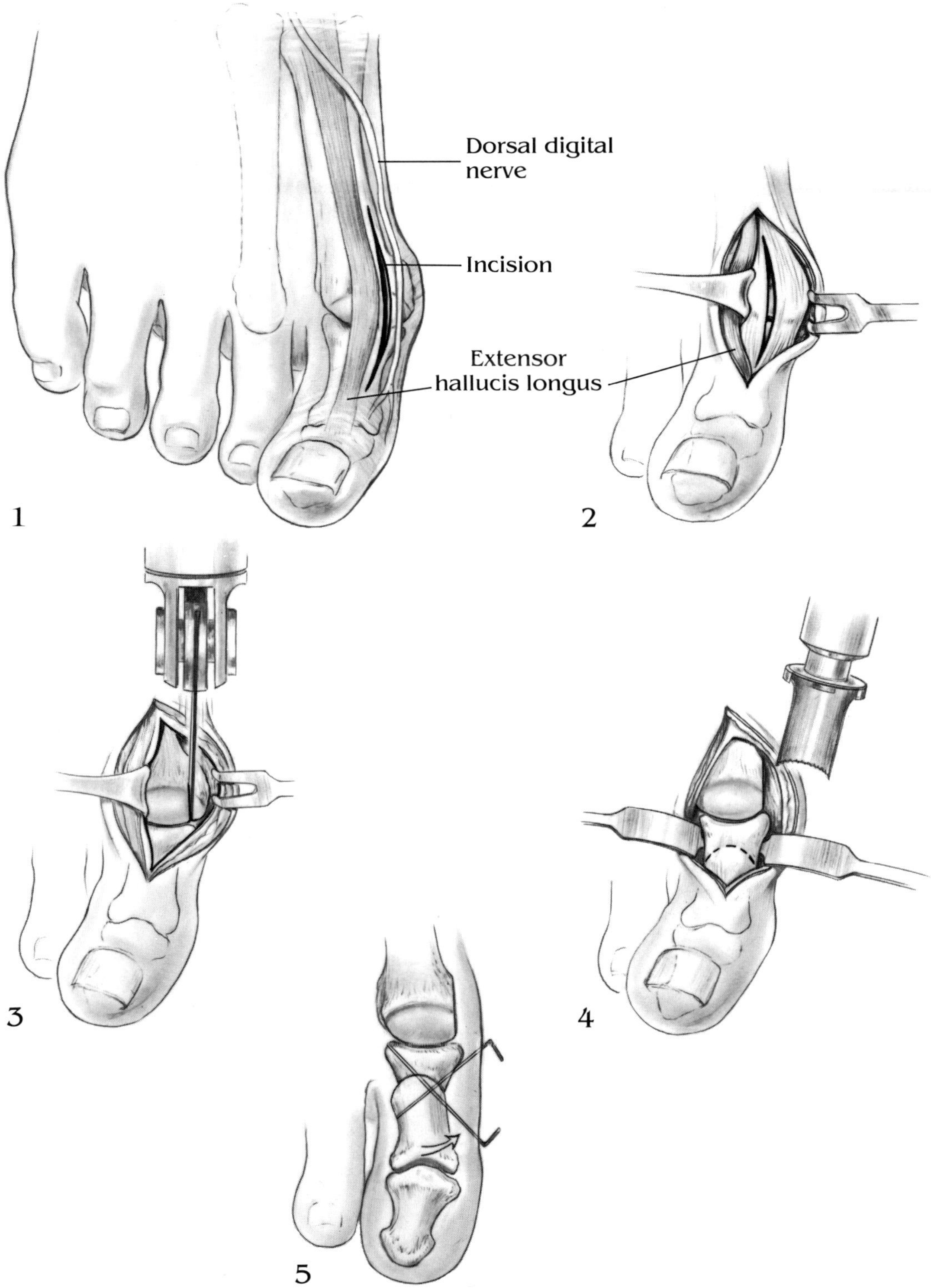
Dorsal digital nerve
Incision
Extensor hallucis longus
1
2
3
4
5

PART 2

Operations for Hallux Rigidus and Hallux Valgus With Arthritis

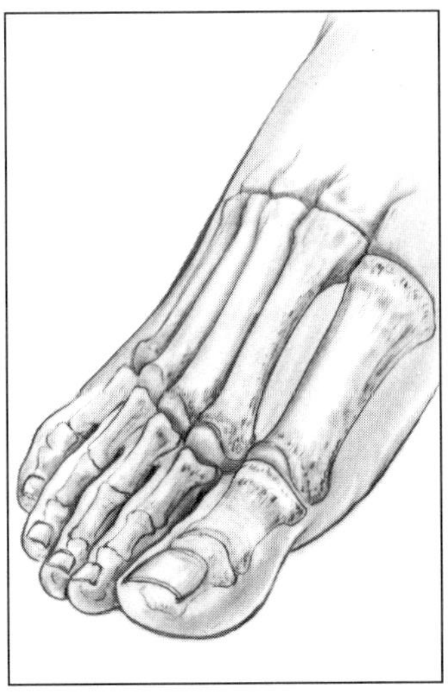

CHEILECTOMY FOR HALLUX RIGIDUS

General Considerations

Hallux rigidus is a disorder characterized by a limitation of motion at the first metatarsophalangeal joint. There is a mechanical block to dorsiflexion caused by the impingement of an exostosis at the dorsal, medial, and lateral aspect of the first metatarsal head against an osteophyte at the base of the proximal phalanx. These osteophytes can be the result of degenerative, traumatic, metabolic, or inflammatory joint disease. Patients note restriction of dorsiflexion and localized pain during the toe-off phase of gait. These individuals therefore tend to shift their weight laterally and toe-off on the lesser metatarsal heads. Initial treatment includes a stiff-soled shoe with a rocker added to the outer sole. This allows the shoe to propel the body forward during push-off and thus avoids the painful grinding of the incongruous articular surfaces. Nonsteroidal anti-inflammatory medications may be helpful. If conservative measures fail, surgical intervention in the form of a cheilectomy is appropriate.

Patient Selection

Indications

1. Active patients with hallux rigidus manifested as restriction of dorsiflexion and localized pain during the toe-off phase of gait
2. Physical examination revealing a prominent exostosis at the dorsum of the metatarsal head, as well as tenderness at the articulation
3. Radiographs revealing arthritic changes localized primarily to the dorsal aspect of the joint
4. Mechanical impingement of the dorsal exostosis against the toe box of the shoe

Contraindications

1. Once the arthritic process has progressed to involve the joint more diffusely, arthrodesis or Keller resection arthroplasty of the joint will be more effective. In this situation, younger, more active individuals are appropriately treated with an arthrodesis. Elderly individuals who engage in limited weight bearing and ambulation may be better served by resection arthroplasty of the joint.
2. Gout may cause restriction of motion, pain, and swelling at the first metatarsophalangeal joint. If hyperuricemia is identified, conservative management with appropriate medications and shoe modifications will often alleviate symptoms.

Surgical Procedure

Operative Technique

1. A dorsal longitudinal incision approximately 5 cm long is made medial to the extensor hallucis longus tendon. It extends from the middle of the first metatarsal to the midpoint of the proximal phalanx (Fig. 1).
2. Incise the subcutaneous tissue along the line of the skin incision, avoiding the dorsal cutaneous nerve. The extensor hallucis longus tendon is retracted laterally.
3. Incise the capsule and periosteum longitudinally and reflect subperiosteally to expose the first metatarsal head and the base of the proximal phalanx (Fig. 2). Hyperflex the hallux to deliver the metatarsal head dorsally.
4. Generously excise the osteophyte dorsally, medially, and laterally with a microsagittal saw to form a smooth dorsal surface flush with the metatarsal shaft (Fig. 3). The goal of the bony decompression is to achieve 60 to 80 degrees of dorsiflexion of the joint.
5. Resect the osteophyte from the base of the proximal phalanx with a power saw or bone cutter (Fig. 4). Smooth the cut surfaces with a rasp (Fig. 5).
6. Close the capsule with interrupted simple 2-0 Vicryl sutures. Reapproximate the skin with interrupted vertical mattress 4-0 nylon sutures.

Postoperative Care

1. A compression dressing is applied.
2. The patient is kept non–weight bearing on crutches for 3 weeks.
3. Sutures are removed at 3 weeks postoperatively, and the patient then begins ambulation in a soft, flexible rubber-soled shoe.
4. Slow, progressive range-of-motion exercises are begun once the sutures are removed.

Technical Pitfalls

1. Inadequate removal of bone may prevent adequate dorsiflexion.
2. Removal of excessive bone from the metatarsal head may lead to dorsal subluxation of the proximal phalanx.
3. Excessive stripping of the capsule and release of the volar plate may lead to avascular necrosis of the metatarsal head.

Potential Complications

1. Recurrence of dorsal exostosis
2. Further progression of articular degeneration leading to recurrent symptoms
3. Loss of motion secondary to periarticular scarring due to inadequate postoperative exercise regimen
4. Avascular necrosis of the metatarsal head

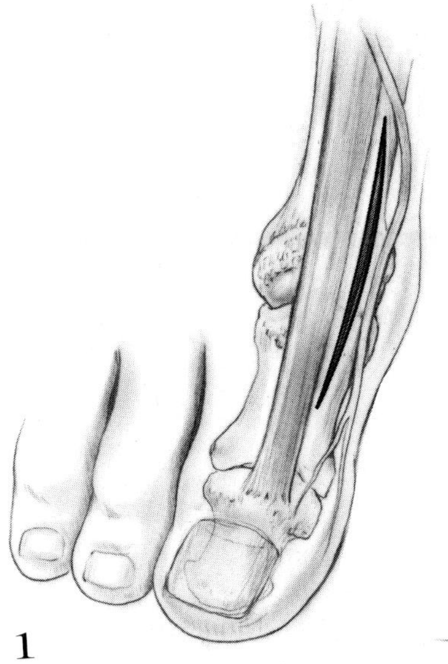

1

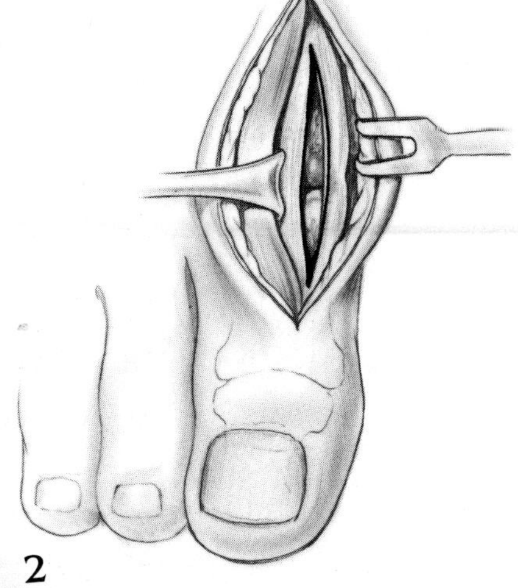

2

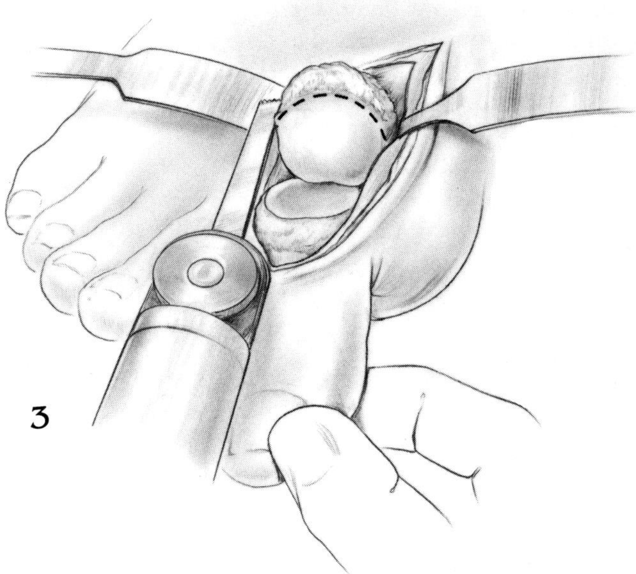

3

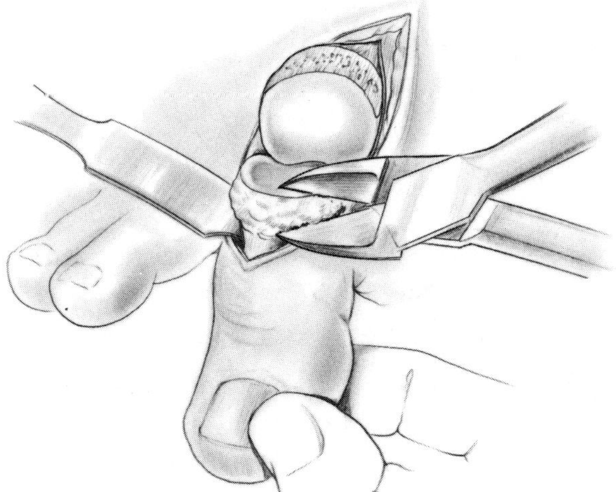

4

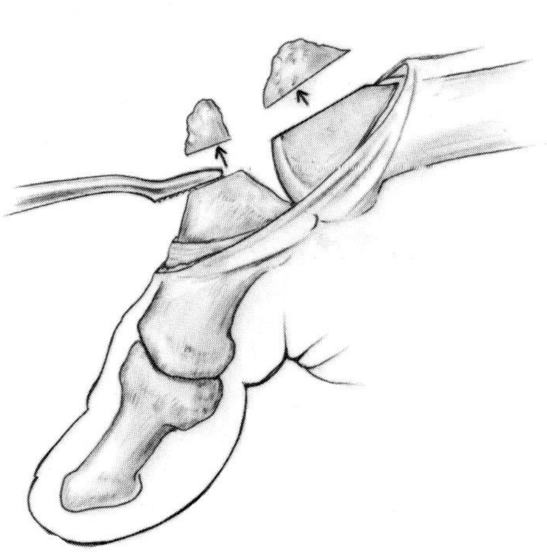

5

ARTHRODESIS OF THE FIRST METATARSOPHALANGEAL JOINT

General Considerations

Arthrodesis of the first metatarsophalangeal joint serves to eliminate painful motion of that joint often associated with intra-articular arthritis. Arthrosis of the metatarsophalangeal joint of the hallux may occur as a localized manifestation of a systemic process and is also seen associated with severe hallux rigidus that has progressed to encompass the entire joint. Long-standing hallux valgus may also be associated with significant intra-articular degenerative changes. Patients note limitation of motion of the joint, as well as pain during the toe-off phase of gait. Physical examination reveals tenderness at the joint line, as well as an abnormal gait in which the patient tends to toe-off on the lateral border of the foot. Nonoperative treatment with an inflexible, rocker-soled shoe and anti-inflammatory medications may provide relief in some patients. If conservative measures fail, arthrodesis is particularly appropriate for young individuals with an active life-style. Numerous surgical techniques have been described in the literature. This technique utilizes a "cup-and-cone" configuration of the bones and fixation with a compression screw.

Patient Selection

Indications

1. Hallux rigidus associated with diffuse degenerative changes throughout the first metatarsophalangeal joint
2. Arthritis of the metatarsophalangeal joint of the hallux
3. Rheumatoid arthritis or other systemic inflammatory arthropathies associated with involvement of the hallux
4. Metabolic disorders such as gout with secondary arthrosis
5. Long-standing hallux valgus deformity associated with intra-articular arthritis
6. Salvage of an arthritic joint secondary to avascular necrosis of the head of the first metatarsal after prior surgery or trauma, particularly in a young, active individual who engages in significant weight-bearing activities

Contraindications

1. Elderly debilitated patients with a limited ambulatory status
2. Patients whose general medical condition may lead to increased risk of complications
3. Inadequate neurologic or vascular status in the distal peripheral extremity

Surgical Procedure

Operative Technique

1. A medial longitudinal incision is made just plantar to the midline from the neck of the proximal phalanx, extending proximally to end 2.5 cm proximal to the metatarsal head (Fig. 1).
2. The capsule is incised longitudinally (Fig. 2). The distal half of the first metatarsal and the proximal half of the proximal phalanx are exposed subperiosteally by sharp dissection.
3. The articular surface of the first metatarsal head is removed with a power saw. This is achieved by means of a cut perpendicular to the longitudinal axis of the metatarsal shaft (Fig. 3).
4. The distal end of the first metatarsal is fashioned to a blunt point with a power saw (Fig. 4). The distal end is then reamed with a female reamer to create a cone-shaped configuration (Fig. 5). If a reamer is not available, a power burr may be used to shape the end of the metatarsal.

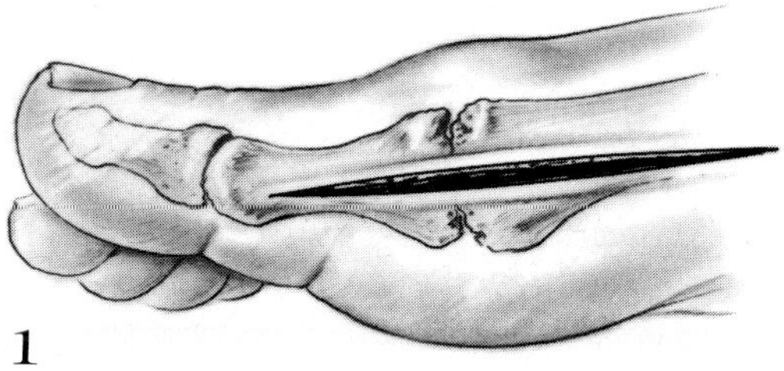

1

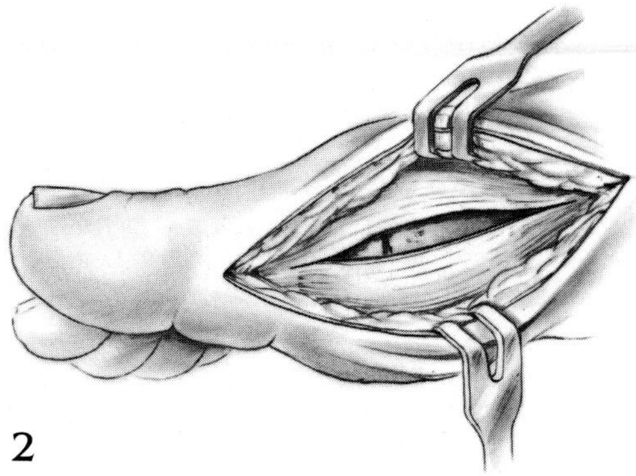

2

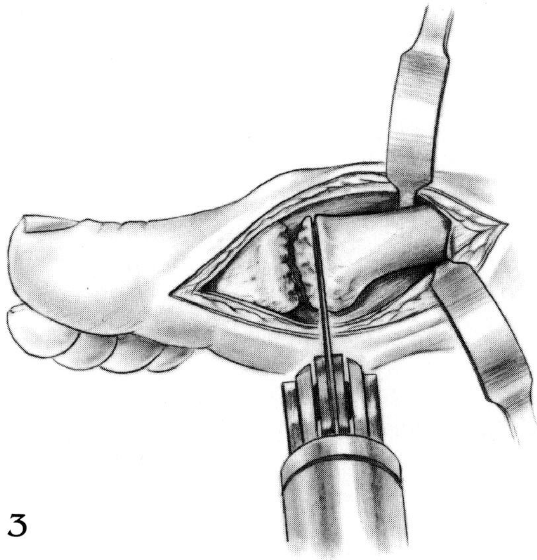

3

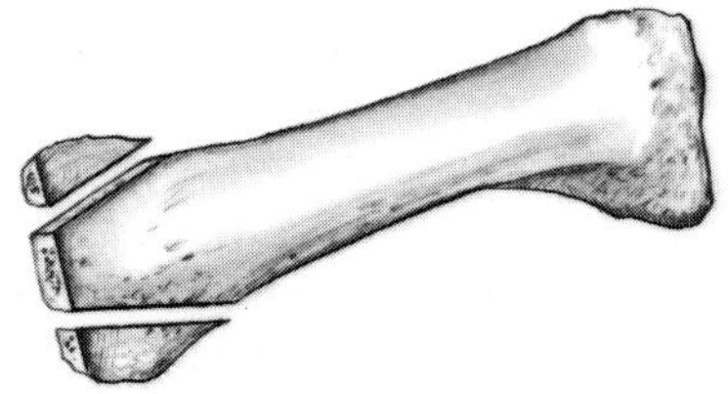

4

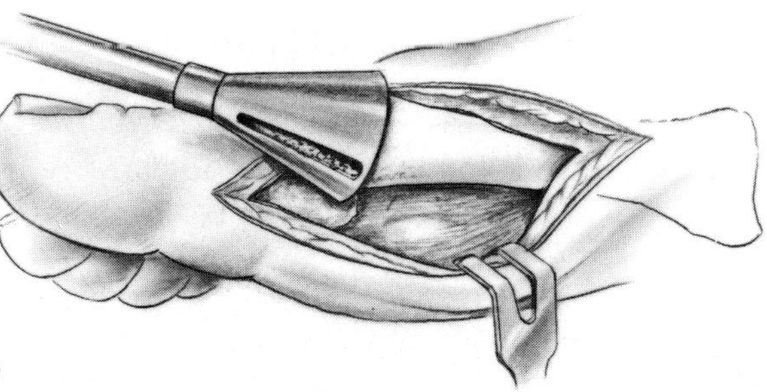

5

5. A hole is drilled centrally in the base of the proximal phalanx (Fig. 6). The base is then reamed with a male reamer or decorticated with a power burr to fashion the end of the bone into a cup configuration (Fig. 7).
6. The cut surfaces are positioned so that the hallux lies in 15 to 20 degrees of dorsiflexion and 15 to 20 degrees of valgus compared with the first metatarsal shaft (Figs. 8 and 9). The position may be held temporarily with Kirschner wires.
7. Fixation is accomplished by means of a compression screw. A hole is drilled from the medial plantar aspect of the base of the proximal phalanx into the intermedullary canal of the metatarsal with a 2.5-mm drill bit. Tap the entire drill path with a 3.5-mm tap. A recess is cut for the screw head with a countersink, and a 4.0-mm intramedullary cancellous screw is inserted (Fig. 9).
8. The capsule is closed with interrupted simple 2-0 Vicryl sutures. Close the skin with interrupted vertical mattress 4-0 nylon sutures.

Postoperative Care

1. A sterile Robert Jones compression dressing with a stirrup splint is applied for 48 hours.
2. A short-leg cast is applied for 6 weeks.
3. Sutures are removed and the cast changed at 3 weeks after surgery.
4. The patient is kept non–weight bearing on crutches for 6 weeks or until radiographs reveal osseous union.

Technical Pitfalls

1. Excessive dorsiflexion of the fusion may lead to impingement of the interphalangeal joint and distal phalanx against the toe box of the shoe.
2. Patients who have some degree of hallux valgus interphalangeus may require less than 15 to 20 degrees of valgus deviation of the great toe to avoid abutment of the second toe.
3. A larger cancellous screw or supplementary Kirschner wire fixation may be required to ensure rotary alignment of the hallux and osseous union.
4. Inadequate valgus deviation or dorsiflexion of the hallux may lead to difficulties during the toe-off phase of gait.

Complications

1. Nonunion or delayed union of the fusion site
2. Excessive valgus deviation of the hallux leading to abutment of the second toe
3. Clawing of the interphalangeal joint, which may be associated with the excessive dorsiflexion of the hallux
4. Some restriction of shoewear, typically seen because the patient is limited to a specific heel height depending on the extent of the dorsiflexion of the hallux at the fusion site

---

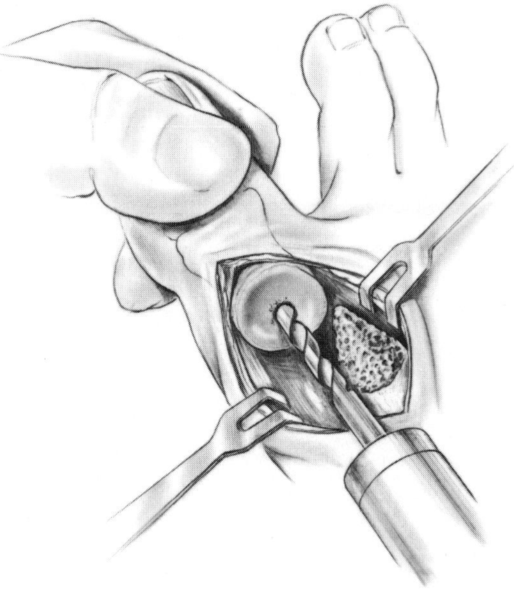

6

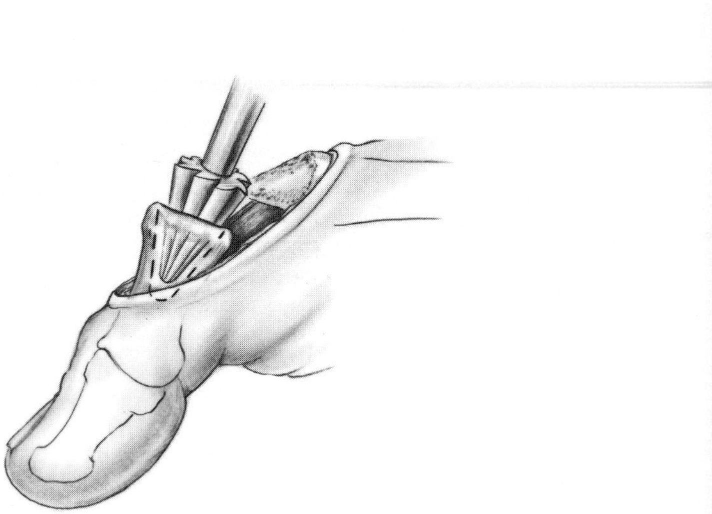

7

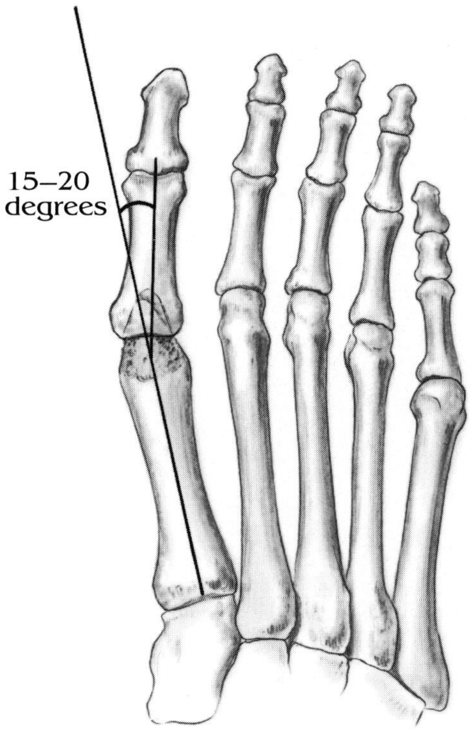

8

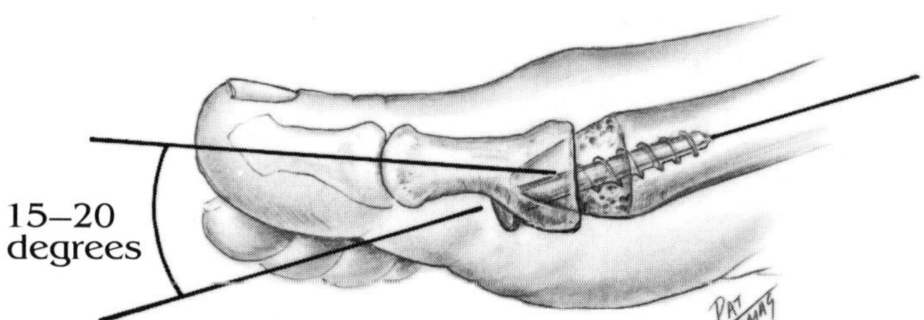

9

KELLER RESECTION ARTHROPLASTY

The Keller resection arthroplasty of the first metatarsophalangeal joint is used to correct severe hallux rigidus and hallux valgus deformities associated with arthrosis of the metatarsophalangeal articulation. This procedure is generally reserved for elderly individuals with limited weight-bearing or ambulatory status.

Patient Selection

Indications

1. Hallux valgus accompanied by metatarsus primus varus with a prominent medial eminence and arthritic changes at the first metatarsophalangeal joint
2. End-stage hallux rigidus with extensive diffuse arthritic involvement throughout the articulation
3. Rheumatoid or related arthropathies and metabolic disorders associated with involvement of the hallux and with joint destruction at the metatarsophalangeal joint
4. Salvage after trauma or other surgical procedures complicated by avascular necrosis or arthritis of the joint, manifested by pain on motion, tenderness at the joint line, and radiographic evidence of degenerative changes

Contraindications

1. Patients younger than 60 years
2. Patients with an active life-style requiring a rigorous ambulatory status
3. Presence of lateral metatarsalgia with pain and hyperkeratotic lesions at the plantar aspect of the metatarsal heads
4. Inadequate neurologic or vascular status or other systemic medical disorders that would contraindicate surgery

Surgical Procedure

Operative Technique

1. A dorsomedial incision is made from the neck of the proximal phalanx to 2 cm proximal to the exostosis (Fig. 1). The subcutaneous tissue is divided along the line of the skin incision, and the skin and subcutaneous tissues are reflected minimally to visualize the capsule.
2. A medial longitudinal capsular incision is made plantar to the skin incision (Fig. 2). The capsule and periosteum are reflected subperiosteally to expose the base of the proximal phalanx and the medial aspect of the metatarsal head.
3. Excise the exostosis parallel to the medial border of the foot with a power saw (Fig. 3). Smooth the cut surface with a rasp.
4. Expose the base of the proximal phalanx circumferentially. Excise the proximal one third of the proximal phalanx perpendicular to its longitudinal axis with the power saw (Fig. 4).
5. If the capsule is redundant, remove a plantar ellipse (Fig. 5). Close the capsule with 2-0 Vicryl interrupted simple sutures inserted obliquely from dorsoproximal to plantar distal while holding the hallux in 5 degrees varus and plantarflexion (Fig. 6).
6. Close the skin with interrupted vertical mattress 4-0 nylon sutures.

Postoperative Care

1. A sterile compression dressing with adhesive tape corrective strapping is applied to hold the hallux in the corrected position.
2. Ambulation on the heel is permitted in a postoperative wooden-soled shoe.
3. The dressings and corrective strapping are changed every 1 to 2 weeks for a total of 6 weeks after surgery.
4. The sutures are removed at 3 weeks postoperatively.

Technical Pitfalls

1. Removal of too much bone from the base of the first proximal phalanx may lead to excessive shortening of the great toe.
2. Cutting of the flexor hallucis longus tendon may lead to a severe cock-up toe.

Potential Complications

1. Shortening of the hallux (expected)
2. Decreased power in the great toe (expected)
3. Transfer metatarsalgia
4. Cock-up toe

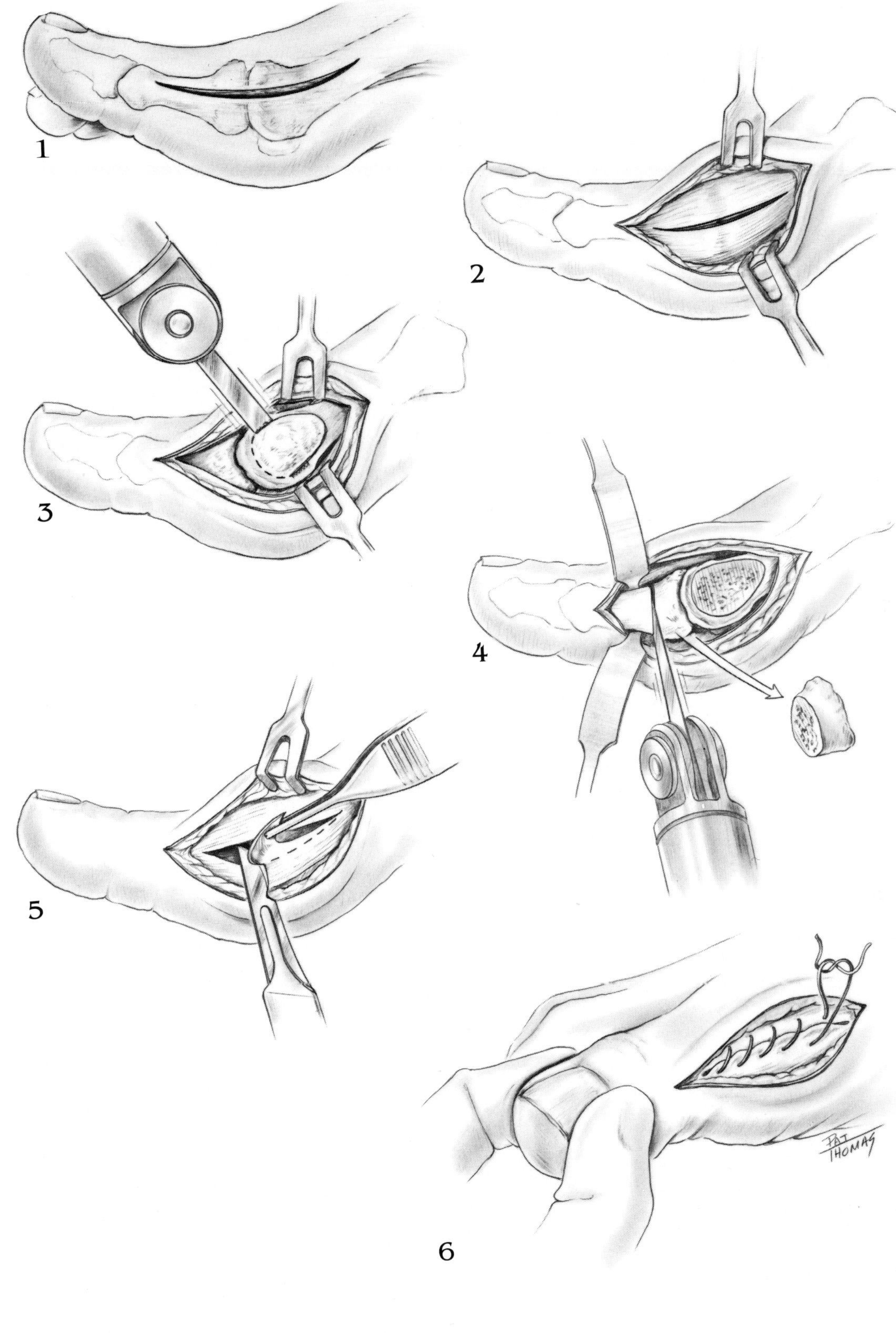
1
2
3
4
5
6

PART 3

Excision Hallux Sesamoids

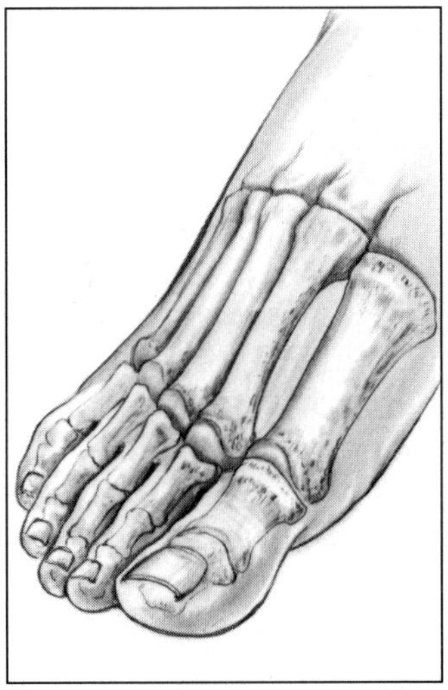

EXCISION MEDIAL HALLUX SESAMOID; EXCISION LATERAL HALLUX SESAMOID

General Considerations

Various pathologic disorders may affect the hallux sesamoids. These small osseous structures, which lie beneath the first metatarsal head, can be affected by any of several systemic disorders. In addition, traumatic injuries to the sesamoid are common, and nonunion of sesamoid fractures may be a source of chronic symptoms. Arthritis at the sesamoidometatarsal articulation may be seen in patients with long-standing hallux valgus deformities. Avascular necrosis of the hallux sesamoids, referred to as *osteochondritis*, may affect either the medial or the lateral sesamoid.

Any of these disorders may lead to localized pain associated with weight bearing. The physical examination will reveal localized tenderness, and the patient's pain can be reproduced with dorsiflexion of the great toe as the flexor hallucis brevis is pulled taut, leading to compression of the sesamoid against the metatarsal head. Radiographs and bone scans may be helpful in identifying the specific pathologic disorder present.

Conservative modalities of treatment are often effective. These include the use of a rubber-soled shoe to decrease impact loading on the area. The addition of a soft, flexible insert with a sulcus elevation to float the hallux sesamoid and first metatarsal head is often effective in relieving the pain associated with weight bearing. Anti-inflammatory medications and other symptomatic measures may also be helpful. In those patients with chronic recurrent sesamoiditis or chronic pain associated with any one of the afflictions of the sesamoid, surgical extrication may be helpful. It is most important to identify which of the two sesamoids is involved. Excision of one sesamoid bone is fairly well tolerated, but excision of both sesamoids should be avoided if possible.

Patient Selection

Indications

1. Chronic recurrent pain on weight bearing and interference with the ability to ambulate secondary to pathologic disorders of the sesamoid
2. Painful nonunion of a fractured sesamoid
3. Avascular necrosis of the sesamoid

Contraindications

1. Elderly patients may obtain relief of symptoms with inserts designed to float the sesamoids off the inner sole of the shoe.
2. Patients with afflictions of both the medial and lateral sesamoids may be best treated with conservative modalities, as surgical excision of both sesamoids may be complicated by a cock-up deformity of the hallux.
3. Professional athletes and dancers may note alterations in the biomechanics of stance phase and other activities after sesamoid excision.

EXCISION MEDIAL HALLUX SESAMOID

Surgical Procedure

Operative Technique: Excision of the Medial Hallux Sesamoid

1. A midline medial longitudinal incision 5 cm long is made, extending from the midpoint of the proximal phalanx to the midpoint of the metatarsal (Fig. 1). The subcutaneous tissue is incised along the line of the skin incision.
2. Incise the joint capsule longitudinally (Fig. 2). Reflect the capsule and periosteum from the metatarsal subperiosteally.
3. By applying traction to the plantar soft tissues, the medial sesamoid may be exposed (Fig. 3).
4. Carefully shell out the medial sesamoid subperiosteally with a scalpel (Fig. 4), avoiding disruption of the conjoined tendon.
5. Repair the defect in the conjoined tendon with a pursestring suture of 2-0 Vicryl (Fig. 5a). An alternate technique of repair consists of two simple sutures inserted at right angles to each other (Fig. 5b).
6. Close the capsule with interrupted simple 2-0 Vicryl sutures. The skin incision is closed with interrupted vertical mattress 4-0 nylon sutures.

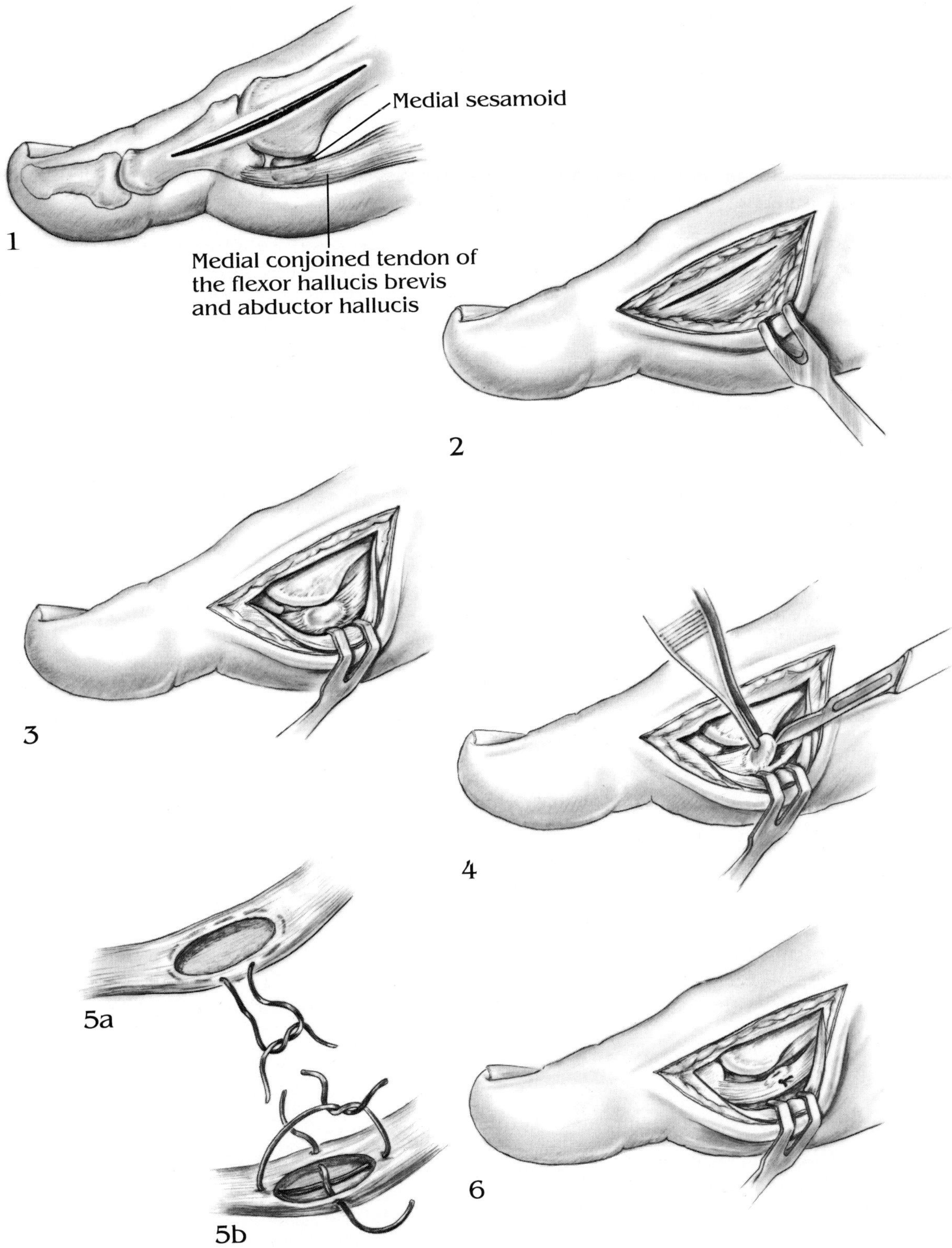
Medial sesamoid
1
Medial conjoined tendon of
the flexor hallucis brevis
and abductor hallucis
2
3
4
5a
5b
6

EXCISION LATERAL HALLUX SESAMOID

Operative Technique: Excision of the Lateral Hallux Sesamoid

1. A plantar longitudinal incision 2.5 cm long is made, centered over the lateral hallux sesamoid and medial to its longitudinal axis (Fig. 1). The subcutaneous tissue is incised along the line of the skin incision, avoiding the digital nerve, which lies at the lateral aspect of the lateral hallux sesamoid.
2. Make a longitudinal incision to split the flexor hallucis brevis muscle and the joint capsule (Fig. 2).
3. Expose the lateral hallux sesamoid subperiosteally (Fig. 3).
4. Extirpate the sesamoid by sharp dissection with a scalpel (Fig. 4).
5. Repair the flexor hallucis brevis muscle with a pursestring or other reapproximating suture of 2-0 Vicryl (Fig. 5).
6. Reapproximate the subcutaneous tissue with interrupted simple 3-0 Vicryl sutures. Close the skin with interrupted vertical mattress 3-0 nylon sutures (Fig. 6).

Postoperative Care

1. A Robert Jones compression dressing may be applied for the first 48 hours.
2. A short-leg cast is applied for 6 weeks.
3. Sutures are removed and the cast changed at 3 weeks after surgery.
4. The patient is kept non–weight bearing for 4 weeks.
5. A slow, gradual return to weight-bearing activity is then allowed.

Technical Pitfalls

1. Care should be taken to avoid injury to the branches of the digital nerve that lie at the medial aspect of the lateral hallux sesamoid during excision of this bone.
2. Adequate reapproximation of the conjoined tendon is necessary to avoid deformity of the hallux.

Complications

1. Cock-up deformity of the hallux may occur after excision of one, and especially after excision of both, sesamoids.
2. Hallux varus may occur after excision of the lateral sesamoid.
3. Hallux valgus may occur after excision of the medial sesamoid.
4. Neuroma may occur secondary to nerve injury or entrapment after lateral sesamoid excision.

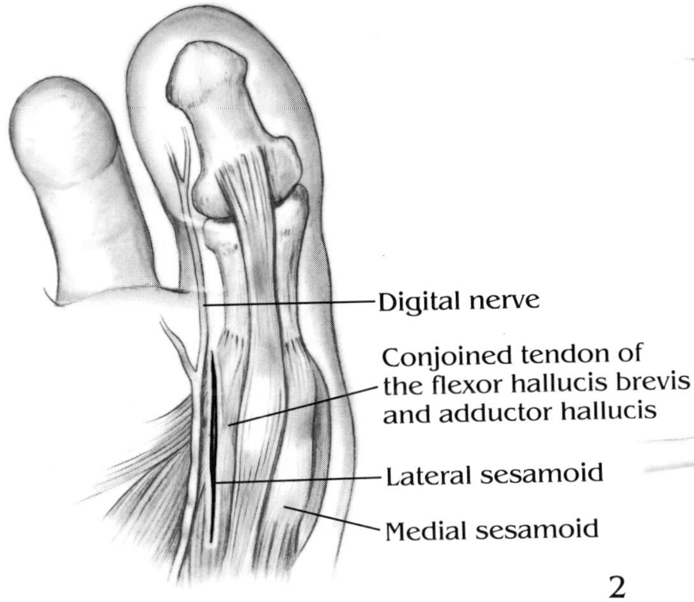
Digital nerve
Conjoined tendon of the flexor hallucis brevis and adductor hallucis
Lateral sesamoid
Medial sesamoid

1

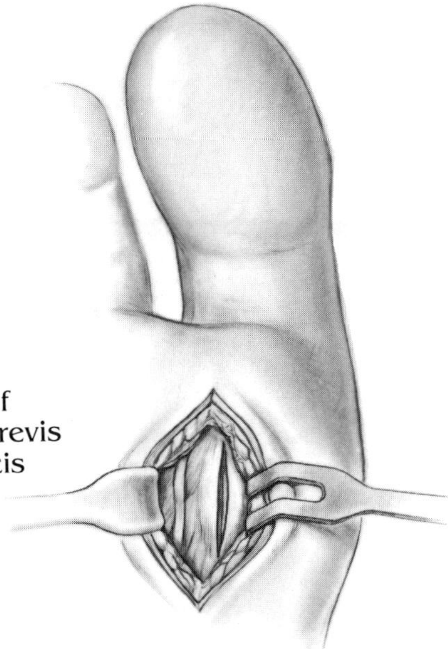

2

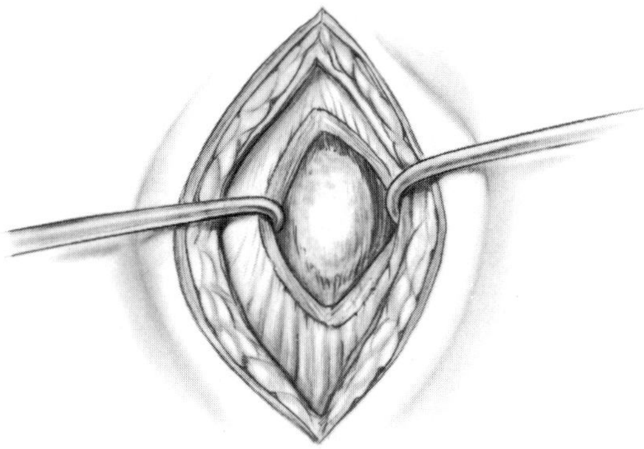

3

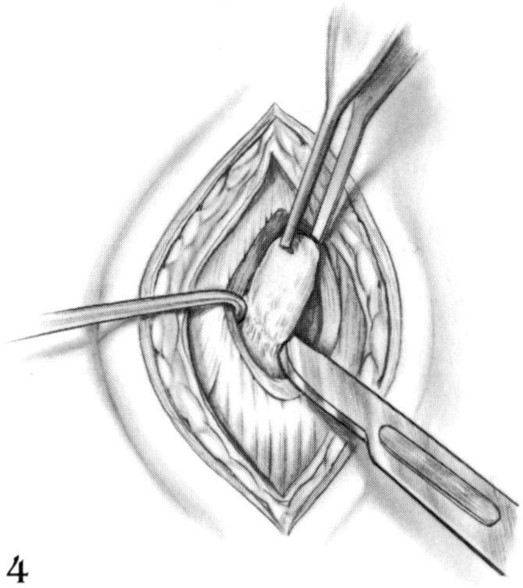

4

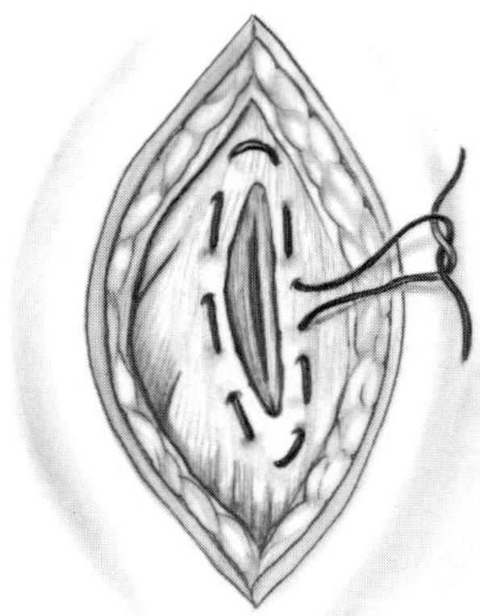

5

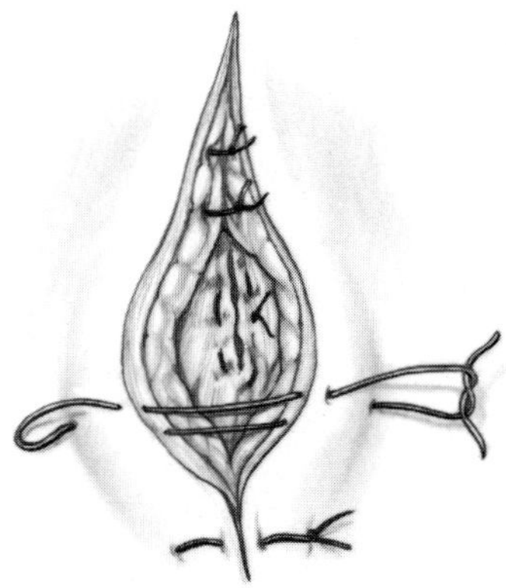

6

PART 4

Osseous Decompression First and Fifth Metatarsal Head

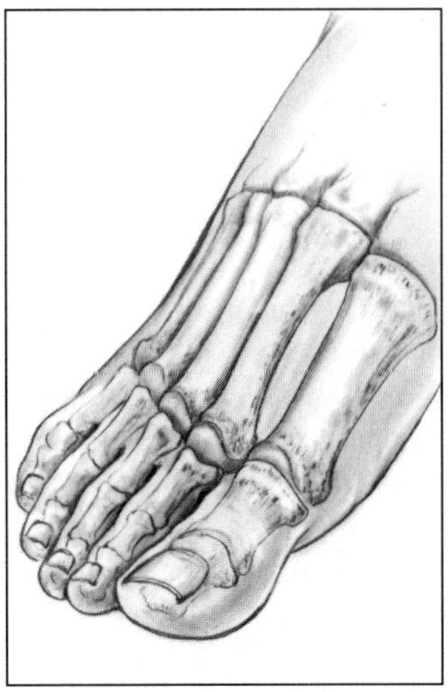

EXCISION OF A PROMINENT MEDIAL EMINENCE OF THE FIRST METATARSAL HEAD; EXCISION OF A PROMINENT LATERAL EMINENCE OF THE FIFTH METATARSAL HEAD

General Considerations

The complex of disorders known as hallux valgus includes a prominent bony eminence at the medial aspect of the first metatarsal head. A bunionette deformity includes a prominent bony eminence at the lateral aspect of the fifth metatarsal head. Although these forefoot deformities often require extensive soft tissue surgery, as well as metatarsal osteotomies, there are situations in which isolated excision of the bony prominence is appropriate.

Metatarsus primus varus and hallux valgus lead to uncovering of the medial aspect of the first metatarsal head, which thus becomes prominent at the medial border of the forefoot. This leads to mechanical impingement against the toe box of the shoe. A bunionette deformity with metatarsus quintus valgus leads to prominence of the lateral aspect of the fifth metatarsal head, also causing mechanical impingement and difficulty with shoewear. Patients note pain and swelling about the skin and soft tissues overlying the bony eminence. The physical examination elicits localized tenderness and erythema of the skin overlying the prominent metatarsal head.

Initial treatment includes the use of appropriate shoewear with a high, wide toe box and soft leather uppers to accommodate the deformity. The use of sponge rubber toe caps and various types of toe protectors may be helpful to float the tender area away from the toe box of the shoe. In elderly patients, local mechanical impingement may lead to chronic bursitis with potential breakdown of the skin overlying the prominent areas. Patients with diabetes and other neuropathic disorders are also prone to skin ulceration. These patients may require temporary use of open-toed shoewear and limitation of weight bearing until healing occurs. In those patients in whom more extensive surgical correction of deformity is contraindicated because of age, circulatory dysfunction, or diabetes, isolated resection of the prominent bony eminence may be the most appropriate means of treatment.

Patient Selection

Indications

1. Patients with primary complaints related to a prominent medial eminence at the first metatarsal head or a prominent lateral eminence at the fifth metatarsal head
2. Patients who have symptoms related to mechanical impingement over these osseous prominences in whom more extensive correction of deformity is deemed inappropriate
3. Patients in whom appropriate shoewear and protective devices have failed to provide relief of symptoms

Contraindications

1. Patients in whom circulatory dysfunction or neuropathy is so severe that significant concern regarding wound healing potential is present; these patients may be better treated with local protective measures.
2. If skin ulceration and soft tissue infection has already occurred, surgery must be postponed until healing is noted. These patients require local wound care and must avoid mechanical pressure from shoewear. Antibiotic therapy is often required.
3. Patients who are nonambulatory may be better treated with open-toed shoewear or Plastazote sandals.

Surgical Procedure

Operative Technique: Excision of the Prominent Medial Eminence of the First Metatarsal

1. A dorsomedial incision 4 cm long is made from the base of the proximal phalanx to just proximal to the exostosis (Fig. 1). Incise the subcutaneous tissue along the line of the skin incision. Reflect the skin and subcutaneous tissue to expose the capsule.
2. Make a Y-shaped capsular incision based distally with the apex of the "V" portion just proximal to the exostosis (Fig. 1). Reflect the V-shaped flap subperiosteally to expose the prominent medial eminence.
3. Excise the prominent medial eminence parallel to the medial border of the foot with a microsagittal saw (Fig. 2). Smooth the cut surface with a rasp.
4. While holding the hallux in slight overcorrection varus and plantarflexion, close the capsule with a horizontal box tension suture of 2-0 Vicryl (Fig. 3). Close the remainder of the capsule with interrupted simple 2-0 Vicryl sutures. Close the skin with interrupted vertical mattress 4-0 nylon sutures.

Operative Technique: Excision of the Prominent Lateral Eminence of the Fifth Metatarsal

1. A dorsolateral incision is made from the base of the proximal phalanx and extending to just proximal to the exostosis. Incise the subcutaneous tissue along the line of the skin incision and reflect the skin and subcutaneous tissue to expose the joint capsule (Fig. 1, bottom).
2. Make a longitudinal capsular incision just plantar to the skin incision. Reflect the capsule subperiosteally to expose the exostosis.
3. Excise the prominent lateral eminence with a microsagittal saw (Fig. 2, bottom). Smooth the cut surface with a rasp.
4. Close the capsule with interrupted simple 3-0 Vicryl sutures. Close the skin with interrupted vertical mattress nylon sutures.

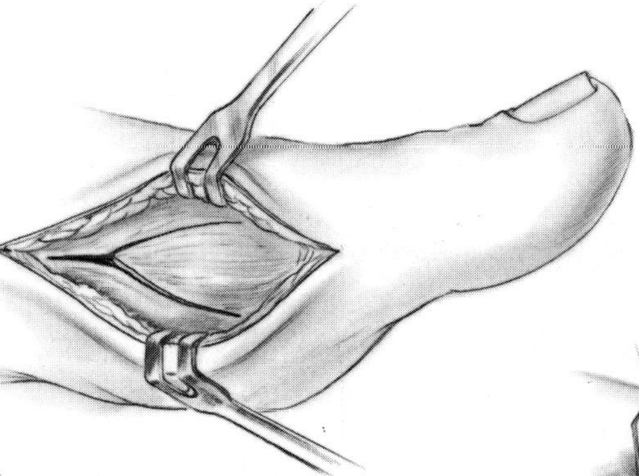

1

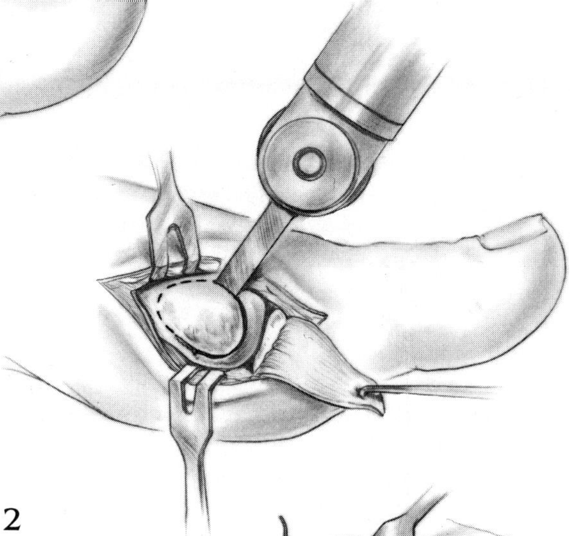

2

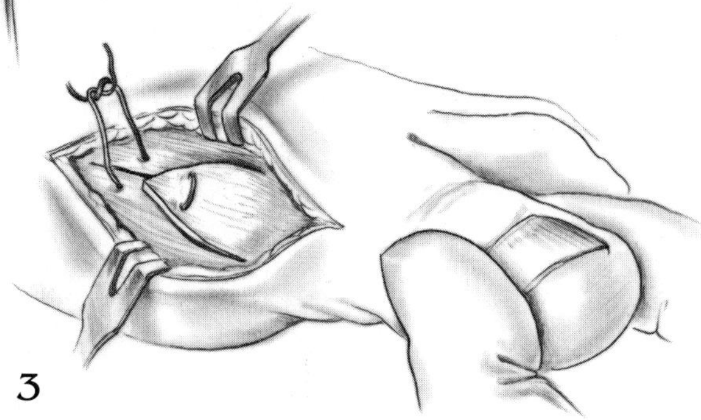

3

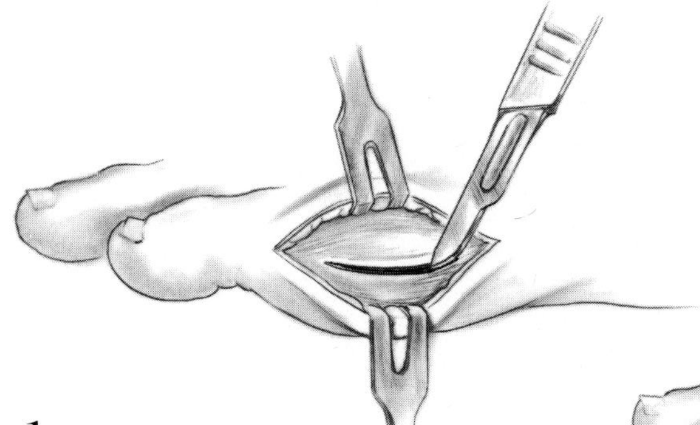

1

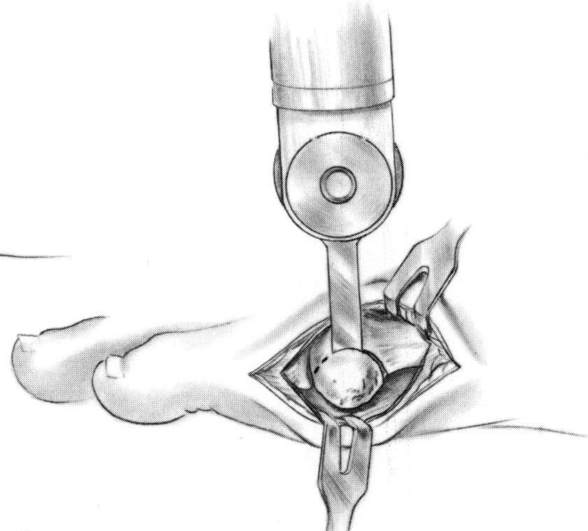

2

Postoperative Care

1. A sterile compression dressing is applied.
2. Partial weight bearing is allowed in a wooden-soled postoperative shoe.
3. Sutures are removed at 3 weeks postoperatively.
4. The patient is allowed a slow, gradual return to weight-bearing activities and wearing shoes within the limits of discomfort.

Technical Pitfalls. Excessive removal of a prominent bony eminence must be avoided, as this may result in instability of the joint. If too large a portion of the first metatarsal head is removed, hallux varus may result. Similarly, excessive removal of the fifth metatarsal head may lead to instability of that joint.

Potential Complications

1. Failure to postpone surgery until the acute bursitis or acute infectious process resolves may lead to delayed wound healing and persistent infection.
2. Recurrence of deformity is possible. The patient should be maintained in reasonable shoewear with a high, wide toe box to prevent further problems.

PART 5

Arthrodesis Interphalangeal Joint Hallux

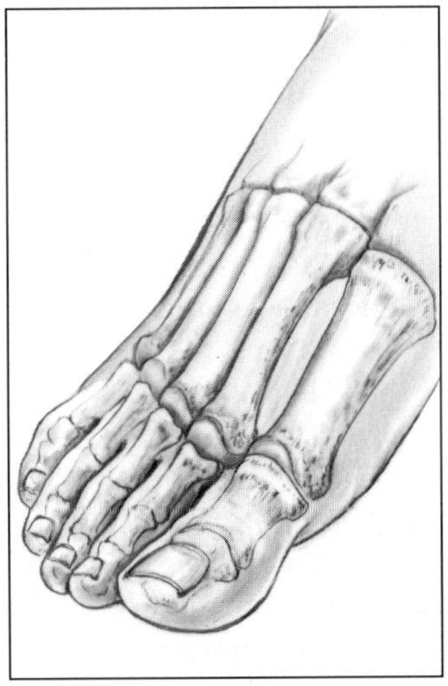

ARTHRODESIS INTERPHALANGEAL JOINT HALLUX

General Considerations

The interphalangeal joint of the hallux may be afflicted with various pathologic disorders. Traumatic arthritis of that joint is commonly seen after a stubbing injury. Other direct mechanisms of injury, such as dropping a heavy object on the dorsum of the hallux, may lead to fracture with subsequent arthrosis. Degenerative joint disease, rheumatoid arthritis, and seronegative systemic inflammatory arthropathy may also affect the interphalangeal joint.

Deformities of the hallux interphalangeal joint may also be seen in clinical practice. Various neuromuscular disorders may lead to deforming forces of the extrinsic or intrinsic muscles about the great toe; this may be manifested as claw or hyperextension deformity. Traumatic injuries to the extrinsic tendons may also lead to muscle imbalance with subsequent deformities. Congenital hallux valgus interphalangeus, as well as deformities secondary to growth plate injuries, may also result in symptoms emanating from this articulation.

Patients describe pain and swelling about the joint. Difficulty in fitting shoes is often described. The hallux plays an important role in weight bearing during the stance phase of gait, and thus many individuals with arthritis or deformity of the interphalangeal joint note interference with their ability to ambulate.

Inspection reveals localized swelling or deformity at the interphalangeal joint, and palpation allows localization of tenderness to that articulation. Range of motion may be decreased, and many patients display pain and crepitus throughout the arc of motion.

Radiographic evaluation includes analysis of anteroposterior, lateral, and oblique cone-down radiographs of the hallux. Deformity is easily identified. Arthrosis is manifested by articular incongruity and a narrowed joint space.

Nonoperative modes of treatment include the use of a rubber-soled shoe to decrease impact loading during the stance phase of gait. The addition of an inflexible tapered rocker sole to the outer sole of the shoe may limit grinding of the incongruous articular surface associated with dorsiflexion during the toe-off phase of gait. Anti-inflammatory medications may help reduce symptoms.

If conservative measures fail, consideration can be given to operative intervention, which consists of localized arthrodesis of the interphalangeal joint. Previously popular surgical techniques included resection of the incongruous articular surfaces and fixation with Kirschner wires. Unfortunately this led to a high rate of pseudarthrosis at that joint. A more recently described technique includes arthrodesis with compression screw fixation. This has proved to be effective in many cases.

Patient Selection

Indications

1. Arthrosis of the interphalangeal joint of the hallux secondary to degenerative joint disease or systemic inflammatory arthropathy
2. Deformity of the interphalangeal joint secondary to neuromuscular disorders, with subsequent muscle imbalance
3. Traumatic discontinuity of the extrinsic tendons to the great toe, leading to deformity with or without arthrosis
4. Traumatic arthritis secondary to stubbing injuries of the hallux
5. Congenital abnormalities leading to deformity of the interphalangeal joint such as hallux valgus interphalangeus
6. Stabilization of the interphalangeal joint required in conjunction with tendon transfers when one or more of the extrinsic tendons about the hallux are removed from their insertion for use elsewhere; examples include arthrodesis of the interphalangeal joint performed in conjunction with transfer of the extensor hallucis longus tendon for correction of the hallux varus deformity

Contraindications

1. Neuropathic disorders that would predispose the patient to increased risks and complications of surgery
2. Patients in whom vascular dysfunction might lead to increased risk of infection or problematic wound healing

Surgical Procedure

Operative Technique

1. Make an L-shaped incision at the dorsum of the hallux. The transverse arm of the incision is placed just distal to the base of the distal phalanx and extends from its lateral to its medial side. The vertical arm extends along the dorsomedial aspect of the proximal phalanx (Fig. 1).
2. Deepen the longitudinal portion of the incision along the medial border of the extensor hallucis longus tendon. Mobilize the extensor hallucis longus tendon and retract it laterally to expose the interphalangeal joint. Incise the capsule and periosteum overlying the interphalangeal joint and reflect subperiosteally (Fig. 2).
3. Resect the joint surfaces perpendicular to the longitudinal axis of the phalanx with a microsagittal saw (Fig. 3). Reapproximate the cut surfaces, and check the position of the arthrodesis (Fig. 4).

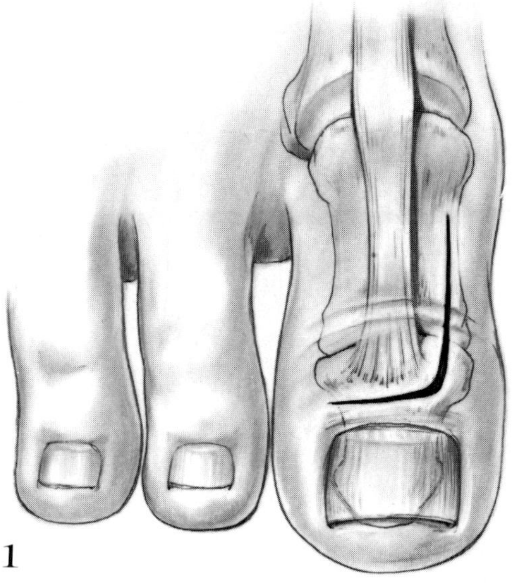

1

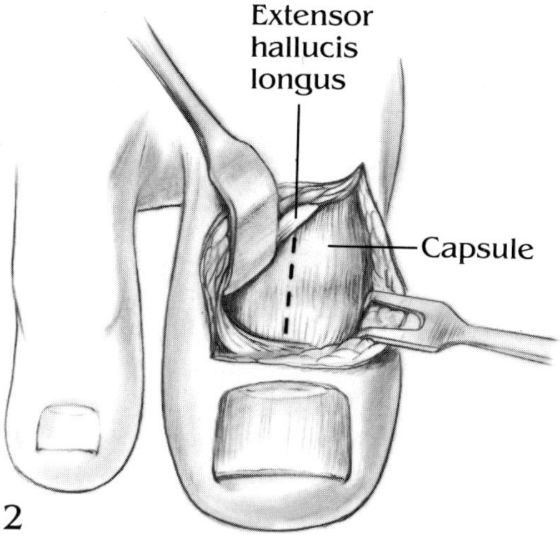

2

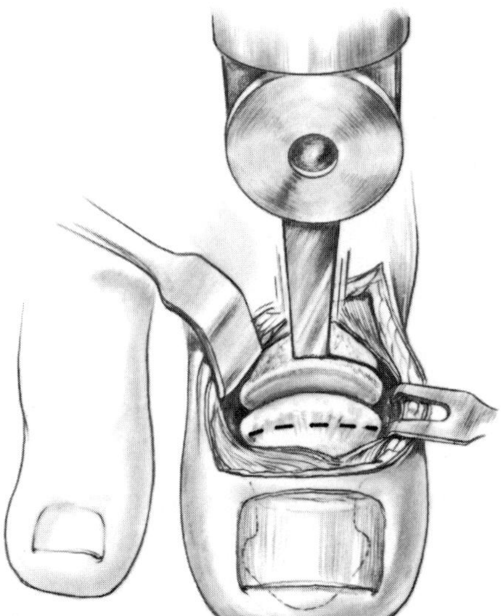

3

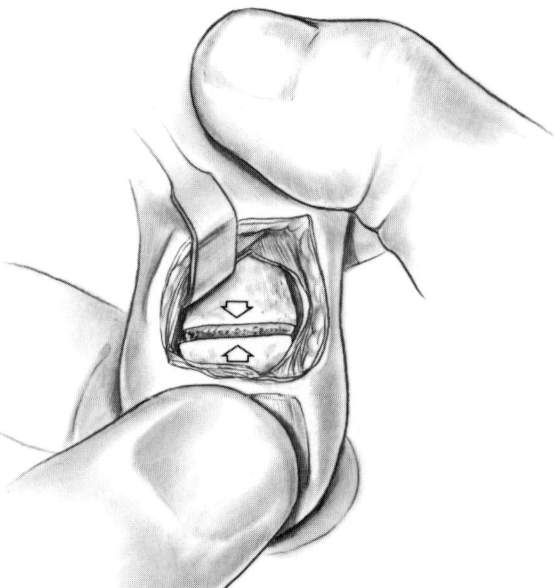

4

4. Make a drill hole from the cut surface distally and longitudinally through the distal phalanx and out the tip of the great toe with a 2.7-mm drill bit (Fig. 5).
5. Reverse the direction of the drill. Place the cut surfaces together, and drill into the proximal phalanx with the 2.0-mm drill bit (Fig. 6).
6. Insert a 4.0-mm cancellous screw by using the drill bit as a guide (Fig. 7). Insert further to obtain firm compression.
7. Close the skin with interrupted simple 4-0 nylon sutures (Fig. 8).

Postoperative Care

1. A sterile dressing is applied.
2. A short-leg ankle boot cast is applied.
3. The patient is kept non–weight bearing on crutches until there is radiographic evidence of union.
4. The cast is changed and sutures removed at 3 weeks after surgery.
5. Once bony union is identified, the patient is allowed a slow, gradual return to weight-bearing activities.

Technical Pitfalls

1. Care should be taken not to disrupt the insertion of the extensor hallucis longus tendon during its mobilization to expose the interphalangeal joint.
2. The skin and subcutaneous tissue are reflected in one flap to decrease the risk of wound necrosis.
3. Care must be taken not to penetrate the metatarsophalangeal joint with the screw.
4. The cut surfaces of the arthrodesis site should be reapproximated prior to fixation to ascertain satisfactory alignment of the hallux.

Complications

1. Wound necrosis secondary to devitalization of skin and subcutaneous tissue may be seen, leading to delayed wound healing. This is most often treated with local wound care with or without prophylactic antibiotics.
2. Pseudarthrosis of the fusion site may occur.
3. Some patients may note tenderness at the tip of the toe because of the proximity of the skin and soft tissue to the screw head. If marked discomfort is noted, consideration must be given to removal of the screw as soon as complete union is documented on radiographs.

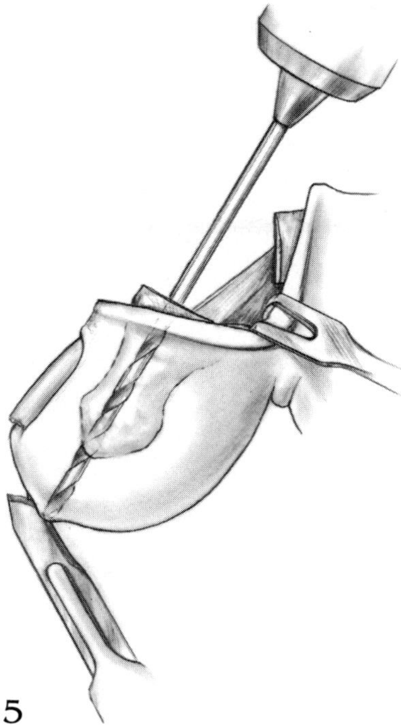

5

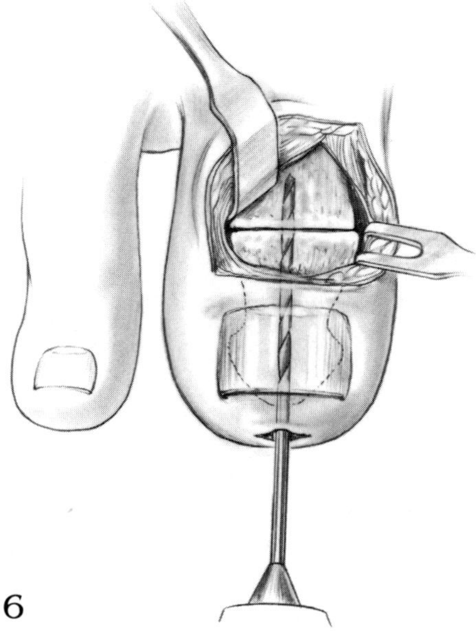

6

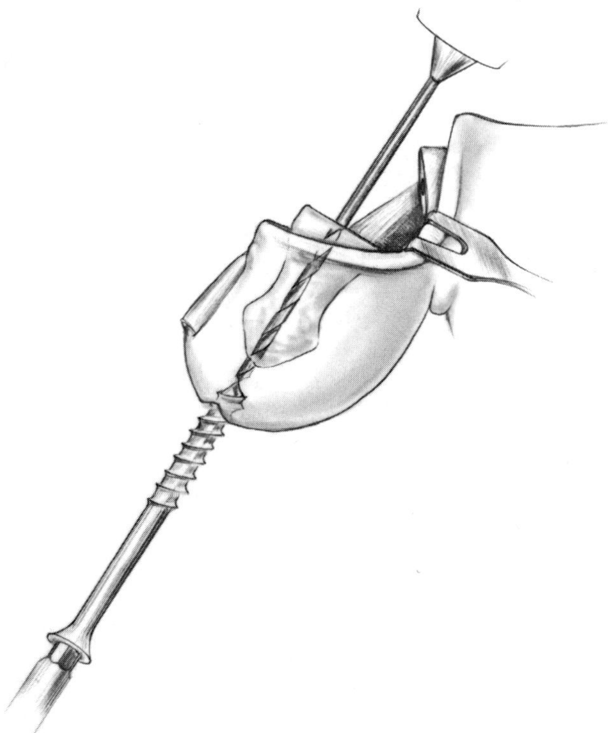

7

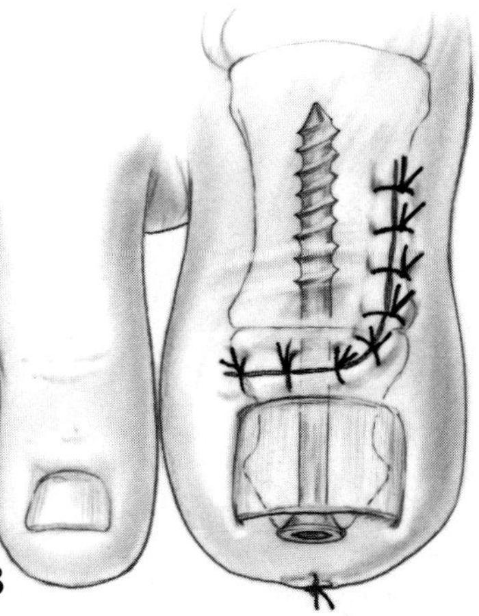

8

PART 6

Operations for Deformities of the Lesser Toes

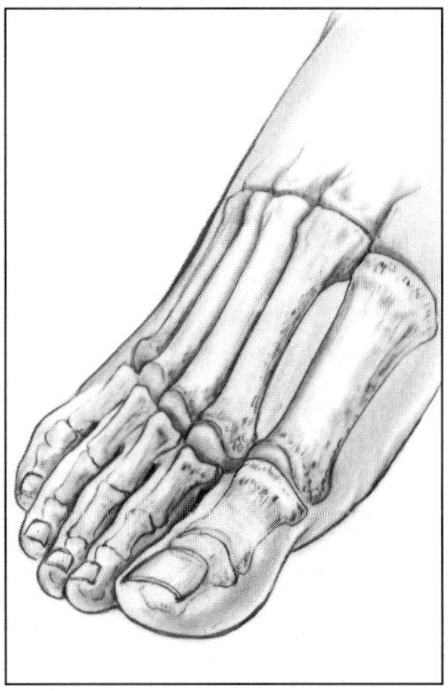

REPAIR HAMMER AND CLAW TOE DEFORMITIES

General Considerations

A hammer toe deformity is characterized by hyperextension at the metatarsophalangeal joint, hyperflexion at the proximal interphalangeal joint, and hyperextension at the distal interphalangeal joint. A claw toe deformity is similar to a hammer toe deformity except that the distal interphalangeal joint is positioned in hyperflexion. Although numerous etiologic factors have been described in the development of these lesser toe deformities, inappropriate shoewear is the most common causative factor. High-heeled shoes propel the feet forward into the narrow, pointed toe box. Axial pressure applied to the tip of the toes leads to buckling, with the resultant deformities as described.

Patients note tender hyperkeratotic lesions over the bony deformities as a result of mechanical impingement by the toe box of the shoe. Significant corns develop at the dorsum of the proximal interphalangeal joint in both deformities. Loads applied to the metatarsal head by the hyperextended phalanx lead to increased pressure at the sole of the foot. Hyperkeratotic lesions may form at the plantar aspect of the metatarsal heads. In the claw toe deformity, apical tip corns occur as the tip of the toe is forced into the inner sole of the shoe. Deformities are flexible at first but later become fixed. Most patients describe difficulty in fitting shoewear.

Initial nonoperative management includes shaving of hyperkeratotic lesions with a scalpel. The patient may decompress corns and calluses by grinding them with a pumice stone. Appropriate shoewear with a high, wide toe box is necessary to accommodate the deformity. The toe box may be stretched in the area of the bony prominence with a ball-and-ring stretcher. Pads or inserts that provide elevation proximal to the metatarsal heads may decrease the hyperextension deformity at the metatarsophalangeal joint and alleviate local metatarsalgia. If the deformities are still flexible, a Buden splint may be effective in maintaining satisfactory alignment of the toe. Toe protectors may be used to float areas of bony prominence away from the toe box of the shoe. Fixed claw toe deformities may be effectively treated with a toe crest to elevate the tip of the toe off the inner sole of the shoe.

If conservative measures fail to provide relief, surgical intervention may be required. Most often tenotomy of the extensor digitorum longus tendon at the level of the metatarsophalangeal joint is required. Dorsal capsulotomy of the metatarsophalangeal joint is also helpful to correct the hyperextension deformity at that articulation.

Typically, the hyperflexion deformity at the proximal interphalangeal joint is fixed. This most often requires resection of the distal portion of the proximal phalanx for correction. In the relatively common situation in which a hallux valgus deformity is associated with a hammered second toe, correction of the great toe deformity is required in addition to the hammer toe repair. Failure to correct the great toe deformity will commonly lead to recurrence of the hammer toe deformity.

Patient Selection

Indications

1. Hammer or claw toe deformity recalcitrant to conservative measures.
2. Some lesser toe deformities seen early may be amenable to soft tissue procedures such as flexor-to-extensor transfers. Most deformities require bony decompression with resection of the distal portion of the proximal phalanx.

Contraindications

1. Patients with diabetic or other neuropathies may be at risk for problematic wound healing after surgical correction of deformities of the lesser toes.
2. Patients with circulatory dysfunction may be at risk for loss of the digit.
3. Deformities secondary to neuromuscular imbalance may be prone to recurrence after surgery.
4. Deformity of the second toe caused by mechanical abutment from a laterally deviated great toe requires correction of the hallux valgus in addition to repair of the hammer toe. Isolated repair of the second toe is commonly associated with recurrence, because the deforming forces that caused the problem have not been corrected.

Surgical Procedure

Operative Technique: Tenotomy of the Extensor Digitorum Longus Tendon and Dorsal Capsulotomy of the Metatarsophalangeal Joint

1. Locate the metatarsophalangeal joint by palpation while performing passive dorsiflexion and plantarflexion of the toe. Perform the extensor tenotomy at that level (Fig. 1).
2. Apply pressure to the dorsum of the involved digit to place the extensor digitorum longus tendon under tension (Fig. 2a).
3. Puncture the skin at the medial margin of the tendon with a No. 11 scalpel blade. Hold the scalpel in such a way that the cutting edge is directed away from the tendon (Fig. 2a).
4. With the dull edge of the blade, lift the skin over the tendon. This places the cutting edge of the blade against the taut tendon at its lateral margin (Fig. 2b).
5. With gentle pressure, transect the tendon at that level (Fig. 2c). If complete release has not been obtained or difficulty has been encountered, the remaining tendon may be delivered from the wound by means of a small curved hemostat placed into the incision. Transection can then be completed.
6. Deepen the incision by using gentle pressure on the scalpel to penetrate the dorsal capsule of the metatarsophalangeal joint (Fig. 3). Transect the capsule transversely to obtain complete correction of the hyperextension deformity. Be careful to avoid injury to the digital neurovascular bundles that run at the medial and lateral aspects of the joint.

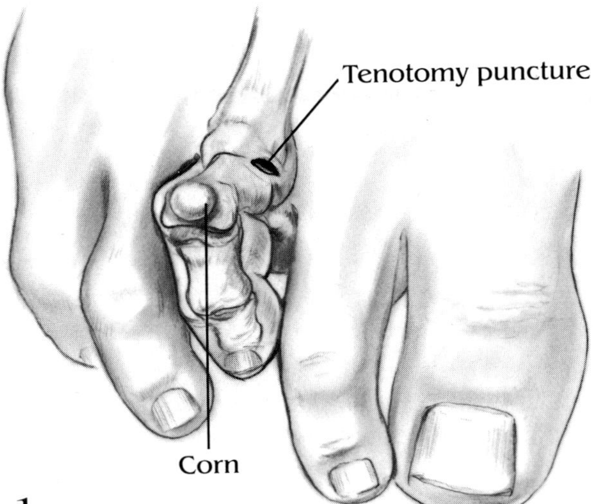

1

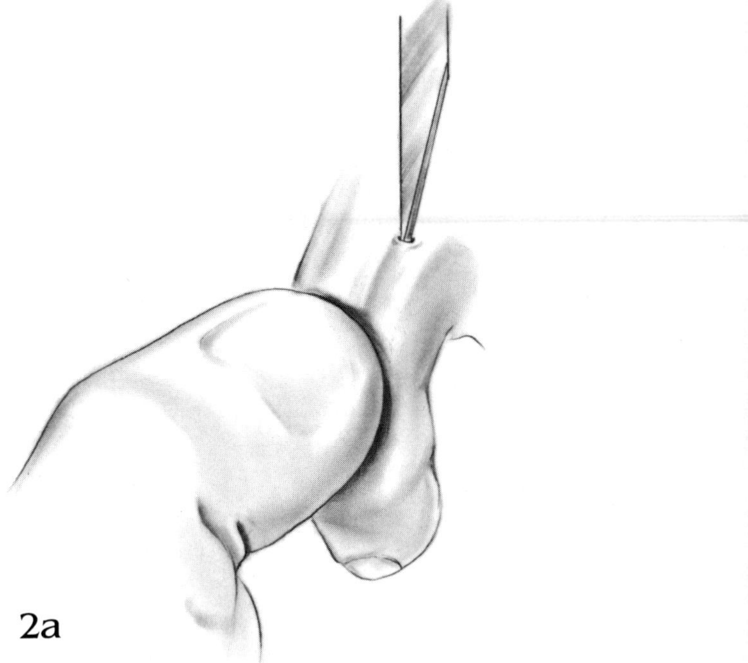

2a

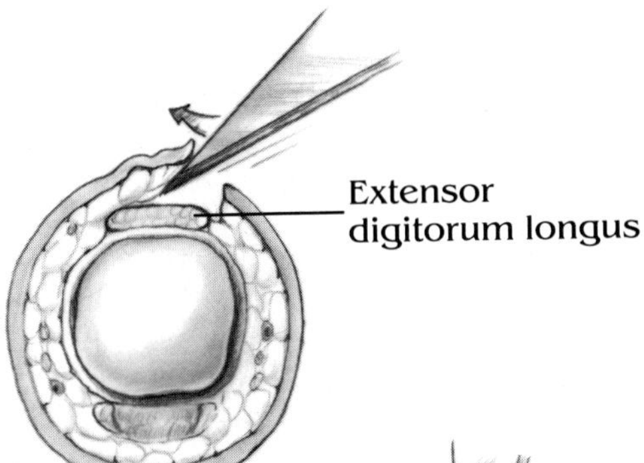

2b

Cross section
at the metatarsal head

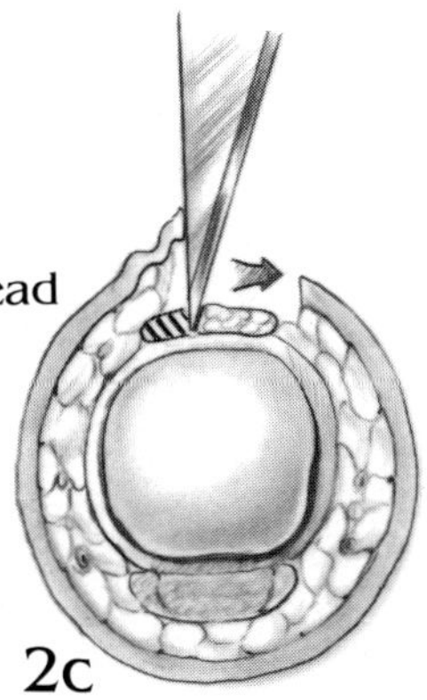

2c

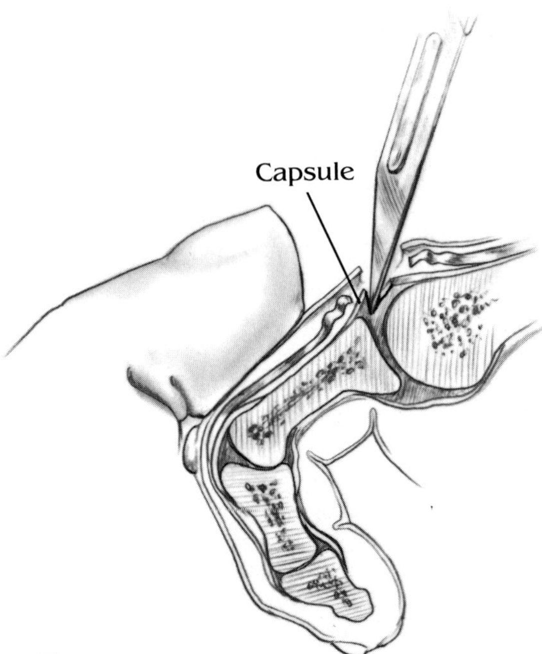

3

Operative Technique: Resection of the Distal Portion of the Proximal Phalanx

1. Make a dorsal longitudinal incision 1½ cm long and centered over the proximal interphalangeal joint of the involved digit (Fig. 4). Incise subcutaneous tissue along the line of the incision.
2. Incise the extensor digitorum longus tendon longitudinally, and retract it medially and laterally (Fig. 5).
3. Incise the capsule of the proximal interphalangeal joint and the periosteum overlying the distal portion of the proximal phalanx longitudinally. Reflect subperiosteally to expose the distal portion of the proximal phalanx (Fig. 6).
4. Resect the distal portion of the proximal phalanx perpendicular to the longitudinal axis of the shaft with a microsagittal saw (Fig. 7).
5. If pin fixation is to be utilized, a 0.045-inch Kirschner wire is inserted from the base of the middle phalanx distally to exit at the tip of the toe. This wire is then drilled retrograde into the intramedullary canal of the shaft of the proximal phalanx while the toe is held in a corrected position.
6. The skin is closed with interrupted vertical mattress or simple 4-0 nylon sutures.

Postoperative Care

1. If pin fixation is used, the tip of the pin is bent to prevent proximal migration. A sterile dressing is applied.
2. If pin fixation is not used, corrective adhesive tape strapping is employed to hold the toe in its corrected position. This corrective strapping must be changed every 1 to 2 weeks for 6 weeks postoperatively until adequate scarring has occurred to maintain correction.
3. Sutures are removed at 3 weeks postoperatively.
4. Partial weight bearing or heel walking in a stiff-soled postoperative shoe is recommended for the first 6 weeks after surgery.

Technical Pitfalls

1. Excessive resection of bone may lead to instability at the proximal interphalangeal joint and result in a floppy toe.
2. Injury to the digital neurovascular structures must be avoided when performing the dorsal capsulotomy at the metatarsophalangeal joint.
3. Inadequate maintenance of postoperative correction by pin fixation or strapping may lead to residual deformity.
4. Subsequent use of inappropriate shoewear may predispose the patient to a recurrence of the deformity.

Complications

1. Recurrence of deformity
2. A floppy toe with an unstable proximal interphalangeal joint
3. Shortening of the toe (expected)

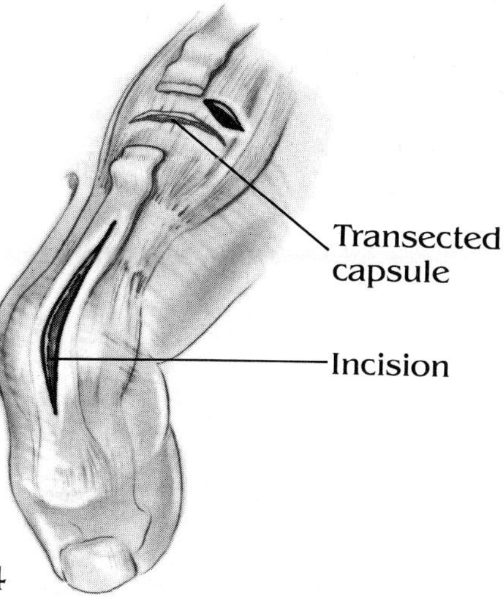
Transected
capsule
Incision

4

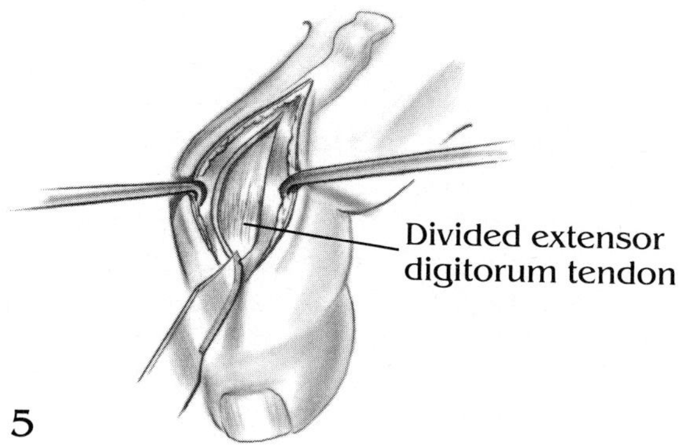
Divided extensor
digitorum tendon

5

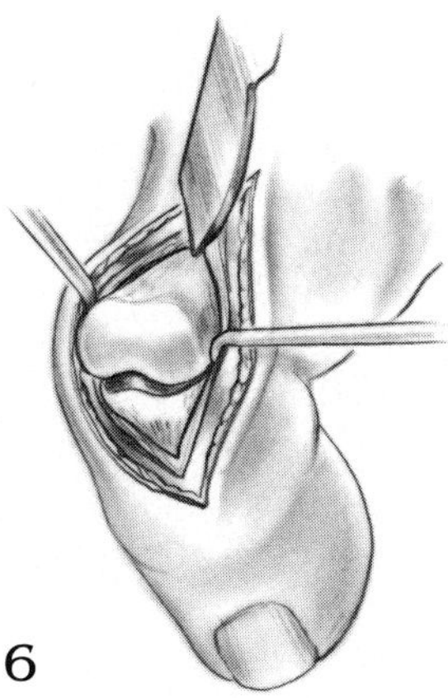

6

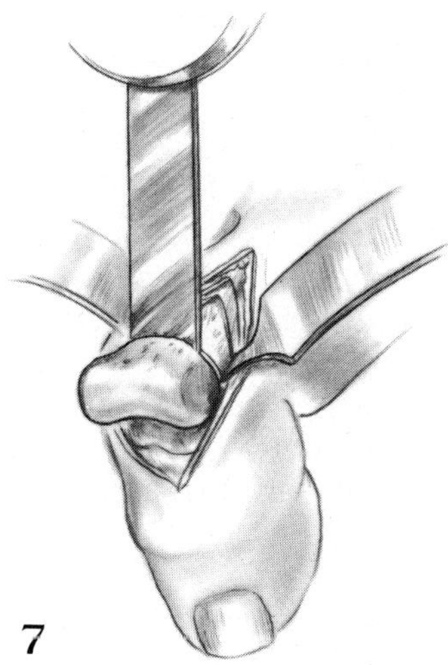

7

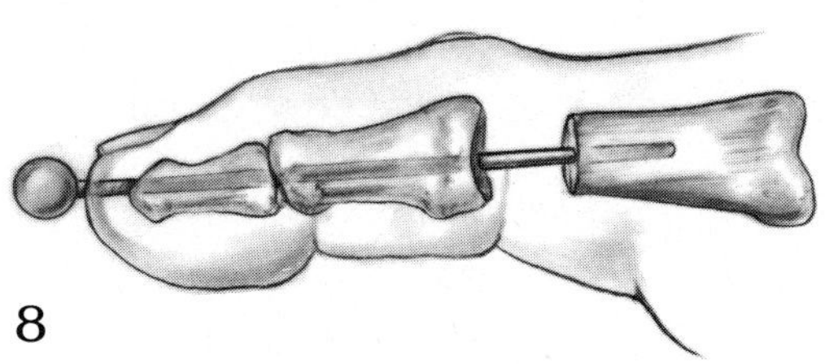

8

REPAIR HAMMER TOE OR CLAW TOE WITH DISLOCATED METATARSOPHALANGEAL JOINT

General Considerations

Long-standing claw toe or hammer toe deformity may be associated with progressive hyperextension at the metatarsophalangeal joint. This may progress to dorsal subluxation or frank dislocation of the base of the proximal phalanx, which comes to lie at the dorsal aspect of the metatarsal head. This abnormality may be seen in conjunction with hallux valgus and mechanical abutment of the hallux against the second toe, leading to an overriding second toe.

Patients note pain over prominent bony eminences at the dorsum of the proximal interphalangeal joint. Metatarsalgia may occur as a result of increased loads applied to the plantar surface of the metatarsal head secondary to pressure from the dislocated proximal phalanx. Patients also note pain and swelling in the dislocated metatarsophalangeal joint. Physical examination reveals a tender, dislocated joint, as well as distal deformities at the interphalangeal joints.

Conservative treatment includes splinting devices to maintain correction of deformities of the great and lesser toes. Adequate shoewear with a high, wide toe box may help accommodate deformities, and elevation proximal to the metatarsal heads by means of pads or inserts may alleviate metatarsalgia. If conservative measures fail to provide relief, consideration can be given to surgical intervention in the form of a complete release of contracted soft tissue structures about the metatarsophalangeal joint, resection of the distal portion of the proximal phalanx, and reduction of the metatarsophalangeal joint with or without pin fixation. Rarely, if reduction is difficult after complete soft tissue release and bony decompression at the interphalangeal joint, resection of the distal portion of the metatarsal head may be required. As with all lesser toe deformities secondary to mechanical abutment from the great toe resulting from hallux valgus, the deformity of the hallux must be corrected regardless of whether the great toe itself is symptomatic. Failure to correct the hallux valgus deformity often leads to recurrence of the lesser toe deformity, as the abnormal causative forces have not been eliminated.

Patient Selection

Indications

1. Patients with a hammer or claw toe deformity associated with a dislocation of the metatarsophalangeal joint
2. Patients with hallux valgus and second toe deformity with dislocation of the metatarsophalangeal joint (surgical correction of both the hallux and the second toe required)

Contraindications

1. Lesser toe deformities without dislocation at the metatarsophalangeal joint are adequately treated with simpler surgical repairs.

Surgical Procedure

Operative Technique

1. A dorsal longitudinal incision 3 cm long is made, centered over the metatarsophalangeal joint (Fig. 1). Subcutaneous tissue is divided along the line of the skin incision.
2. Identify the extensor digitorum tendon, and incise it transversely at the level of the metatarsophalangeal joint. Identify the extensor digitorum brevis tendon. Transect this tendon at the same level (Fig. 2).
3. Identify the dorsal capsule of the metatarsophalangeal joint. Incise it transversely. Release soft tissue structures circumferentially and subperiosteally from the medial and lateral aspects of the base of the proximal phalanx and the metatarsal head. Make certain to release the medial and lateral collateral ligaments (Fig. 3).
4. Release the volar plate from its insertion at the neck of the metatarsal head with a periosteal elevator (Fig. 4).

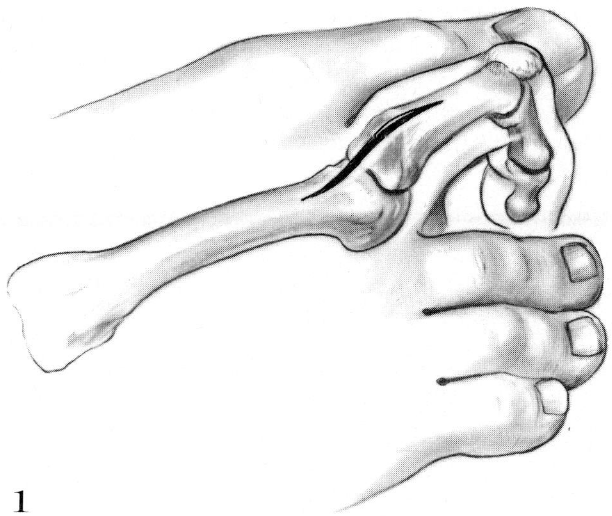

1

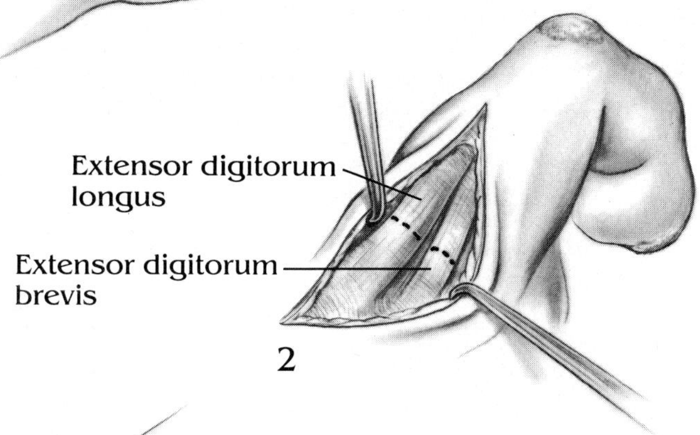
Extensor digitorum
longus
Extensor digitorum
brevis

2

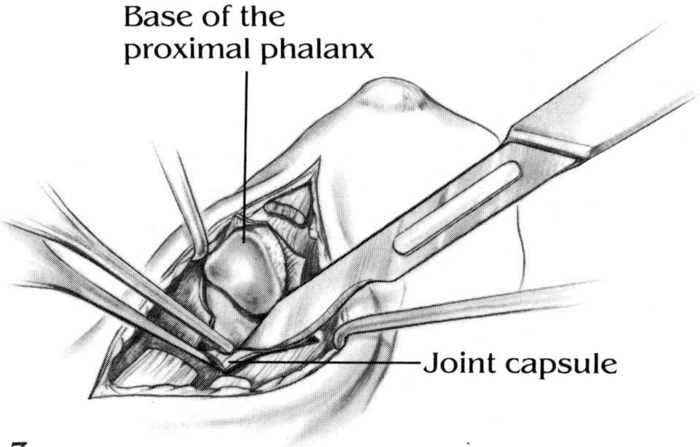
Base of the
proximal phalanx
Joint capsule

3

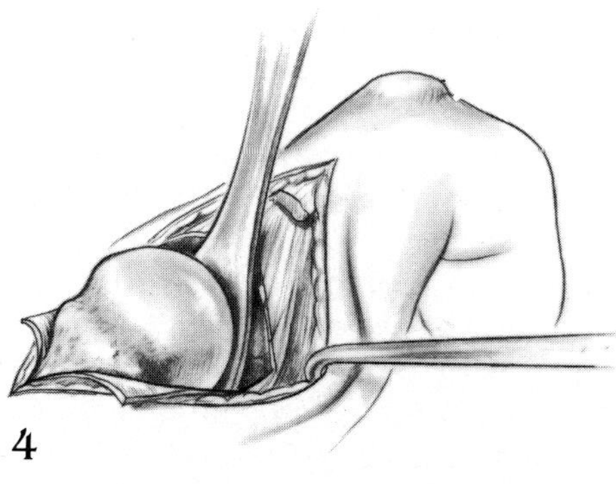

4

5. If required, because of deformity at the interphalangeal joint or to facilitate reduction at the metatarsophalangeal joint, resect the distal portion of the proximal phalanx through a second dorsal longitudinal incision centered over the proximal interphalangeal joint. Shortening of the phalanx distally allows for more effective reduction at the metatarsophalangeal joint level (Fig. 5).
6. If reduction is still difficult, consideration may be given to resection of the distalmost portion of the metatarsal head. The distal articular surface of the involved metatarsal head is resected perpendicular to the longitudinal access of the shaft with a microsagittal saw (Fig. 6).
7. Reduce the metatarsophalangeal joint. If the base of the proximal phalanx tends to subluxate dorsally, pin fixation is appropriate. Insert a 0.045-inch or 0.062-inch Kirschner wire from the base of the proximal phalanx, across the interphalangeal joint, and out the tip of the toe while holding the interphalangeal joint in corrected position. Drill the Kirschner wire in a retrograde fashion into the metatarsal while holding the metatarsophalangeal joint reduced (Fig. 7).
8. Close the skin with interrupted vertical mattress 4-0 nylon sutures.

Postoperative Care

1. If pin fixation was not required, then adhesive strapping is applied to hold the toe in satisfactory alignment. Strapping is changed weekly.
2. Sutures are removed at 3 weeks postoperatively.
3. The patient is allowed protected ambulation (partial weight bearing, or heel walking).
4. The pin is left in place for 4 to 6 weeks or until enough scar formation has occurred to enable maintenance of reduction.

Technical Pitfalls

1. Inadequate soft tissue release may lead to recurrence of dislocation.
2. Failure to excise the distal portion of the proximal phalanx may make reduction at the metatarsophalangeal joint difficult. Recurrent dislocation may occur unless effective shortening of the digit is accomplished.
3. Failure to correct concomitant hallux valgus deformity leads to a high incidence of recurrence of a second toe deformity.

Potential Complications

1. Recurrence of deformity
2. Floppy toe secondary to excessive shortening
3. A stiff metatarsophalangeal joint (especially if it is necessary to resect the distal articular surface of the metatarsal head). The patient should be forewarned about a significant loss of motion at that articulation.

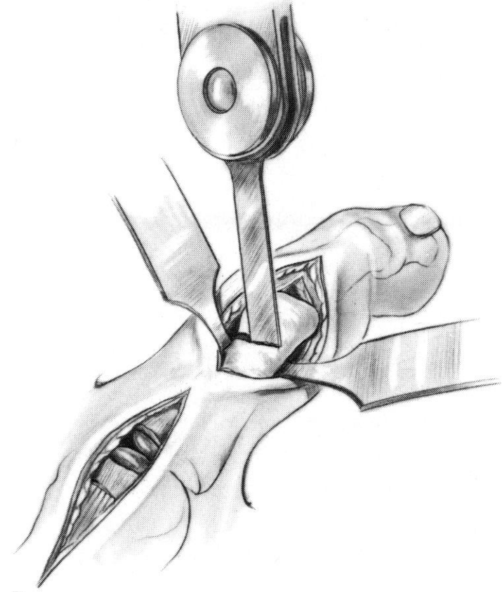

5

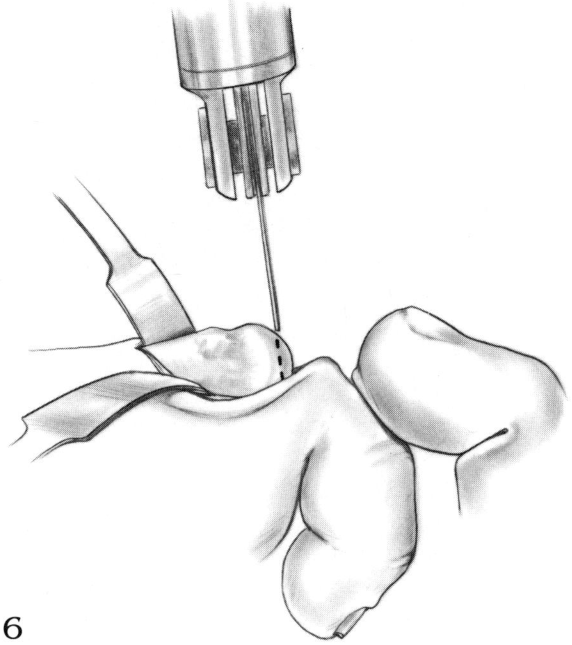

6

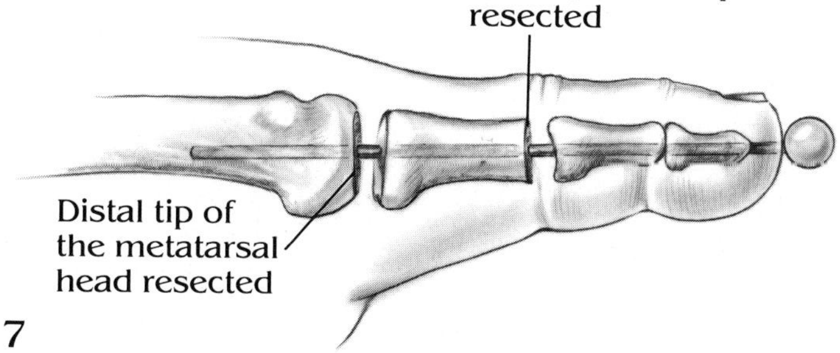
Distal portion
of the proximal phalanx
resected
Distal tip of
the metatarsal
head resected

7

REPAIR MALLET TOE DEFORMITY

General Considerations

A mallet toe deformity is characterized by isolated hyperflexion at the distal interphalangeal joint. Although this deformity may be caused by trauma with avulsion of the extensor digitorum longus tendon from its insertion, the most common etiology is axial loading of the phalanx by the distal portion of the toe box of the shoe. High-heeled shoes propel the foot forward into the toe box, resulting in axial loads applied to the phalanx. Shoes that are too short also provide abnormal mechanical pressure, which may lead to a mallet toe deformity.

Patients note localized pain at the tip of the involved digit. The physical examination reveals hyperflexion at the distal interphalangeal joint, as well as an apical tip corn. This is a hyperkeratotic lesion caused by loads applied to the tip of the toe as the hyperflexed digit is forced into the inner sole of the shoe. Deformities of the toenail may also occur with flattening caused by pressure. Initial treatment includes the use of a toe crest to elevate the distal tip of the distal phalanx off the inner sole of the shoe. A toe crest may also be incorporated within a soft flexible insert to accomplish the same goal. Appropriate shoewear is important.

If conservative measures fail, consideration can be given to surgical intervention in the form of a resection of the distal portion of the middle phalanx. In severe cases, the entire middle phalanx may be excised.

Patient Selection

Indications

1. Mallet toe deformity with localized pain and a hyperkeratotic lesion at distal tip of the distal phalanx
2. Failure of conservative measures

Contraindications

1. Hyperflexion at the distal interphalangeal joint associated with hyperflexion at the proximal interphalangeal joint may be better treated with resection of the distal portion of the proximal phalanx.
2. In patients with circulatory dysfunction, operative intervention may place the digit at risk.
3. Diabetic and neuropathic patients may be better treated with nonoperative therapies.

Surgical Procedure

Operative Technique

1. A dorsal longitudinal incision 1½ cm long is made, centered over the distal interphalangeal joint (Fig. 1). The subcutaneous tissue is divided along the line of the skin incision.
2. The extensor digitorum longus is incised longitudinally and retracted medially and laterally (Fig. 2).
3. The capsule overlying the distal interphalangeal joint and the periosteum overlying the middle phalanx are incised longitudinally and reflected subperiosteally to expose the distal portion of the middle phalanx.
4. The distal portion of the middle phalanx is resected with a microsagittal saw by means of a cut made perpendicular to the long axis of the shaft (Fig. 3).
5. If pin fixation is elected, a 0.045-inch Kirschner wire is passed from the base of the distal phalanx out the tip of the toe (Fig. 4). It is then driven retrograde into the intermedullary canal of the remnant of the middle phalanx (Fig. 5).
6. The wound is copiously irrigated with triple antibiotic solution, and the skin is closed with interrupted simple 4-0 nylon sutures.

Postoperative Care

1. A sterile dressing is applied.
2. If pin fixation has not been utilized, a mallet toe strapping bandage, using adhesive tape to hold the toe in the corrected position, is applied. This strapping is changed weekly or biweekly for 6 weeks until adequate healing has occurred.
3. Sutures are removed at 3 weeks after surgery. The pin is removed in 4 to 6 weeks as soon as adequate scar formation has occurred.
4. Heel walking in a stiff-soled postoperative shoe is allowed.

Technical Pitfalls

1. In cases in which severe hyperflexion at the distal interphalangeal joint is present and in patients with a small middle phalanx, resection of the entire middle phalanx may be required to obtain adequate correction.

Potential Complications

1. Shortening of the digit
2. Loss of flexion and extension power of the digit
3. Recurrence of deformity

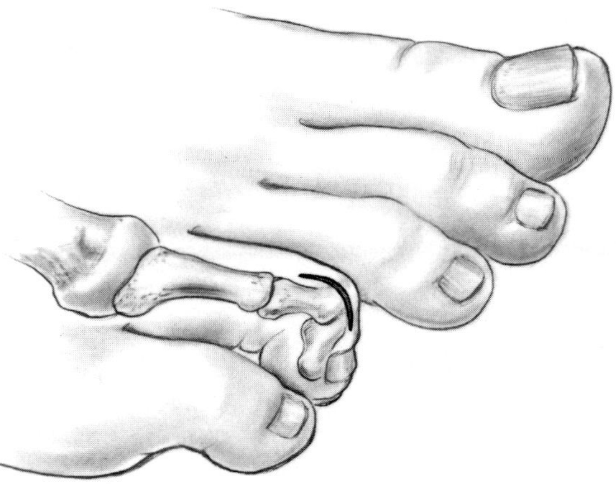

1

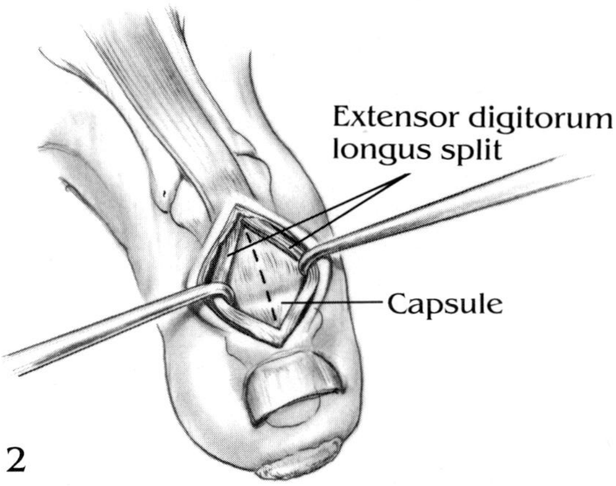

2

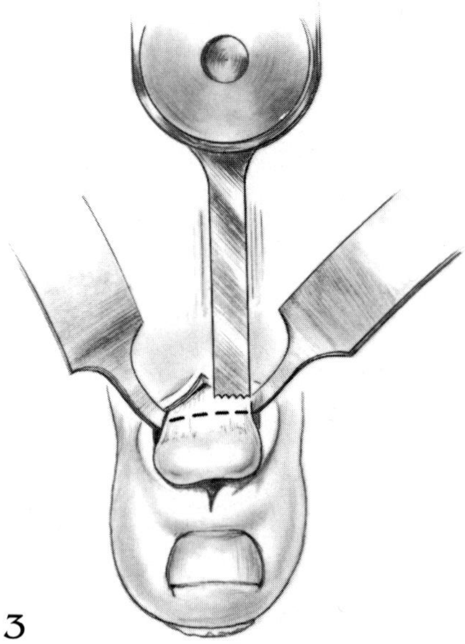

3

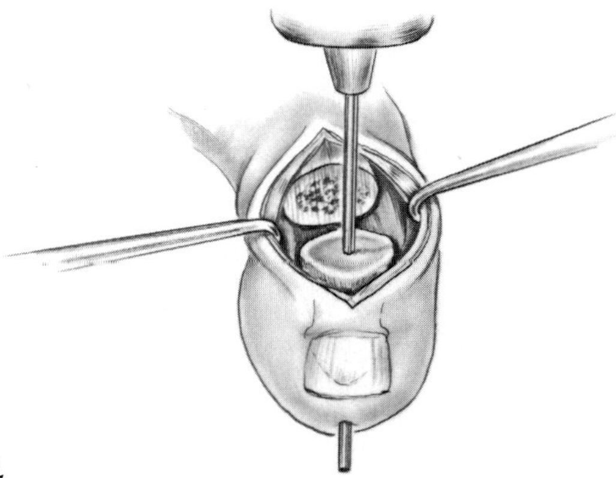

4

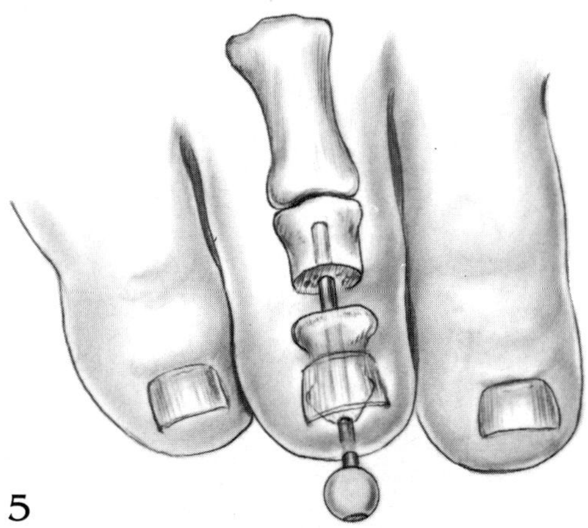

5

PART 7

Operations for Interdigital Soft Corns

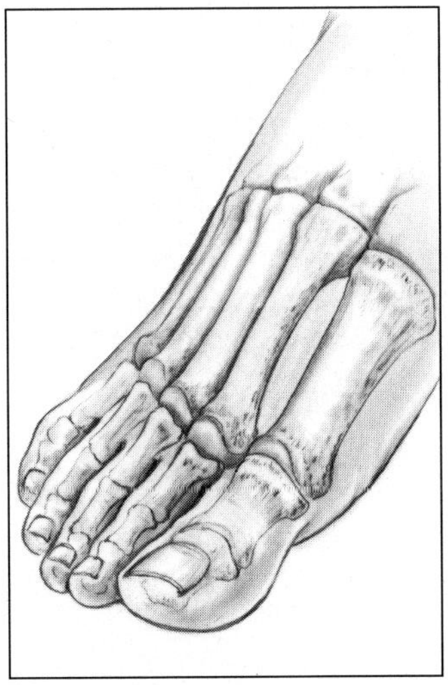

INTERDIGITAL SOFT CORN FOURTH WEB SPACE

General Considerations

Mechanical impingement of a bony condyle against a portion of a phalanx of an adjacent toe may lead to an interdigital soft corn (heloma molle) (Fig. 1). The most common site of an interdigital soft corn is the fourth web space. Often the medial aspect of the head of the proximal phalanx of the fifth toe impinges against the lateral portion of the base of the proximal phalanx of the fourth toe. This mechanical impingement leads to the formation of a hyperkeratotic lesion at the base of the fourth web space. Maceration of the skin may also be seen.

Patients note localized pain associated with the formation of an interdigital soft corn. Nonoperative treatment includes the use of lamb's wool or a soft rubber toe separator placed between the digits. These devices are used in conjunction with wide-toe-box shoes to alleviate mechanical pressure.

If symptoms persist despite these measures, surgical intervention is warranted. Preoperative planning includes the use of an anteroposterior radiograph of the foot to identify the specific bony prominences causing the problem. Most often surgical correction requires resection of the distal portion of the proximal phalanx of the fifth toe, as well as excision of the lateral condyle at the base of the proximal phalanx of the fourth toe. To remove the hyperkeratotic lesion, excision of the damaged skin at the base of the web space is performed. Subsequent to this, the offending bony prominences are resected. Closure is accomplished by means of subtotal syndactylization of toe 4 to toe 5. This technique also provides increased stability of the fifth toe after resection of the distal portion of the proximal phalanx.

Patient Selection

Indications

1. Interdigital soft corn of the fourth web space
2. Interdigital soft corn associated with a dorsolateral corn on the fifth toe

Contraindications

1. Isolated interdigital soft corns located more distally on the digit may be better treated with isolated condylectomy through a slightly curved incision made longitudinally along the margin of the corn. The offending bony condyle is exposed subperiosteally by sharp dissection and is excised with a microsagittal saw.
2. Neurologic, vascular, or other medical disorders may necessitate a more limited surgical intervention. Isolated condylectomy or simple excision of the distal portion of the proximal phalanx may be appropriate.

Surgical Procedure

Operative Technique

1. With a surgical marking pen, outline a web incision from the base of the web dorsally to the proximal interphalangeal joint (Fig. 2). The outline is extended on the plantar aspect of the web of the fifth toe to encompass the interdigital corn. The fifth toe is then placed adjacent to the fourth toe to transfer the marking.
2. The web is incised along the outline. The skin at the base of the web space is excised, but subcutaneous tissue is left intact (Fig. 3).
3. The subcutaneous tissue is incised longitudinally in the region of the distal half of the proximal phalanx of the fifth toe and the base of the proximal phalanx of the fourth toe. The incision is deepened to bone, and the offending bony structures are exposed subperiosteally (Fig. 4).
4. The distal portion of the proximal phalanx of the fifth toe is excised perpendicular to the longitudinal axis of the shaft with a microsagittal saw (Fig. 5). The lateral condyle at the base of the proximal phalanx of the fourth toe is excised with a power saw. The cut surfaces are smoothed with a rasp.
5. The wound is closed in the form of a subtotal syndactylization with interrupted 3-0 chromic sutures (Figs. 6a and 6b).

Postoperative Care

1. A sterile dressing is applied.
2. Ambulation in an open-toed wooden-soled shoe is allowed.
3. At 3 weeks postoperatively the patient is allowed a gradual progressive return to weight bearing in a wide-toe-box shoe within the limits of discomfort.
4. If wound necrosis or delayed wound healing is noted, soaking in dilute povidone-iodine (Betadine) three times a day for 20 minutes is recommended until healing is complete.

Potential Complications

1. Excessive weight bearing may lead to wound necrosis, delayed wound healing, or diathesis of the syndactyly.
2. Resection of the distal portion of the proximal phalanx of the fifth toe without syndactylization may lead to relative instability of that toe.

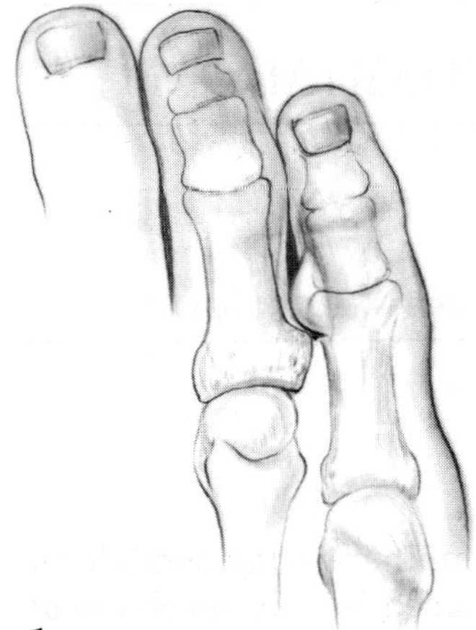

1

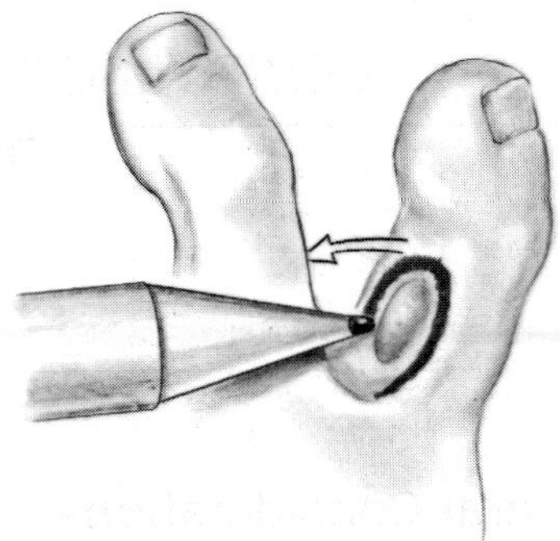

2

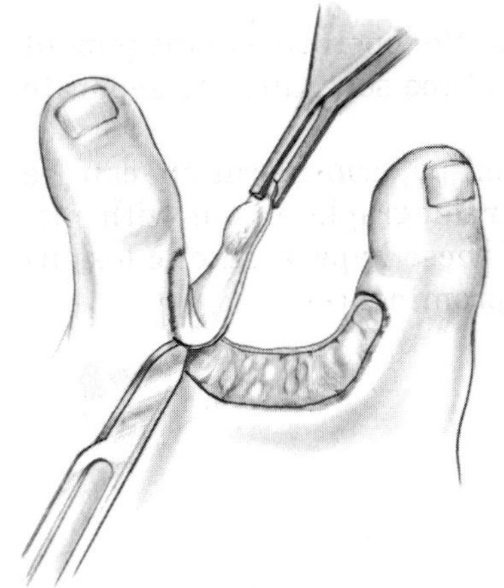

3

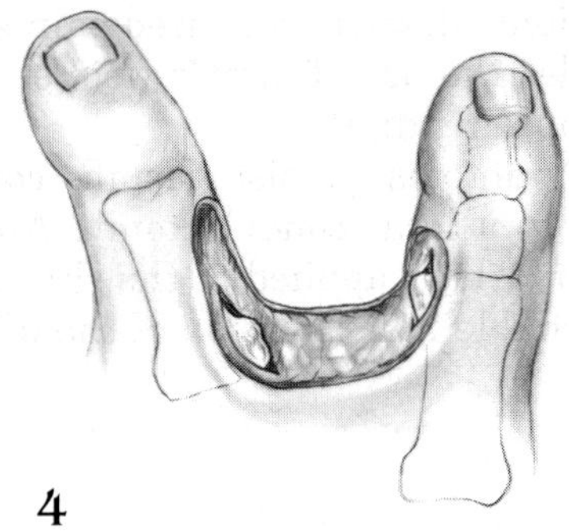

4

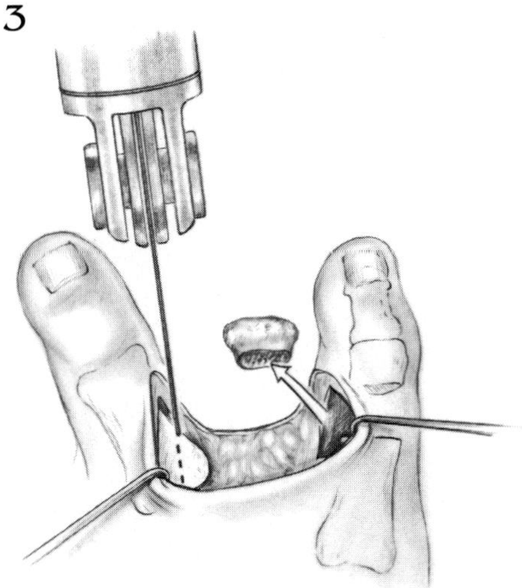

5

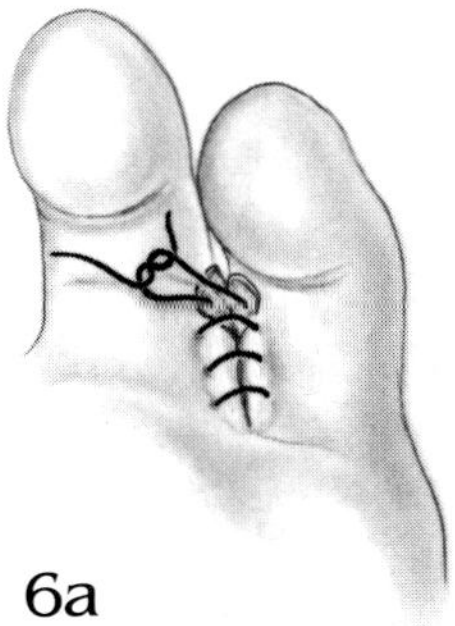

6a

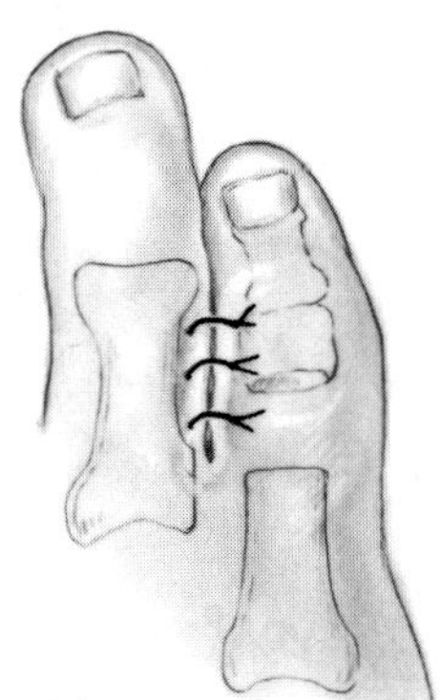

6b

CONDYLECTOMY FOR INTERDIGITAL SOFT CORNS

General Considerations

Interdigital soft corns may occur overlying any prominent bony condyle in any web space. These hyperkeratotic lesions are caused by the mechanical pressure of the bony prominence of one toe against that of the adjacent toe. Although such lesions are commonly seen at the base of the fourth web space, as described in the previous chapter, they may also occur proximally or distally in any web space.

Patients describe localized pain and tenderness. Nonoperative management includes the use of lamb's wool or various types of toe separators to separate the opposing digits.

If symptoms persist despite conservative therapy, consideration can be given to a local condylectomy. Anteroposterior radiographs taken with metallic markers applied to the skin at the level of these hyperkeratotic lesions may enable identification of the offending bony prominences.

Patient Selection

Indications. The primary indication is an interdigital soft corn not responsive to nonoperative treatment.

Contraindications. Patients with neurologic or vascular dysfunction may be better treated with conservative measures.

Surgical Procedure

Operative Technique

1. A longitudinal incision is made along the dorsal margin of the interdigital corn. The incision is centered over the offending bony condyle(s) (Fig. 1). Subcutaneous tissue is divided along the line of the skin incision.
2. Incise deep tissue, including the capsule and periosteum, longitudinally, and reflect subperiosteally to visualize the offending bony condyle(s) (Fig. 2).
3. Resect the prominent bony eminences with a microsagittal saw (Fig. 3).
4. Smooth the cut surface with a rasp (Fig. 4).
5. Close the skin with interrupted simple 4-0 nylon sutures.

Postoperative Care

1. A sterile dressing is applied.
2. Heel walking in a stiff-soled postoperative shoe is allowed.
3. Sutures are removed at 3 weeks after surgery.

Technical Pitfalls. Inadequate bony resection may lead to persistence of symptoms or recurrence of the lesion after surgery.

Potential Complications

1. Persistence of symptoms due to inadequate bony resection.
2. Recurrence of interdigital soft corn is possible.

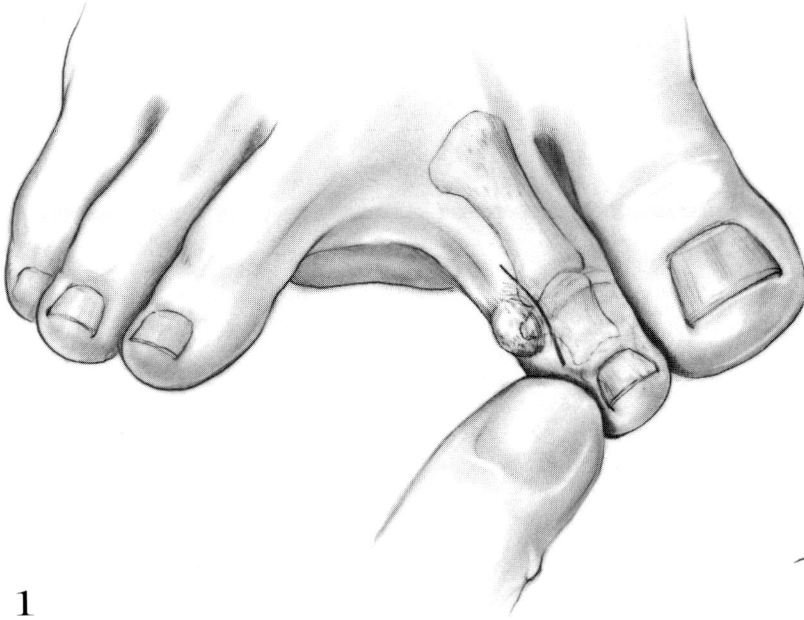

1

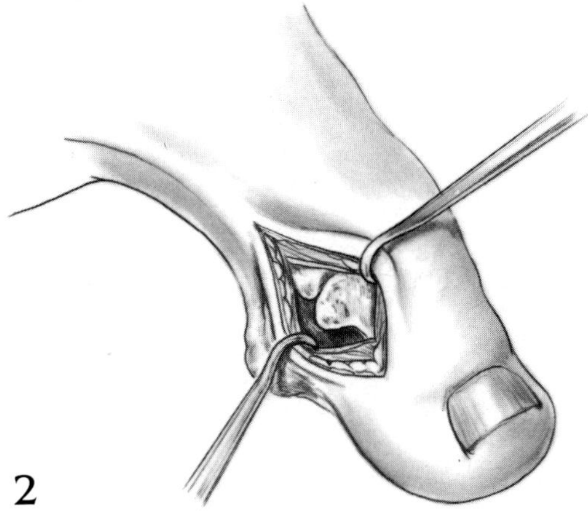

2

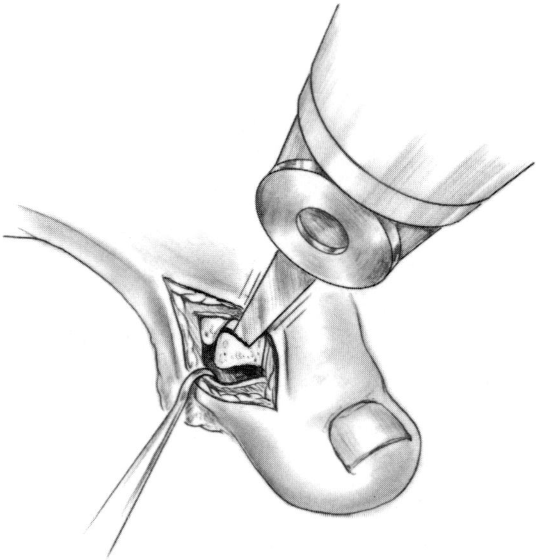

3

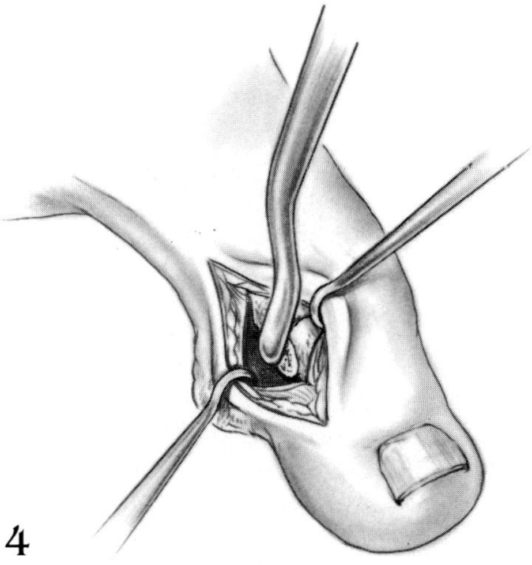

4

PART 8

Operations for Disorders of the Fifth Toe

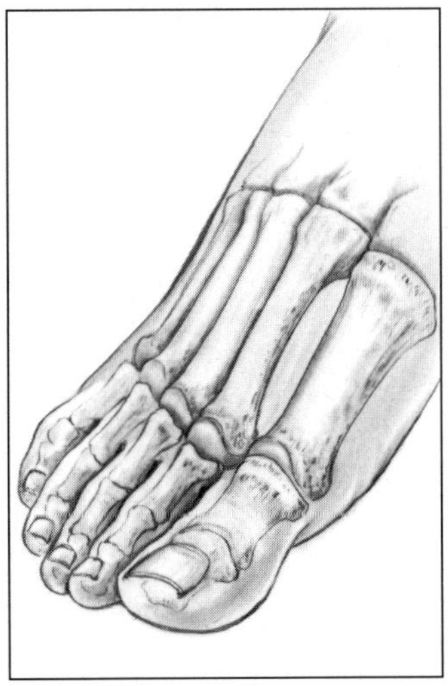

REPAIR CONGENITAL OVERRIDING FIFTH TOE

General Considerations

An overlapping fifth toe is a congenital abnormality in which the fifth toe comes to override the fourth toe (Fig. 1). The digit is rotated, and the metatarsophalangeal joint becomes contracted in its abnormal position.

Patients describe difficulty with shoewear, and there is often mechanical impingement of the overlapping fifth toe against the toe box of the shoe. Erythema and maceration of the skin may be present. Impingement of the fifth toe against the fourth toe may lead to interdigital lesions.

Nonoperative methods of treatment include the use of lamb's wool to separate the digits. Shoes with a high, wide toe box may help accommodate the deformity. If conservative modalities fail, surgical intervention may be appropriate. Various types of bony and soft tissue procedures have been described for correction of this common abnormality. Resection of the proximal portion of the proximal phalanx of the fifth toe combined with syndactylization of toes 4 to 5 has proved to be a reliable procedure for this deformity.

Patient Selection

Indications. The indication is a congenital overriding fifth toe.

Contraindications. Less severe abnormalities may be amenable to correction with a Ruiz-Mora procedure or other soft tissue operations.

Surgical Procedure

Operative Technique

1. Outline a triangular web incision with the marking pen (Fig. 2). The incision extends from the base of the web just dorsal to the midline to the level of the proximal interphalangeal joint. The incision then extends plantarward to the base of the web along the fifth toe.
2. Place the fourth and fifth toes together in their corrected position to transfer the marking (Fig. 2).
3. Excise the skin along the outline (Fig. 3).
4. Extend the incision as a dorsal longitudinal incision from the base of the web proximally between the metatarsal heads (Fig. 3a). Reflect the skin and subcutaneous tissue laterally over the base of the proximal phalanx. Alternatively, a second incision may be made overlying the base of the proximal phalanx. This is a dorsal longitudinal incision centered at the metatarsophalangeal joint (Fig. 3b).

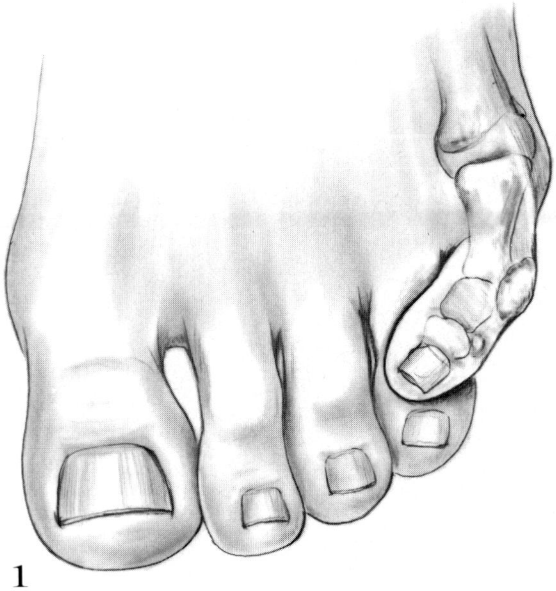

1

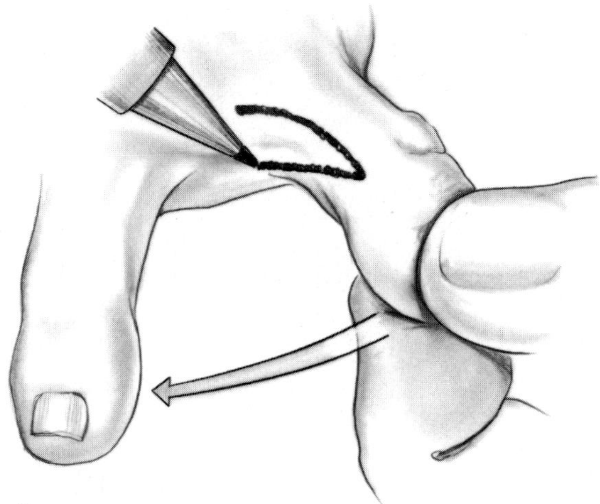

2

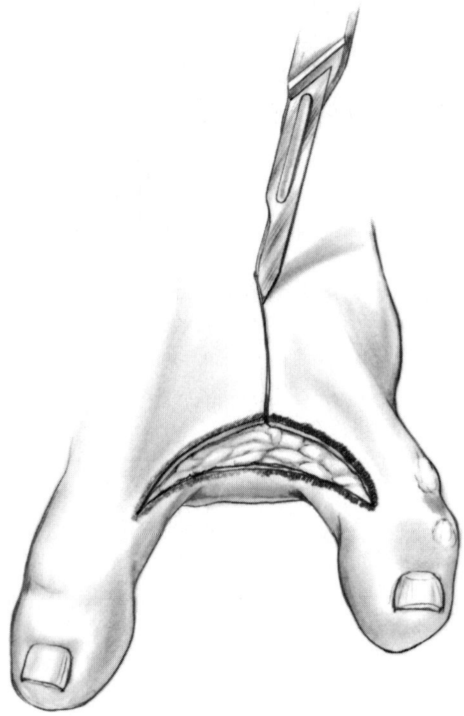

3a

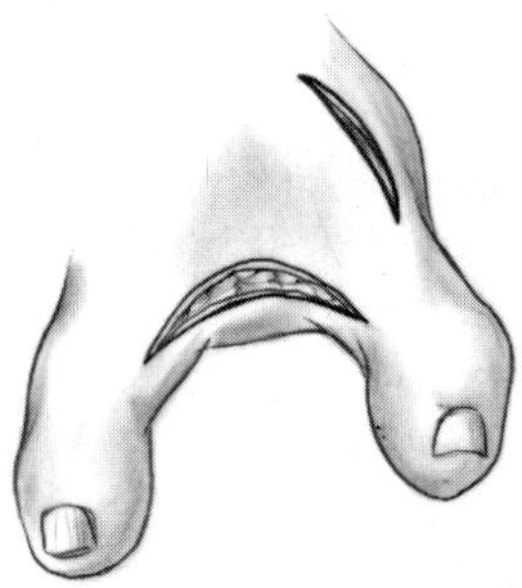

3b

5. The extensor digitorum longus tendon is transected (Fig. 4).
6. The capsule overlying the metatarsophalangeal joint and the periosteum overlying the proximal portion of the proximal phalanx are incised longitudinally and reflected subperiosteally to expose the base of the proximal phalanx.
7. Excise the proximal portion of the proximal phalanx with a microsagittal saw. The cut is made perpendicular to the longitudinal axis of the shaft (Fig. 5).
8. Close the incision as a subtotal syndactylization with interrupted buried simple 3-0 chromic sutures (Fig. 6a). The proximal extension of the incision between the metatarsal heads or the alternate dorsal longitudinal incision may be closed with interrupted vertical mattress nylon sutures (Fig. 6b).

Postoperative Care

1. A sterile compression dressing is applied.
2. Although some physicians allow heel walking in a stiff-soled postoperative shoe, non–weight bearing may be helpful to allow adequate healing of the syndactylization.
3. Nonabsorbable sutures may be removed at 2 to 3 weeks postoperatively.
4. If wound healing is delayed at the site of the syndactylization, the patient should soak the foot in dilute povidone-iodine (Betadine) three times per day for 15 minutes until healing is complete.

Technical Pitfalls

1. Early postoperative weight bearing may be associated with diathesis of the syndactyly.
2. An adequate diamond-shaped area of skin and subcutaneous tissue must be incised. Redundant skin may lead to recurrence of deformity despite syndactylization.

Potential Complications

1. Diathesis of the syndactyly
2. Recurrence of deformity

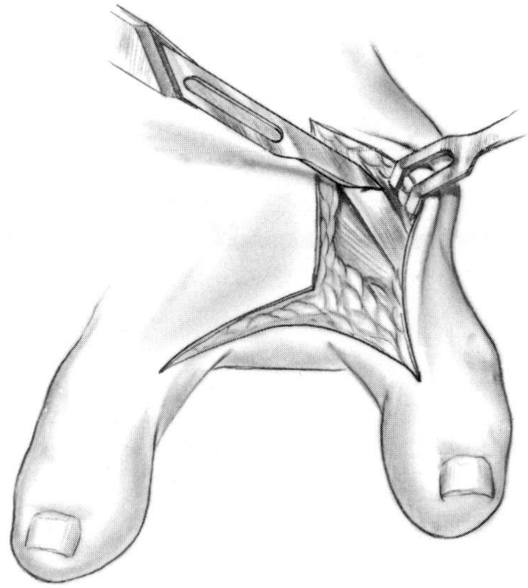

4

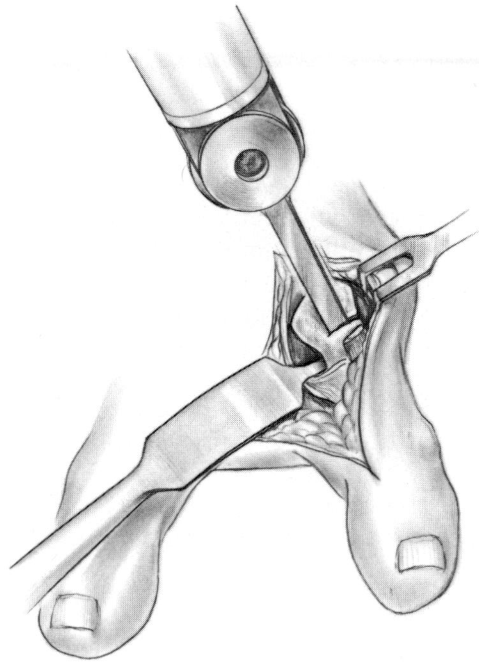

5

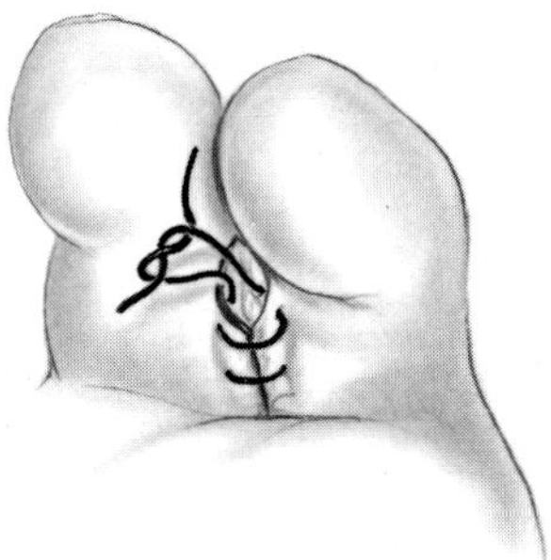

6a

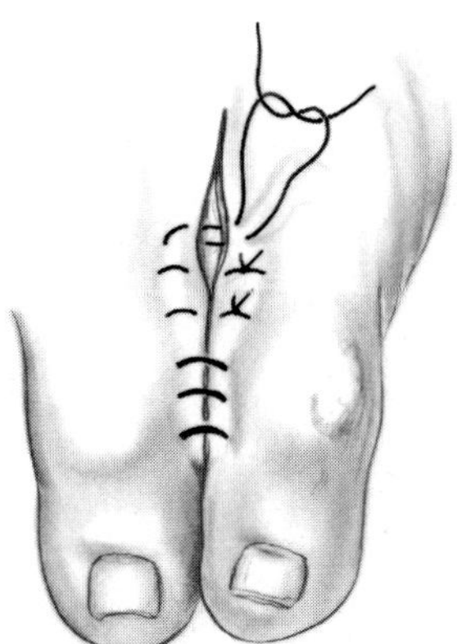

6b

CHEVRON OSTEOTOMY FIFTH TOE

General Considerations

The bunionette deformity consists of metatarsus quintus valgus, medial deviation of the fifth toe, and a prominent bony eminence at the lateral aspect of the fifth metatarsal head. This disorder may occur in conjunction with a hallux valgus deformity, in which case the patient is said to have a *splay foot.* Nonoperative treatment includes the use of appropriate shoewear with a high, wide toe box to accommodate the deformity. Surgical alternatives include excision of the prominent lateral eminence as an isolated procedure. In more significant deformities, particularly in those cases associated with metatarsus quintus valgus, metatarsal osteotomy may be advantageous. The Chevron osteotomy allows for narrowing of the forefoot width, excision of the prominent lateral eminence, and correction of the metatarsus quintus valgus, as well as the medial deviation of the fifth toe.

Patient Selection

Indications

1. Young active patients with a bunionette deformity
2. A bunionette deformity that includes significant metatarsus quintus valgus

Contraindications

1. Mild bunionette deformities may be amenable to excision of the prominent lateral eminence without metatarsal osteotomy.
2. Elderly patients and those at risk for wound healing problems may be better served with simple excision of the prominent eminence, if surgery is required.
3. Severe metatarsus quintus valgus not amenable to correction with a distal osteotomy may require an oblique osteotomy performed further proximally in the diaphysis.

Surgical Procedure

Operative Technique

1. A dorsolateral incision approximately 3 cm long is made from the midpoint of the proximal phalanx to 1 cm proximal to the exostosis (Fig. 1). The subcutaneous tissue is divided along the line of the skin incision. The skin and subcutaneous tissue are reflected to visualize the capsule.
2. A lateral longitudinal capsular incision is made plantar to the skin incision (Fig. 2). Capsule is reflected subperiosteally to expose the head and neck of the 5th metatarsal.
3. Excise the exostosis parallel to the lateral border of the foot with a microsagittal saw (Fig. 3).
4. Make a transverse V-shaped osteotomy distally with a microsagittal saw (Fig. 4).
5. Push the metatarsal head medially approximately 2 mm (Fig. 5).
6. Fix the osteotomy with an oblique 0.045-inch Kirschner wire inserted through a separate stab incision. The pin is inserted from dorsal distal to plantar proximal (Fig. 6). Cut off and bend the pin above the skin.
7. Excise the bony projection at the lateral aspect of the fifth metatarsal shaft with the microsagittal saw (Fig. 6). Close the capsule with interrupted simple 3-0 Vicryl sutures. Close the skin with a running subcuticular suture of 3-0 prolene.

Postoperative Care

1. A soft compression dressing is applied for 48 hours.
2. A short-leg walking cast is used for 3 weeks.
3. The sutures and pin are removed at 3 weeks.
4. A wooden-soled shoe is used for 3 weeks.

Technical Pitfalls

1. Excessive soft tissue stripping should be avoided.
2. Excessive resection of the prominent lateral eminence should be avoided.
3. Excessive medial translocation of the distal fragment may lead to an unstable osteotomy.

Potential Complications

1. Nonunion of the osteotomy
2. Postoperative displacement

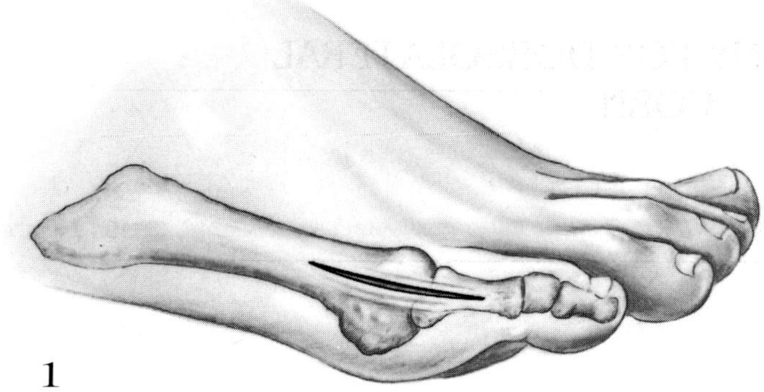

1

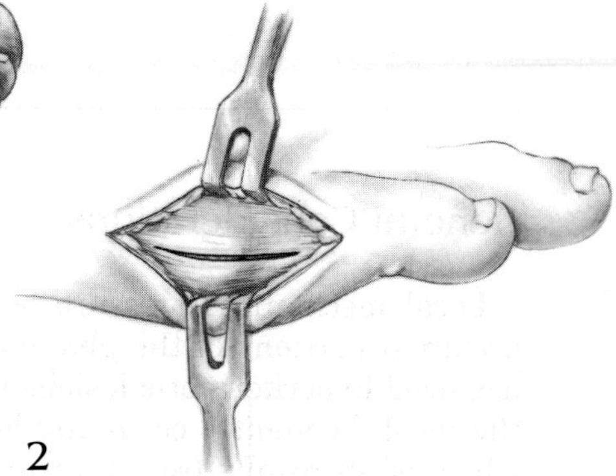

2

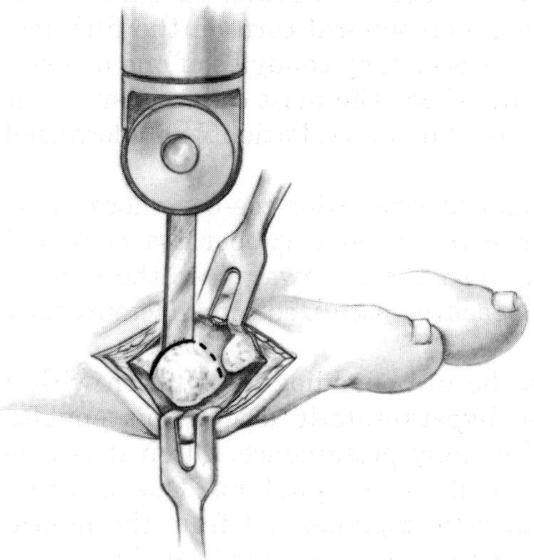

3

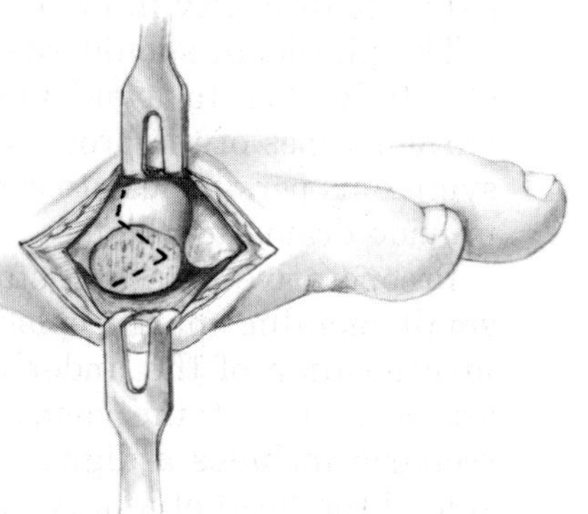

4

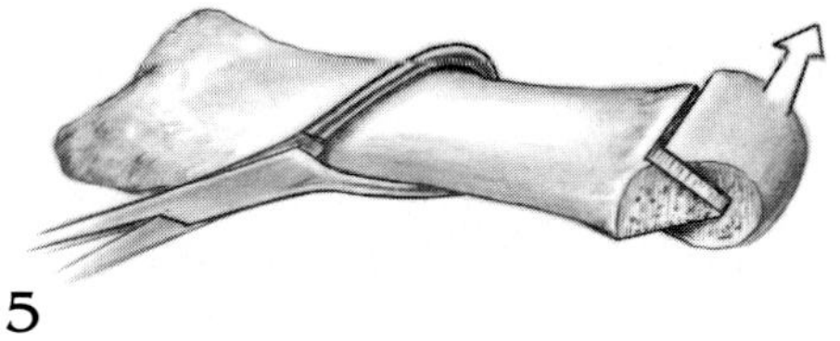

5

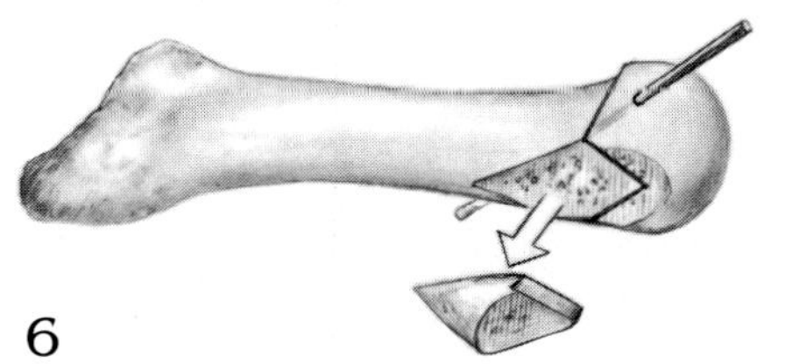

6

CONDYLECTOMY FOR DORSOLATERAL CORN

General Considerations

Local mechanical pressure between the osseous condyles at the distal or proximal portions of the phalanges and the forepart of the shoe may lead to localized hyperkeratotic lesions known as *hard corns* (heloma durum). One of the most frequently occurring lesions is a dorsolateral corn on the fifth toe, which often results from pressure of the lateral bony condyles of one or more of the phalanges against the toe box of the shoe. The most common site is at the lateral condyle of the head of the proximal phalanx. Patients note localized pain and difficulty in fitting shoewear.

The physician should advise the patient to wear wide-toe-box shoes made of soft leather to avoid mechanical pressure. Sponge rubber toe caps and various types of toe protectors may help float the toe away from the shoe. If symptoms persist despite conservative measures, localized condylectomy may provide dramatic relief.

Preoperative planning often includes the use of radiographs taken with a small metallic marker placed over the hyperkeratotic lesion; this enables identification of the underlying offending bony prominence. Often it is necessary to resect the condyles from more than one phalanx. One common scenario includes a digital corn secondary to impingement from the lateral side of the head of a proximal phalanx and the ipsilateral side of the base of the middle phalanx. In this situation, both prominent condyles should be removed.

Patient Selection

Indications. The indication is a dorsolateral corn of the fifth toe.

Contraindications

1. A common clinical situation is one in which the dorsolateral corn is seen in conjunction with an interdigital corn in the fourth web space. This often requires resection of the distal portion of the fifth proximal phalanx with or without a lateral condylectomy of the base of the fourth proximal phalanx, often with syndactylization of toe 4 to toe 5.
2. A dorsolateral corn of the fifth toe that has recurred after prior condylectomy is best treated with resection of the distal portion of the proximal phalanx with or without syndactylization of toe 4 to toe 5.
3. Large dorsolateral corns on the fifth toe may require resection of the head of the proximal phalanx with or without lateral condylectomy at the base of the middle phalanx.
4. Neurologic or vascular disorders may increase the risk of infection and wound healing problems.

Surgical Procedure

Operative Technique

1. A slightly curved dorsolateral incision is made longitudinally just medial to the corn. The incision extends from the middle phalanx to the midpoint of the proximal phalanx (Fig. 1). Subcutaneous tissue is incised along the line of the skin incision.
2. Deepen the incision to bone through subcutaneous tissue and the extensor tendon (Fig. 2). Expose the lateral condyle at the head of the proximal phalanx and the lateral condyle at the base of the middle phalanx subperiosteally.
3. Excise the lateral condyle at the head of the proximal phalanx and the lateral condyle at the base of the middle phalanx with a microsagittal saw (Fig. 3). Smooth the cut surface with a rasp (Fig. 4).
4. If necessary, close deep tissues with interrupted simple 3-0 Vicryl sutures. Close the skin with interrupted vertical mattress or simple 4-0 nylon sutures (Fig. 5).

Postoperative Care

1. A sterile dressing is applied to the digit.
2. The patient is allowed to ambulate in a stiff-soled postoperative shoe.
3. The sutures are removed at 2 to 3 weeks after surgery.
4. The patient is allowed a gradual progressive return to weight bearing and wide-toe-box shoes within the limits of discomfort.

Technical Pitfalls

1. Resection of bone may be inadequate. It is often helpful to obtain preoperative radiographs with metallic markers overlying the hyperkeratotic lesion to identify all offending osseous structures.

Potential Complications. Recurrence of the lesion is possible.

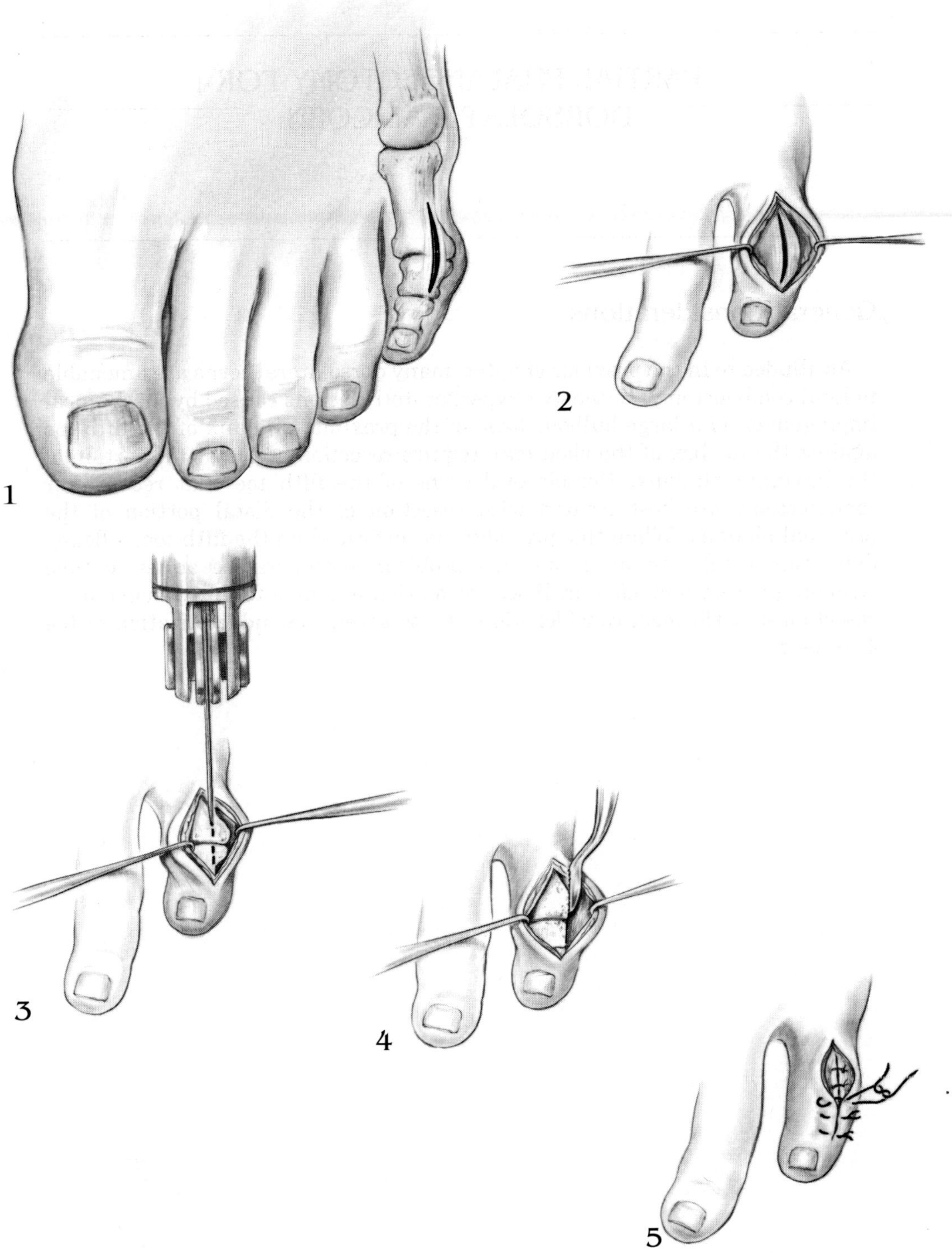
1
2
3
4
5

PARTIAL PHALANGECTOMY FOR DORSOLATERAL CORN

General Considerations

As alluded to in the previous chapter, many dorsolateral corns are amenable to local condylectomy. Extensive hyperkeratotic lesions caused by mechanical impingement of a large bulbous head of the proximal phalanx of the fifth toe against the toe box of the shoe may require resection of the distal portion of the proximal phalanx. Dorsolateral corns of the fifth toe that recur after condylectomy are best treated with resection of the distal portion of the proximal phalanx. When this procedure is performed on the fifth toe, a floppy digit may result. To minimize this problem, postoperative adhesive tape strapping is recommended until scar formation is complete. If extensive bony resection is performed, consideration can be given to syndactylization of toe 4 to toe 5.

Patient Selection

Indications

1. Dorsolateral corn of the fifth toe secondary to an enlarged distal portion of the proximal phalanx of the fifth toe
2. Recurrent dorsolateral corn after condylectomy

Contraindications

1. Many dorsolateral corns are amenable to more limited bony resection in the form of local condylectomy.
2. Extensive bony resection may require syndactylization of toe 4 to toe 5.
3. Patients with a dorsolateral corn on the fifth toe associated with an interdigital corn in the fourth web space may require more extensive surgical intervention. This is treated by resection of the distal portion of the proximal phalanx of the fifth toe combined with lateral condylectomy at the base of the fourth toe in addition to syndactylization of toe 4 to toe 5. (See "Interdigital Soft Corns of the Fourth Web Space.")

Surgical Procedure

Operative Technique

1. A dorsal longitudinal incision 1½ cm long is made, centered over the proximal interphalangeal joint (Fig. 1). The subcutaneous tissue is divided along the line of the skin incision.
2. Incise the extensor digitorum longus tendon longitudinally, and retract medially and laterally (Fig. 2).
3. Incise the capsule overlying the proximal interphalangeal joint and the periosteum overlying the distal portion of the proximal phalanx longitudinally, and reflect subperiosteally.
4. Excise the distal portion of the proximal phalanx using a microsagittal saw with a cut made perpendicular to the longitudinal axis of the shaft (Figs. 3a and 3b).
5. Close the skin with interrupted vertical mattress or simple 4-0 nylon sutures.

Postoperative Care

1. A sterile dressing is applied. Adhesive tape strapping is applied to hold the fifth toe in the corrected position.
2. Adhesive tape strapping is continued for 6 weeks after surgery to ensure adequate scar tissue formation.
3. Sutures are removed at 2 to 3 weeks after surgery.
4. Heel walking in a stiff-soled postoperative shoe is allowed.

Technical Pitfalls. Excessive bony resection may create instability at the proximal interphalangeal joint, leading to a floppy toe. If this is problematic, consideration could be given to syndactylization of toe 4 to toe 5.

Potential Complications

1. A floppy toe secondary to an unstable proximal interphalangeal joint
2. Shortening of the toe (expected)

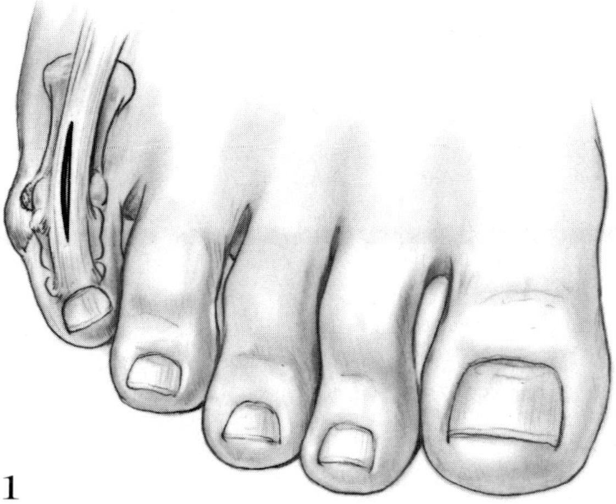

1

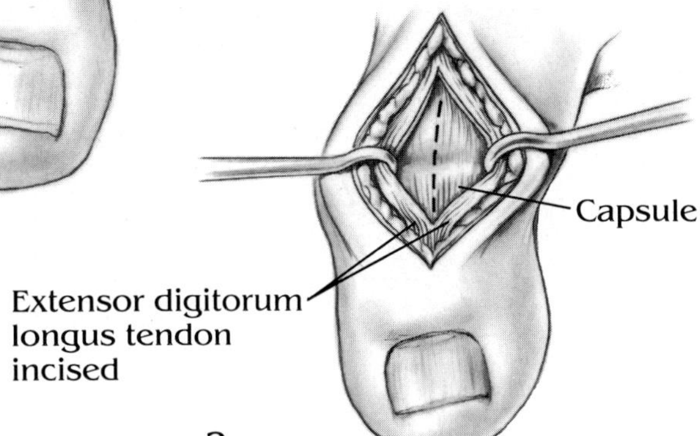

2

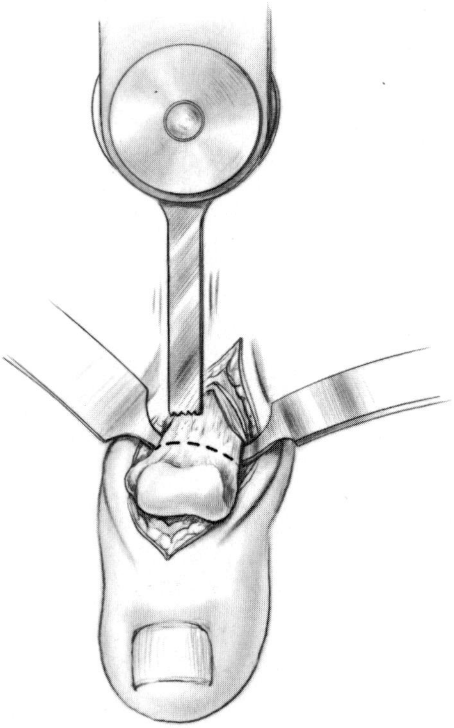

3a

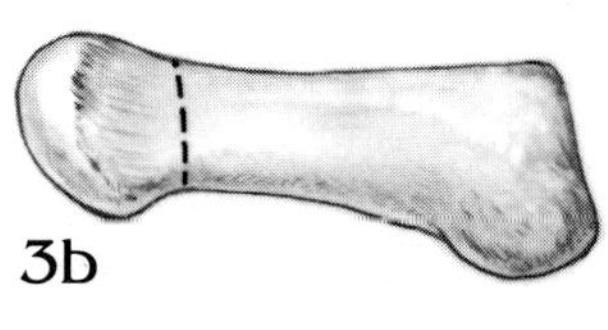

3b

PART 9

Operations for Disorders of the Metatarsophalangeal Region

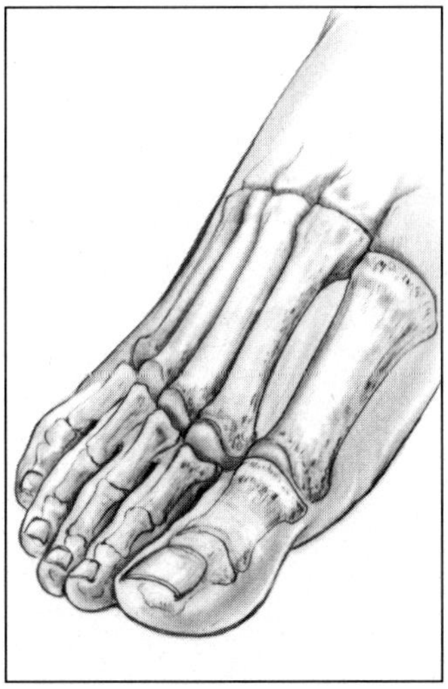

EXCISION INTERDIGITAL NEUROMA

General Considerations

An interdigital neuroma is an enlargement of one of the common digital nerves of the foot at the level of the metatarsal heads. Neuromas are unilateral in 90% of cases, and the most common site of occurrence is the third digital nerve lying in the third web space. The second digital nerve may be involved, but this is less common. Excision of a neuroma is an effective method of treating this common disorder if conservative measures fail to provide relief of symptoms. The dorsal longitudinal approach is recommended.

Patient Selection

Indications

1. Young active patients with pain in the third web space associated with numbness and paresthesias of the third and fourth toes
2. Symptoms resistant to conservative measures (i.e., metatarsal pads, nonsteroidal anti-inflammatory medications, and injections of anesthetic and steroid)

Contraindications

1. Elderly, debilitated patients
2. The presence of vascular disorders, diabetes, or other problems that increase the risks associated with operative intervention

Surgical Procedure

Operative Technique

1. A dorsal longitudinal incision is made from 2.5 cm proximal to the web space and extending distally between the third and fourth metatarsals; it ends at the junction of the web and the sole of the foot (Fig. 1). Subcutaneous tissue is incised along the line of the skin incision. Deepen the incision between the metatarsal heads with blunt dissection.
2. Insert a neuroma retractor to apply tension to the intermetatarsal ligament (Fig. 2).
3. The intermetatarsal ligament is incised along its course to expose the neuroma and decompress the web space (Fig. 3).
4. Dissect surrounding fat and blood vessels away from the neuroma. Grasp the neuroma with forceps and pull distally.
5. Transect the neuroma proximal to the metatarsal heads (Fig. 4). Dissect distally and transect the neuroma distal to its bifurcation into its terminal branches (Fig. 4, inset).
6. Reapproximate the subcutaneous tissue with interrupted simple 3-0 Vicryl sutures. Close the skin with interrupted vertical mattress 4-0 nylon sutures (Fig. 5).

Postoperative Care

1. A compression dressing is applied.
2. Heel walking in a stiff-soled postoperative shoe is recommended for 3 weeks.
3. Sutures are removed at 3 weeks after surgery.

Technical Pitfalls

1. The nerve must be transected proximal to the metatarsal heads to avoid formation of a stump neuroma with recurrence of symptoms.
2. Incomplete release of the intermetatarsal ligament may lead to persistent symptoms.

Potential Complications

1. A stump neuroma may form at the site of transection.
2. Permanent numbness of toes 3 and 4 is expected but may be poorly tolerated in a small percentage of patients.

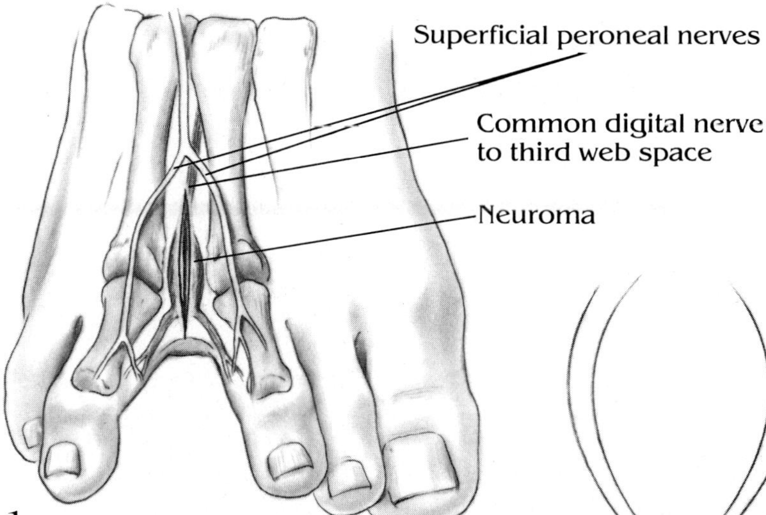
Superficial peroneal nerves
Common digital nerve
to third web space
Neuroma

1

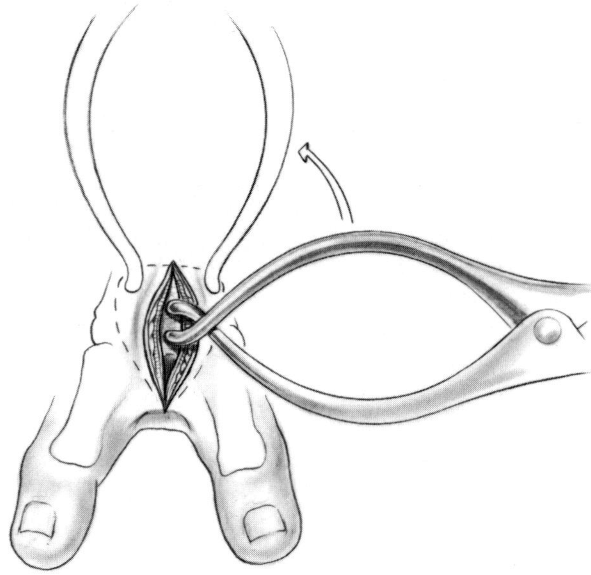

2

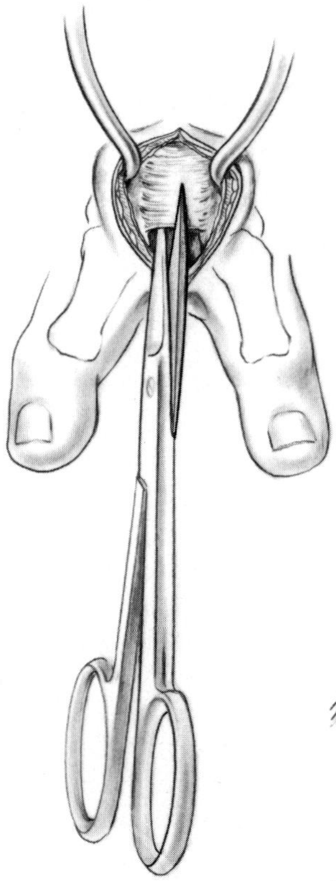

3

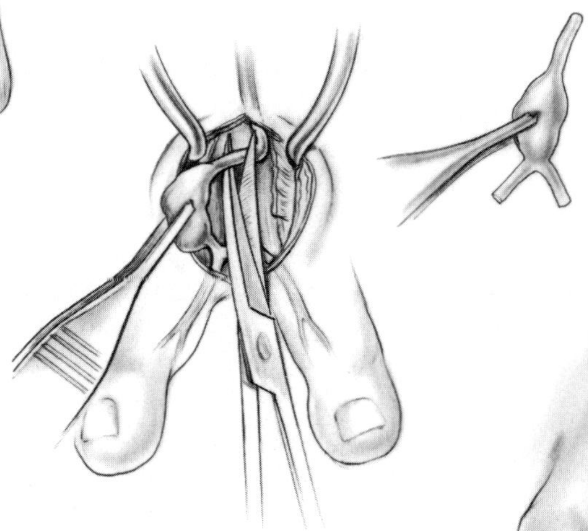

4

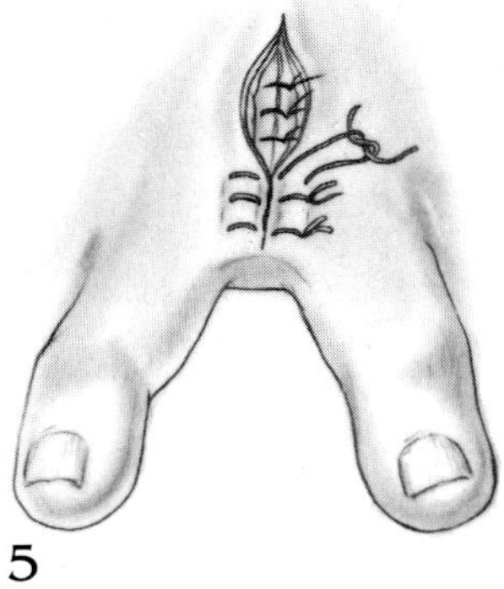

5

PLANTAR CONDYLECTOMY FOR INTRACTABLE PLANTAR KERATOSES

General Considerations

Metatarsalgia is defined as pain beneath the metatarsal heads. This common problem may be caused by any of a variety of pathologic disorders. With age, collagen tissue throughout the body atrophies. The fat pad under the metatarsal heads decreases in height, and increased pressure is borne by the bones, which become prominent under the skin at the plantar surface of the foot. Intractable plantar hyperkeratotic lesions form because of increased weight-bearing pressures in these regions. This abnormality is common after 40 years of age, and women seem to be affected more frequently than men. Predisposing factors include high-heeled shoes, which increase weight-bearing pressure at the level of the metatarsal head.

Patients note aching pain at the plantar aspect of the forefoot. Tender hyperkeratotic lesions form under the metatarsal heads. Physical examination reveals localized hyperkeratotic lesions. Increased loads owing to a hyperextension deformity at the metatarsophalangeal joint may be associated with claw or hammer toe deformities.

Nonoperative treatment includes rubber-soled shoes to decrease impact loading. Soft metatarsal pads applied proximal to the metatarsal head may decrease weight-bearing pressure and thus alleviate symptoms. Calluses may be shaved by the physician, and patients may attempt decompression of the hyperkeratotic lesion by grinding with a pumice stone. The vast majority of lesions are adequately treated by conservative modalities.

If nonoperative management fails to provide relief of symptoms and the hyperkeratotic lesion can be localized under a specific metatarsal head, then consideration can be given to plantar condylectomy popularized by R. A. Mann and H. L. DuVries. Preoperative x-ray evaluation with a radiopaque marker placed over the hyperkeratotic lesion may be helpful in identifying the offending bony condyle. If the hyperkeratotic lesion is associated with a hammer or claw toe deformity, correction of that abnormality may lead to decreased loads applied by means of correction of the hyperextension deformity at the metatarsophalangeal joint. In addition, if the involved metatarsal appears to be long relative to adjacent metatarsals, resection of the distal tip of the metatarsal, in addition to plantar condylectomy, may be appropriate.

Patient Selection

Indications. The primary indication is isolated intractable plantar keratosis underlying one of the lesser metatarsal heads that fails to respond to conservative modes of treatment.

Contraindications

1. Hyperkeratotic lesions secondary to malunion of metatarsal fractures may be better treated with corrective metatarsal osteotomies at the apex of the deformity.
2. Diffuse plantar callosities underlying multiple metatarsal heads are better treated nonoperatively.
3. Diffuse plantar metatarsalgia secondary to pes cavus deformity may be better treated by means of correction of the forefoot equinus further proximally.
4. Because of the high incidence of recurrence of hyperkeratotic lesions and the marked frequency of transfer lesions, these abnormalities are best treated with conservative care utilizing soft flexible inserts with elevation proximal to the metatarsal heads to float the metatarsal heads off the inner sole of the shoe.

Surgical Procedure

Operative Technique

1. A dorsal longitudinal incision 3 cm long is made, centered over the metatarsophalangeal joint (Fig. 1). Subcutaneous tissue is divided along the line of the skin incision.
2. The extensor hallucis longus tendon is identified and retracted laterally. The capsule overlying the metatarsophalangeal joint and the periosteum overlying the neck of the metatarsal and the base of the proximal phalanx are incised longitudinally (Fig. 2). The capsule and periosteum are reflected subperiosteally to expose the head and neck of the metatarsal.
3. The collateral ligaments are reflected from both sides of the metatarsal head. The volar plate is detached from the undersurface of the metatarsal head with a periosteal elevator (Fig. 3).
4. The proximal phalanx is firmly plantarflexed, allowing exposure of the plantar aspect of the metatarsal head.
5. The plantar aspect of the metatarsal head is resected flush with the metatarsal shaft using a small osteotome (Fig. 4).
6. If necessary, the distal tip of the articular surface of the metatarsal is resected perpendicular to the long axis of the shaft with a small osteotome (Fig. 5).
7. The joint is then reduced. The skin is closed with interrupted vertical mattress 4-0 nylon sutures.

Postoperative Care
1. A sterile dressing is applied.
2. Heel walking in a stiff-soled postoperative shoe is permitted.
3. Sutures are removed 2 to 3 weeks after surgery.
4. Gentle range-of-motion exercises are encouraged.

Technical Pitfalls
1. Resection of excessive bone from the tip of the metatarsal may lead to instability of the metatarsophalangeal joint.
2. Excessive removal of bone from either the distal aspect or the plantar surface of the metatarsal head may lead to transfer metatarsalgia, with a shift in weight-bearing pressures to adjacent metatarsal heads.
3. Inadequate resection of bone from the plantar surface of the metatarsal may lead to persistent residual symptoms.

Potential Complications
1. Transfer metatarsalgia with hyperkeratotic lesions beneath adjacent metatarsal heads may occur.
2. Stiffness and loss of joint motion at the metatarsophalangeal joint are quite common after surgery.

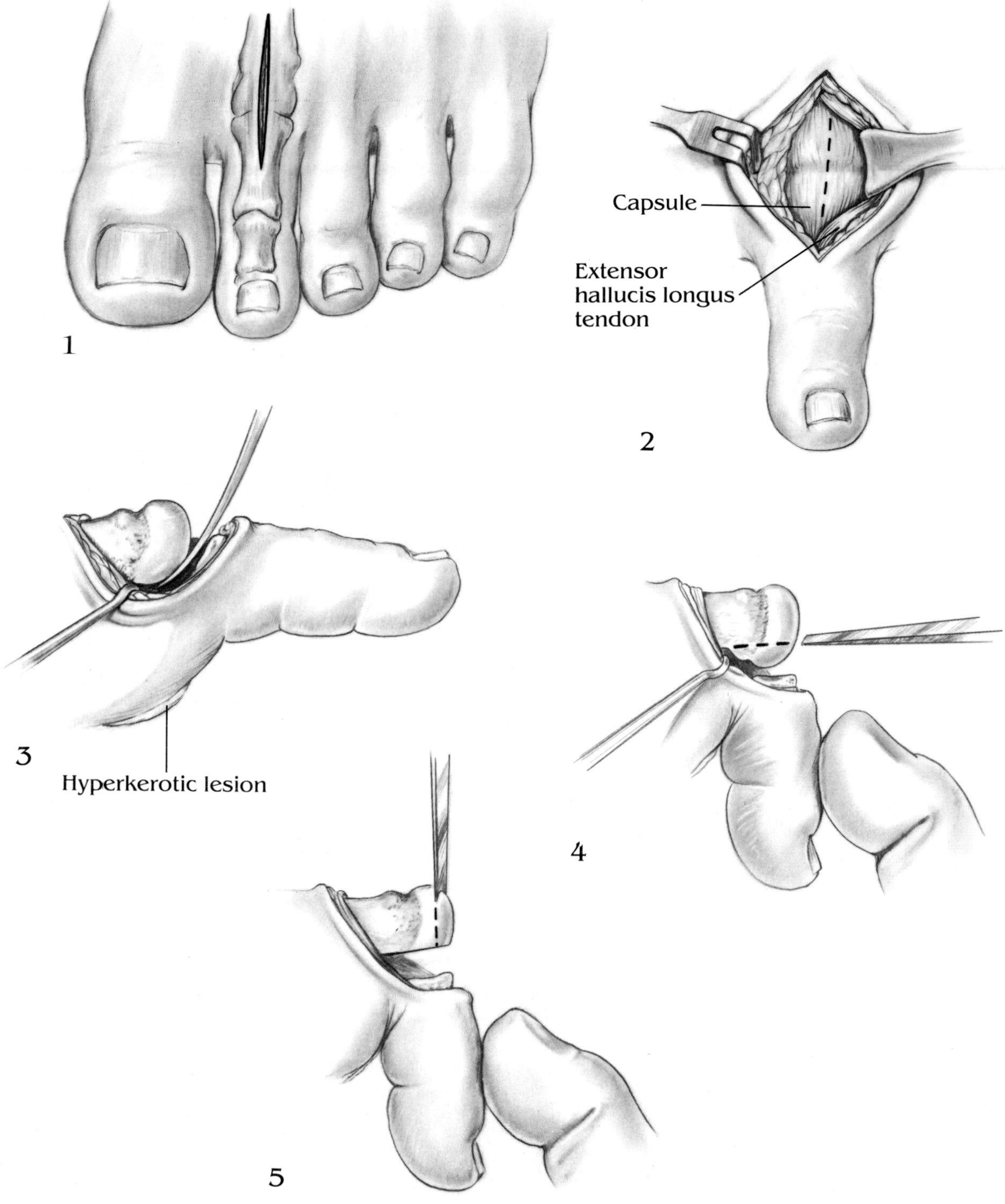
1
Capsule
Extensor hallucis longus tendon
2
3
Hyperkerotic lesion
4
5

DEBRIDEMENT ARTHROPLASTY FOR AVASCULAR NECROSIS METATARSAL HEAD

General Considerations

Osteochondrosis of the metatarsal head (Freiberg's infarction) consists of avascular necrosis of the subchondral bone with secondary revascularization and reparation. Typically the metatarsal head collapses and becomes quite misshapen. This process tends to occur most commonly in the second metatarsal head, although avascular necrosis of other metatarsal heads has been described. Most often this process has its onset during the second decade of life.

The acute phase is characterized by pain, swelling, and limitation of motion of the involved metatarsophalangeal joint and generally subsides with conservative treatment. The use of rubber-soled shoes will decrease impact loading during the stance phase of gait. A soft flexible insert to provide elevation proximal to the metatarsal heads may help alleviate weight-bearing pressures in the region of the injury. For severe cases, a short-leg cast and the use of crutches (non–weight bearing) may be appropriate. If pain and swelling persist, consideration can be given to debridement arthroplasty of that joint with synovectomy.

In many cases the acute symptoms subside, but arthritic changes progress, causing patients to become symptomatic later on in life. Degenerative changes of the involved articulation, with further loss of joint space and osteophyte formation, may occur. Again, conservative treatment with inserts and appropriate shoewear, as well as anti-inflammatory medications, may be helpful. If symptoms persist, debridement arthroplasty may be attempted.

Debridement arthroplasty of the joint includes removal of osteochondral fragments, debridement of irregular areas of avascular bone, and reshaping of the metatarsal head with resection of any existing osteophytes. If extensive hypertrophic synovium is present, a synovectomy is performed. Concomitant arthritic change at the base of the proximal phalanx is commonly seen, for which debridement of the arthritic osteophyte at the base of the phalanx is also performed. If severe arthritic changes are present, local debridement arthroplasty may not provide complete relief of symptoms. In this situation resection of the proximal portion of the proximal phalanx and syndactylization of toe 2 to toe 3 may be appropriate.

Patient Selection

Indications

1. Avascular necrosis of the metatarsal head with synovitis of the metatarsophalangeal joint that persists despite conservative treatment
2. Degenerative arthrosis at a lesser metatarsophalangeal joint secondary to Freiberg's infarction of the metatarsal head

Contraindications

1. Severe arthritic change may be better treated with resection of the base of the proximal phalanx and subtotal syndactylization of toe 2 to toe 3.
2. Patients with less severe symptoms or a limited activity level may be better treated with conservative measures.

Surgical Procedure

Operative Technique

1. A dorsal longitudinal incision 3 cm long is made, centered over the metatarsophalangeal joint (Fig. 1). Subcutaneous tissue is incised along the line of the skin incision.
2. Identify and retract the extensor digitorum longus tendon. Alternatively, if hyperextension deformity is present at the metatarsophalangeal joint, the extensor digitorum longus tendon may be transected transversely to achieve tenotomy at the level of the joint.
3. Incise the capsule overlying the metatarsophalangeal joint and the periosteum overlying the base of the proximal phalanx and the head of the metatarsal longitudinally (Fig. 2). Reflect the capsule and periosteum subperiosteally to expose the base of the proximal phalanx and the head of the metatarsal.
4. If hypertrophic synovium is noted, perform a synovectomy of the metatarsophalangeal articulation (Fig. 3).
5. Remove osteochondral fragments from the joint (Fig. 3).
6. Hyperflex the toe to expose the entire metatarsal head. Resect the osteophytes about the metatarsal head (Fig. 4). Debride areas of necrotic bone and cartilage.
7. Resect the osteophytes and reshape the base of the proximal phalanx (Fig. 5).
8. Close the skin with interrupted vertical mattress 4-0 nylon sutures.

Postoperative Care

1. A sterile dressing is applied.
2. A compression dressing is applied.
3. Heel walking in a stiff-soled postoperative shoe is permitted.
4. Sutures are removed at 2 to 3 weeks after surgery.
5. Gentle range-of-motion exercises are encouraged.

Technical Pitfalls

1. Adequate resection of areas of avascular bone and hypertrophic osteophyte is required. This allows reshaping of the metatarsal head.
2. If hyperextension deformity is present at the metatarsophalangeal joint, extensor tenotomy, dorsal capsulotomy, and postoperative adhesive strapping in the corrected position are necessary to prevent recurrence of deformity.

Potential Complications

1. Inadequate debridement may result in persistent or recurrent symptoms.
2. Arthritis is likely to progress despite surgical intervention. Additional surgery may be required in the future.

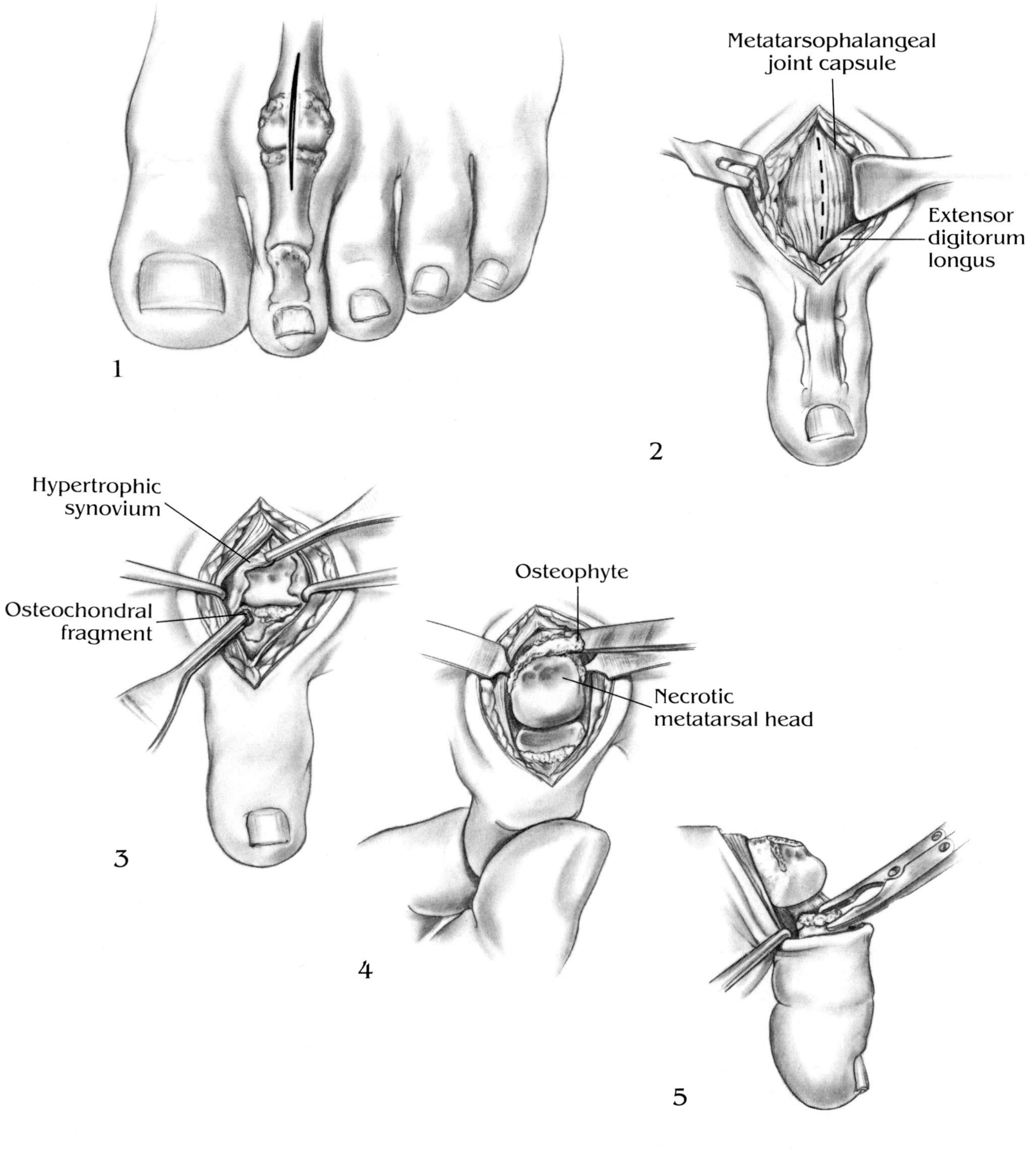

1
Metatarsophalangeal joint capsule
Extensor digitorum longus
2
Hypertrophic synovium
Osteochondral fragment
3
Osteophyte
Necrotic metatarsal head
4
5

PARTIAL PHALANGECTOMY AND SYNDACTYLIZATION FOR ARTHRITIS MTP JOINT

General Considerations

As alluded to in the previous section, extensive degenerative change secondary to avascular necrosis of the metatarsal head may require resection of the proximal portion of the proximal phalanx if debridement arthroplasty of the joint fails to provide relief of symptoms. Resection of the proximal portion of the proximal phalanx often leads to a cock-up deformity of the digit. Syndactylization of toe 2 to toe 3 is required to avoid this problem.

Patient Selection

Indications

1. Avascular necrosis of the metatarsal head with articular degeneration that fails to respond to conservative treatment
2. Recurrent pain, swelling, and limitation of motion at the metatarsophalangeal joint after prior debridement arthroplasty of that joint

Contraindications

1. Debridement arthroplasty is preferable, if feasible.
2. Patients with a relatively limited ambulatory status may be better treated nonoperatively. The use of a soft flexible insert with elevation proximal to the metatarsal heads may help decrease symptoms.

Surgical Procedure

Operative Technique

1. With a marking pen, outline a triangular web incision along the lateral aspect of the second toe. The outline is marked just dorsal to the midline from the base of the web to the level of the proximal interphalangeal joint. The incision is then extended plantarward back toward the base of the web (Fig. 1).
2. Press the second toe against the third toe in a corrected position to transfer the mark (Fig. 2). Excise the skin and subcutaneous tissue along the outline created. Extend the incision proximally as a dorsal longitudinal incision between the metatarsal heads (Fig. 2).
3. Incise the subcutaneous tissue along the incision between the metatarsal heads. Reflect skin and subcutaneous tissue medially to expose the dorsal aspect of the second proximal phalanx and the metatarsal head, if necessary (Fig. 3).
4. Incise the capsule and periosteum longitudinally (Fig. 3). Expose the base of the proximal phalanx subperiosteally. Expose the metatarsal head, if necessary.

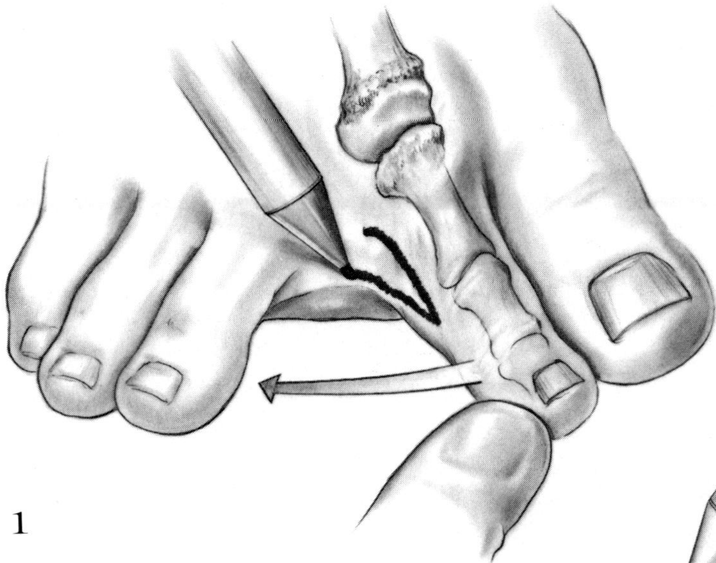
1

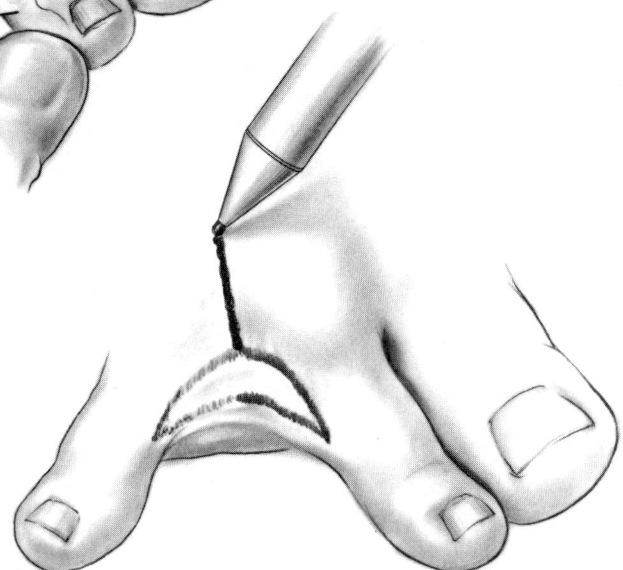
2

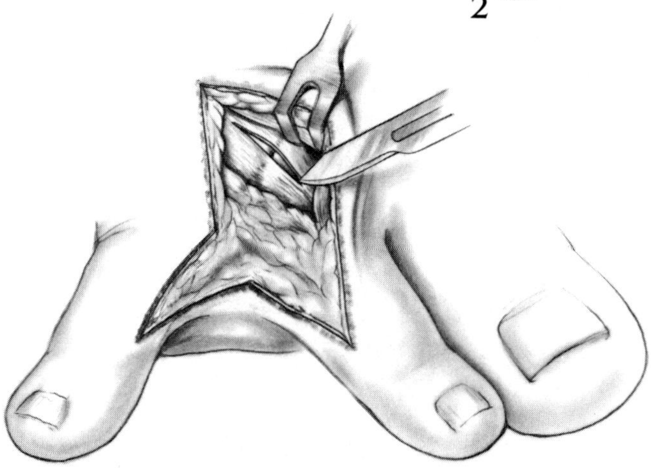
3

5. Excise the proximal portion of the proximal phalanx with a microsagittal saw (Fig. 4).
6. If the metatarsal head is misshapen, excise the osteophyte and reshape the metatarsal head with a rongeur (Fig. 5).
7. Close the web incision with interrupted simple buried 3-0 chromic sutures. Closure is begun on the plantar surface and progresses to the apex of the syndactyly (Fig. 6). Closure then progresses on the dorsum of the digit. Proximal to the web, skin closure may be performed with interrupted vertical mattress 4-0 nylon sutures (Fig. 7).

Postoperative Care

1. A sterile dressing is applied.
2. It may be preferable to require the patient to maintain non–weight bearing status utilizing crutches. This may prevent excessive tension at the site of syndactylization and thus avoid wound healing problems.
3. Sutures are removed at 2 to 3 weeks after surgery.
4. Once healing has progressed, partial weight bearing (heel walking) in a stiff-soled postoperative shoe is appropriate.
5. If delayed wound healing or wound necrosis is noted, the patient should soak the foot in dilute povidone-iodine (Betadine) three times per day for 15 minutes until wound healing is complete.

Technical Pitfalls. Avoidance of excessive weight bearing may be helpful to allow adequate progression of healing of the subtotal syndactylization.

Potential Complications

1. A cock-up deformity is possible as a result of diathesis of the syndactylization. This can often be minimized by avoidance of excessive weight bearing.
2. Delayed wound healing is possible.

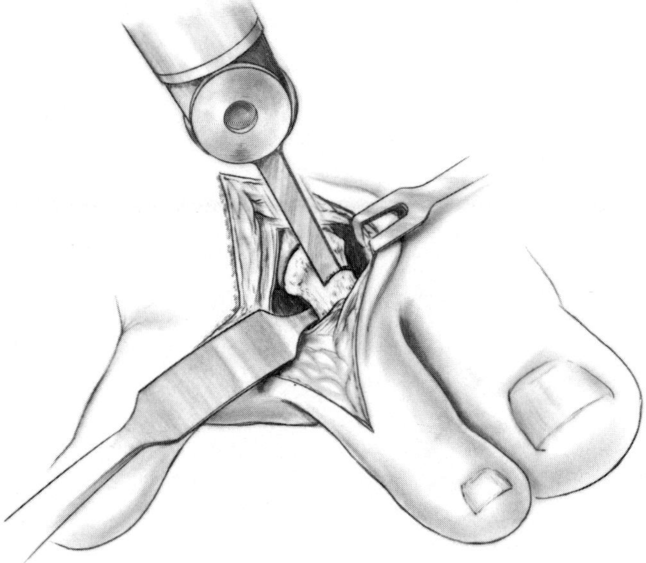

4

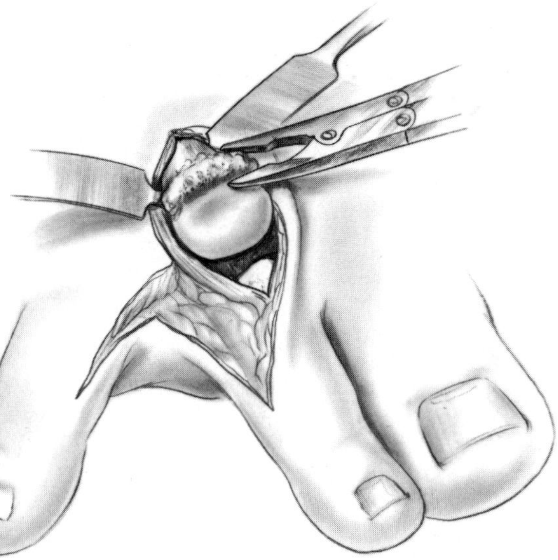

5

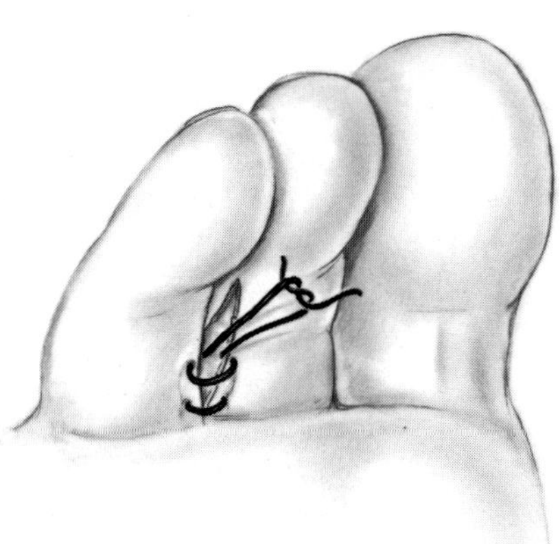

6

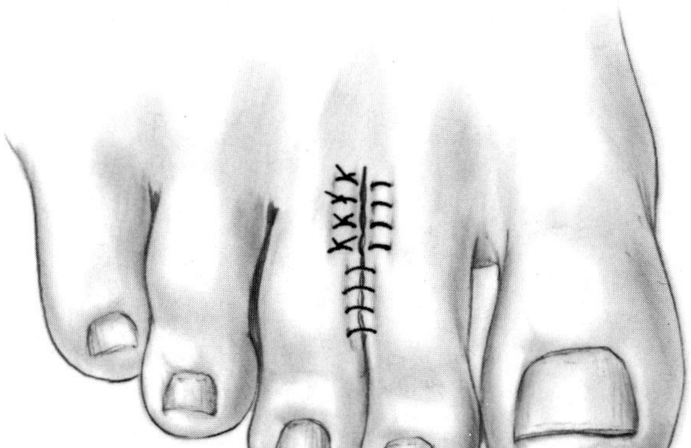

7

PART 10

Operations for Disorders of the Nails and Skin

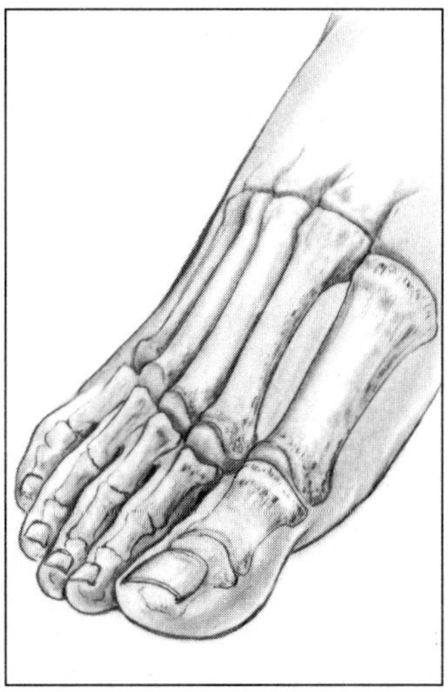

SURGICAL TREATMENT FOR INGROWN TOENAIL AND OTHER NAIL DISORDERS

General Considerations

An ingrown toenail (unguis incarnatus) develops when the nail margin protrudes into the soft lateral nail groove and the surrounding skin, causing a local inflammatory reaction. If the nail penetrates the adjacent soft tissue, a small wound is formed. This wound is susceptible to invasion by fungal and bacterial agents normally present on the skin and nail. This sequence of events may lead to a paronychial infection.

Predisposing factors include shoes with a narrow toe box that compresses the forefoot. Tight socks may also lead to mechanical pressure. If the nail is cut too short, the corners may penetrate the skin when growing outward. Various deformities of the nail plate and nail bed, such as an incurvated nail, may predispose an individual to this disorder.

The most common site is the lateral edge of the hallux nail, although any side of any nail may be involved. Symptoms include pain and swelling, and physical examination reveals localized erythema and tenderness, as well as hypertrophy of the nail lip and formation of granulation tissue along the nail groove. If a paronychial infection has occurred, purulent exudate may be seen.

Initial treatment is conservative. If a spike of nail is seen penetrating the skin, it should be excised. If hypertrophic tissue is present at the skin fold, silver nitrate cauterization may be helpful. Povidone-iodine (Betadine) soaks three times a day for 20 minutes are begun. The physician instructs the patient with regard to nail packing and training, which is performed after each soak. A wisp of cotton is inserted under the distal corner of the nail and then interposed proximally between the nail margin and the adjacent skin fold. If severe gross purulence is noted, the patient is given an oral broad-spectrum antibiotic. Shoes with low heels and a high, wide toe box are advised. If these measures fail, surgical intervention may be appropriate.

WEDGE RESECTION OF THE NAIL MARGIN, MATRIX, AND GROOVE

General Considerations

Wedge resection is most appropriate in cases of a chronic ingrown nail that does not respond to conservative treatment. The procedure should be postponed until the acute infectious process has subsided. It is most effective for recurrent ingrown nails and incurvated nails in which only the nail margin is deformed.

Surgical Procedure

Operative Technique

1. Incise the eponychium from the point where the proposed nail excision meets the eponychium. The incision extends proximally and slightly obliquely away from the nail for a distance of 5 mm (Fig. 1).
2. Expose the root of the nail by elevating the eponychial flaps.
3. Elevate the nail with a small hemostat or elevator. Incise the nail longitudinally from its distal end to its root and remove the fragment (Fig. 2).
4. Incise the nail bed and matrix along the nail incision down to bone. Incise the skin margin to remove an elliptical wedge of tissue down to bone. Remove the wedge en bloc (Fig. 3).
5. Curet the matrix and bed to ensure complete removal of germinal material (Fig. 4).
6. Apply one simple 4-0 nylon suture at the corner of the incision to reapproximate the eponychial flaps.
7. Pack the cavity with Xeroform gauze (Fig. 5). Apply a sterile compression dressing.

Postoperative Care

1. The compression dressing and Xeroform gauze are removed at 24 to 36 hours postoperatively.
2. An adhesive bandage may then be applied.
3. If inflammation occurs, the patient should soak the foot in dilute povidone-iodine (Betadine) for 20 minutes three times per day.
4. An open-toed wooden-soled shoe is worn until the wound is healed.

Technical Pitfalls

1. Failure to remove the nail root
2. Inadequate removal of germinal cells (nail matrix)
3. Failure to postpone surgery until the acute paronychial process has subsided

Potential Complications

1. Delayed wound healing and postoperative inflammation
2. Recurrence with regrowth of a nail horn (onychoma)
3. Unsightly narrowing of the nail

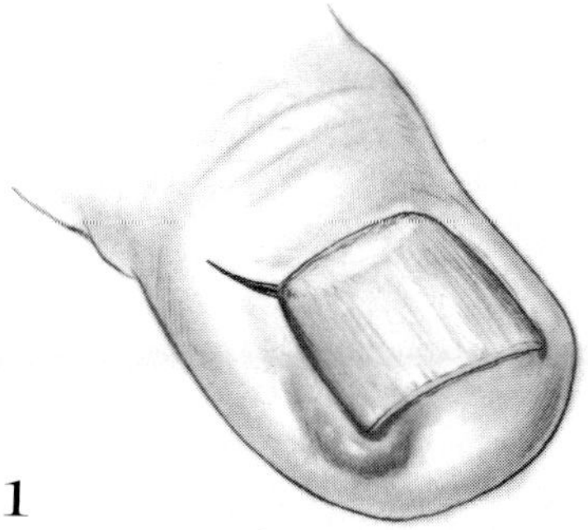

1

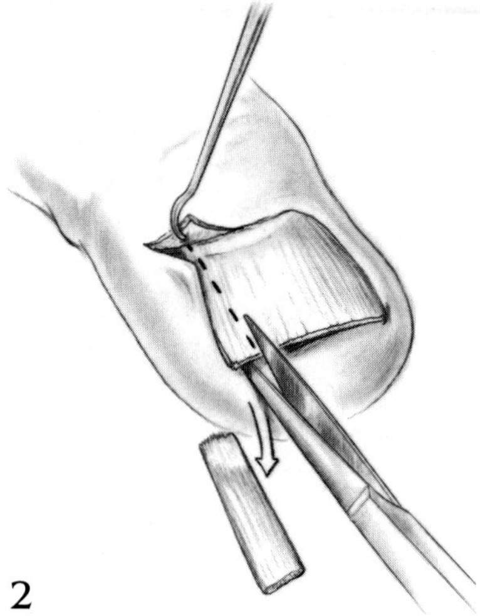

2

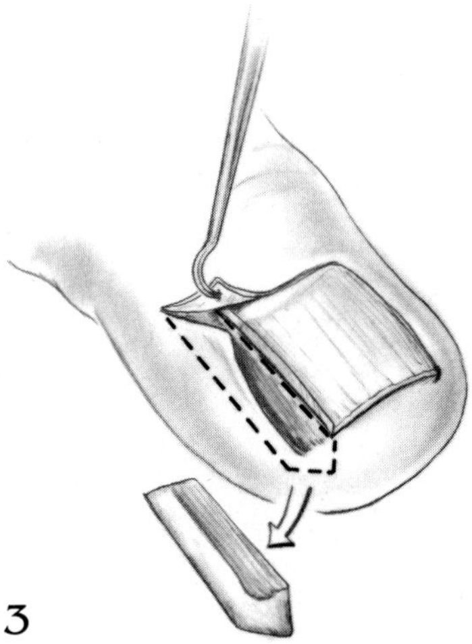

3

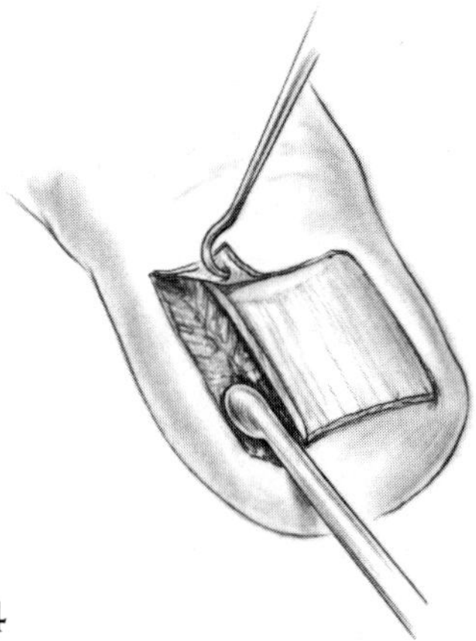

4

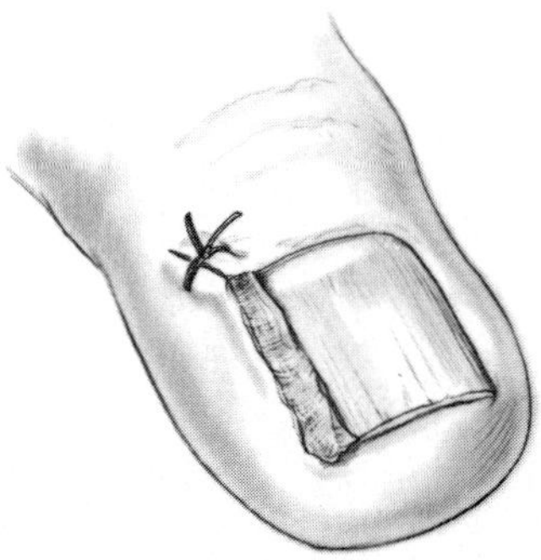

5

ABLATION OF NAIL AND NAIL MATRIX

General Considerations

Ablation of the nail and nail matrix is most effective for patients with a recurrent ingrown nail following prior less radical procedures. It is also appropriate for severe incurvation, onychomycosis, or onychogryphosis.

Surgical Procedure

Operative Technique

1. Make an oblique incision 5 mm long in each corner of the nail from the base of the nail and extending through the eponychium proximally.
2. Elevate the flaps formed with a dental elevator and retract proximally (Fig. 1).
3. Elevate the nail from the underlying nail matrix and bed with an elevator or hemostat. Grasp with a Kocher clamp and avulse the nail (Fig. 2).
4. Just proximal to the eponychium, incise the nail matrix transversely down to the periosteum of the underlying distal phalanx. Incise the matrix transversely just distal to the lunula. Connect these transverse incisions with the medial and lateral longitudinal incisions to remove a rectangular segment including the entire matrix (Fig. 3).
5. Excise all germinal material with a scalpel and curet (Fig. 4).
6. Excise the undersurface of the eponychium (upper root matrix) by sharp dissection (Fig. 5).
7. Insert one simple 4-0 nylon suture in each corner to reapproximate the eponychium.
8. Pack the defect with Xeroform gauze. Apply a compression dressing.

Postoperative Care

1. The compression dressing and gauze are removed at 24 to 36 hours postoperatively.
2. An adhesive bandage is applied.
3. If inflammation occurs, the patient should soak the foot in dilute povidone-iodine (Betadine) for 20 minutes three times per day.
4. An open-toed wooden-soled shoe is worn until the wound is healed.

Technical Pitfalls

1. Inadequate removal of the nail matrix
2. Failure to remove the root of the nail

Potential Complications

1. Delayed wound healing and postoperative inflammation
2. Regrowth of a portion of the nail (nail horn)

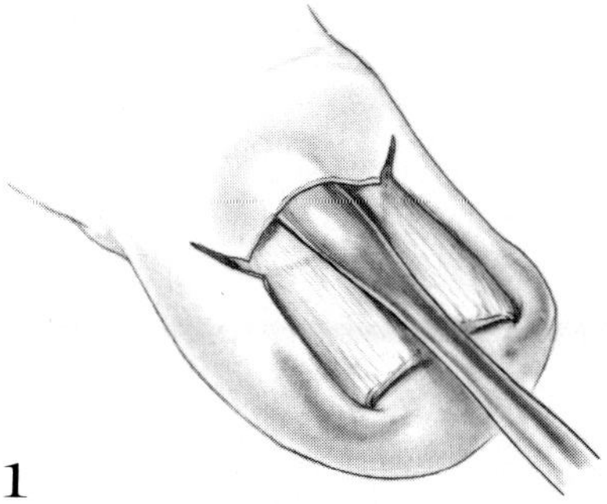

1

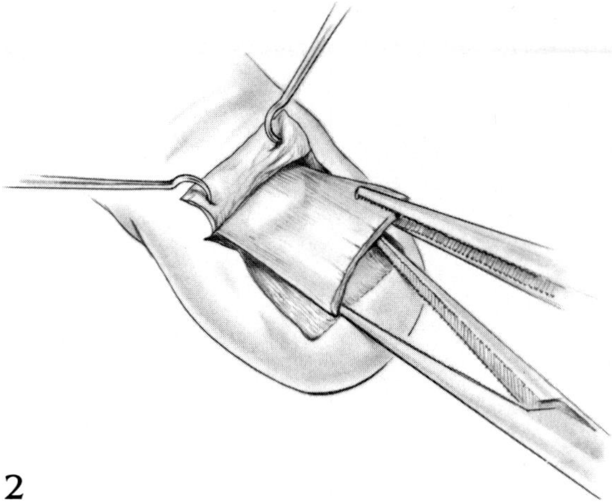

2

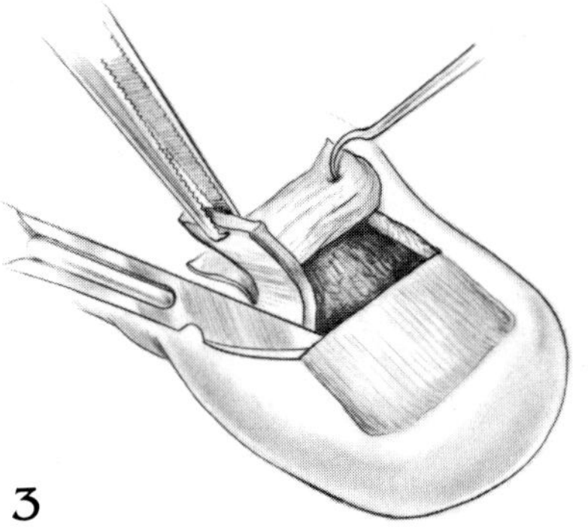

3

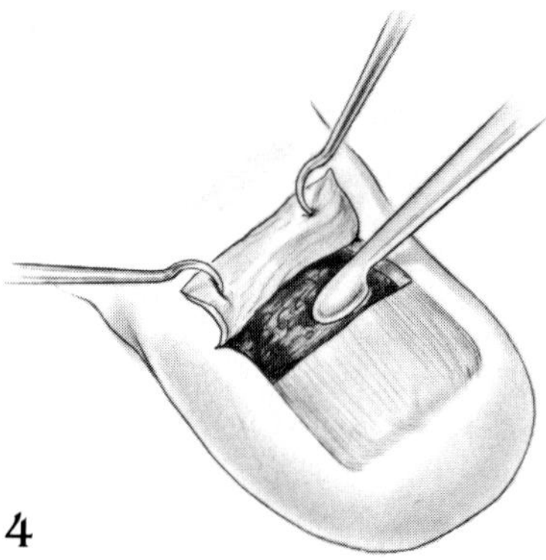

4

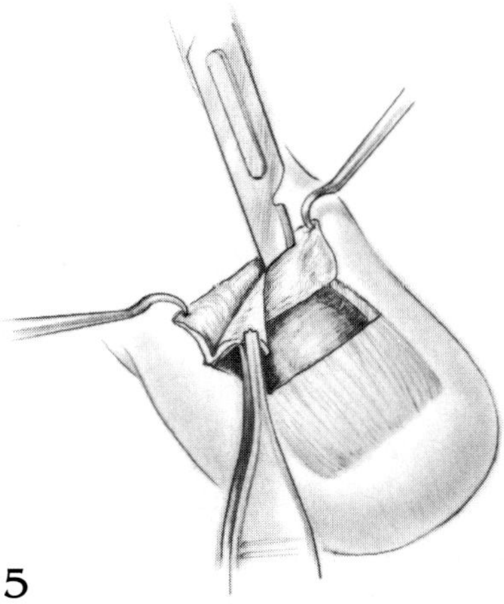

5

TERMINAL SYME PROCEDURE

General Considerations

The terminal Syme procedure is particularly effective for a recurrent ingrown nail after prior attempts at surgical ablation have failed. It is also quite effective for paraungual lesions of the lesser toes (especially the fifth toe) and may be applicable to some subungual tumors.

Surgical Procedure

Operative Technique

1. Make an incision 5 mm proximal to the base of the nail and encircling the entire nail and nail bed (Fig. 1).
2. Excise the nail completely, removing the nail, nail bed, and all soft tissues down to the distal phalanx (Fig. 2).
3. Separate the plantar fat pad from the tuft of the distal phalanx subperiosteally (Fig. 3).
4. Excise the distal portion of the distal phalanx with a microsagittal saw (Fig. 4). Smooth the end of the phalanx with a rasp.
5. Bring the plantar flap over the stump of the phalanx and suture the flap to dorsal skin with interrupted sutures of 3-0 nylon (Fig. 5).
6. Apply a compression dressing.

Postoperative Care
1. The compression dressing is removed at 24 hours.
2. An open-toed wooden-soled shoe is worn until sutures are removed.

Technical Pitfalls
1. Inadequate removal of bone
2. Inadequate tailoring of the plantar flap

Potential Complications
1. Unsightly bulbous stump
2. Formation of an inclusion cyst

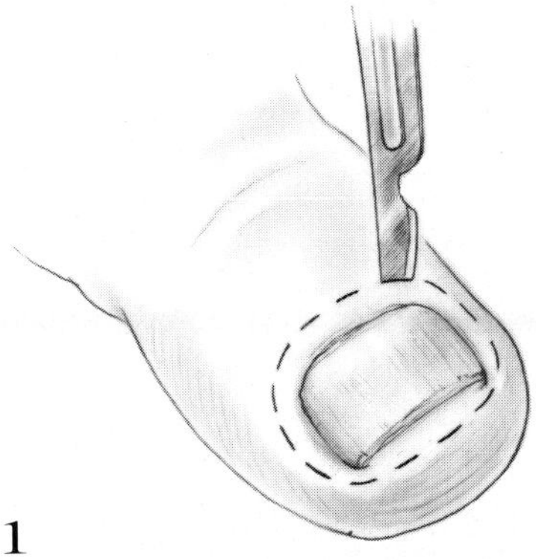

1

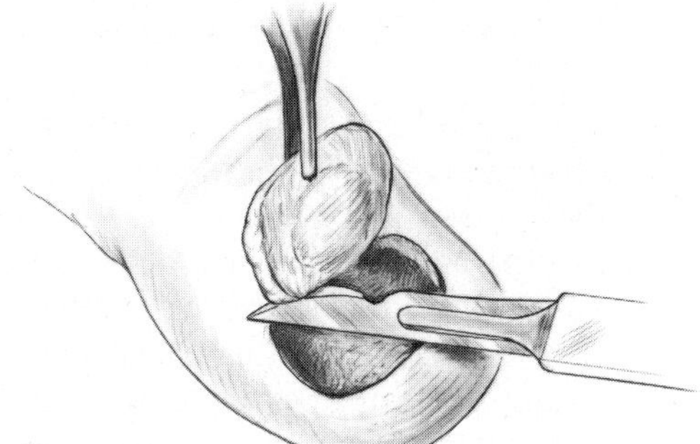

2

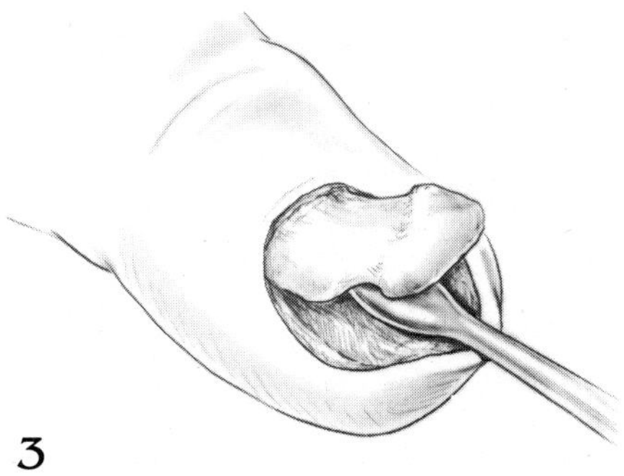

3

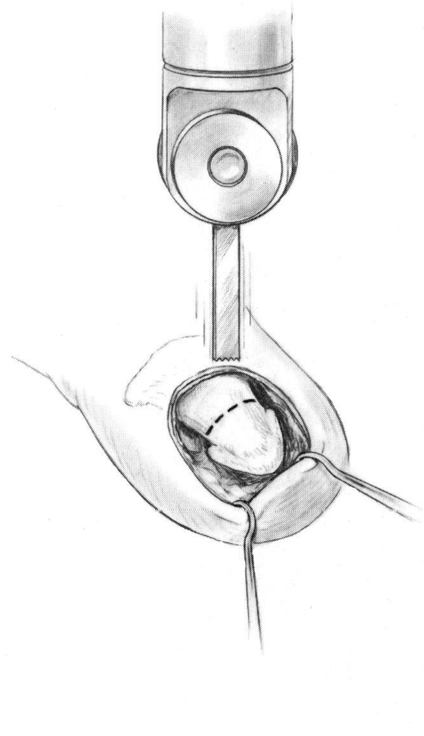

4

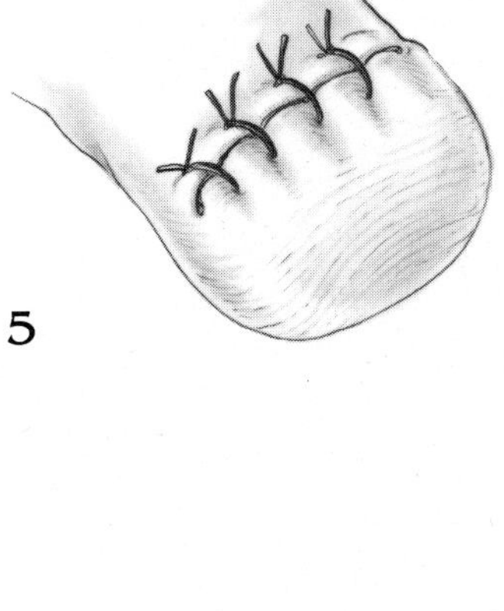

5

CURETTAGE PLANTAR WART

General Considerations

Plantar warts are hard whitish growths, caused by a papovavirus, that often may occur on the sole of the foot. Warts may often be differentiated from other hyperkeratotic lesions by the fact that they are more tender to lateral compression than to direct pressure and may occur on non–weight-bearing areas. Paring will reveal pinpoint bleeding.

Initial treatment consists of daily application of 40% salicylic acid plasters or application of other chemical ablative agents. Surgical curettage may be helpful if conservative measures fail.

Patient Selection

Indications

1. Tender warts that fail to respond to chemical ablation
2. Recurrence of the lesion after attempts at nonsurgical treatment

Contraindications

1. Asymptomatic warts may not require treatment.
2. Mosaic warts are better treated by paring and chemical ablation.
3. Plantar warts in children often regress spontaneously or respond to nonsurgical methods.

Surgical Procedure

Operative Technique

1. Infiltrate the area surrounding the verrucae with local anesthetic.
2. Create a small keyhole window at the junction of the verrucae and normal skin with a No. 11 blade. Avoid cutting into the lesion and penetrating the dermal layer (Fig. 1).
3. Insert a curet into the window and manipulate to find the plane between the verrucae and normal tissue (Fig. 2).
4. Enucleate the wart. Once removed, the base of the lesion is white (Fig. 3).
5. Remove the overhanging edges with small iris scissors (Fig. 4).
6. Gently curet the base of the lesion (Fig. 5).
7. Pack with sterile iodoform gauze soaked in povidone-iodine (Betadine) solution. Apply a sterile dressing.

Postoperative Care

1. The dressing is changed 3 to 5 days after surgery and the wound checked.
2. If exudate is noted, the patient should soak the foot in dilute povidone-iodine (Betadine) twice each day. An adhesive bandage is applied until the operative site is healed.
3. Weight bearing is permitted as tolerated in a wooden-soled shoe.

Technical Pitfalls

1. Penetration of the basilar layers of the skin may increase the likelihood of formation of a tender hyperkeratotic scar.
2. Inadequate removal may lead to recurrence.

Potential Complications

1. Recurrence of the lesion is not uncommon.
2. Formation of a tender scar may occur with healing.

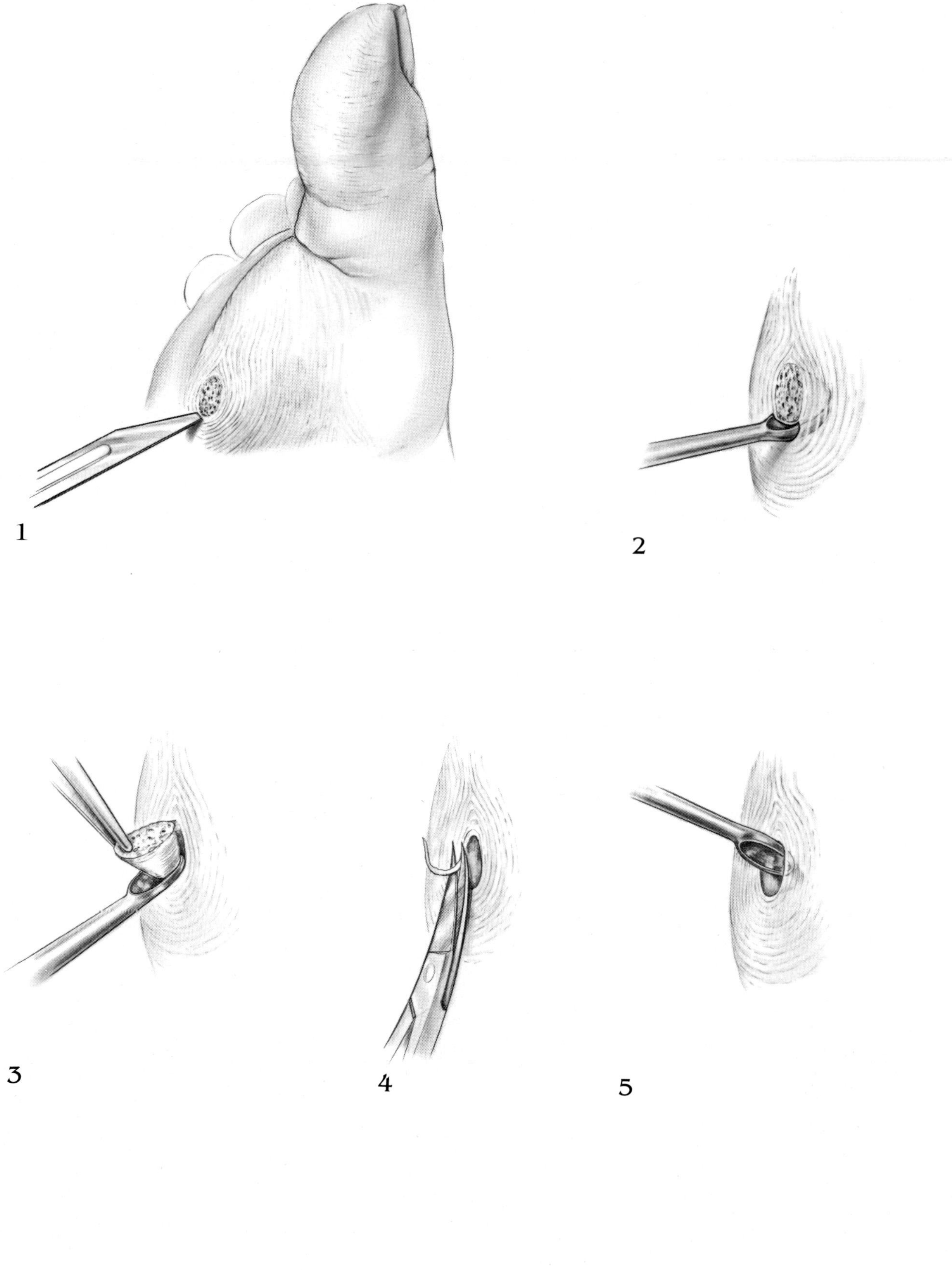
1
2
3
4
5

PART 11

Operations for Rheumatoid Arthritis of the Forefoot

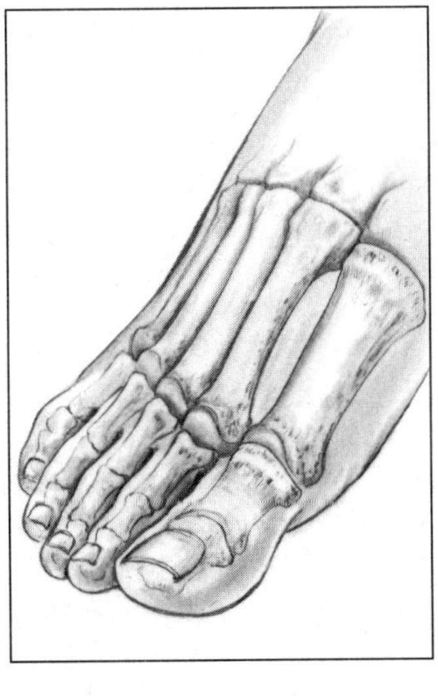

RHEUMATOID FOREFOOT RECONSTRUCTION

General Considerations

Involvement of the foot is the first manifestation of rheumatoid arthritis in 16% of patients. Pathologic disorders of the foot occur in 90% of patients who have been afflicted with rheumatoid arthritis for more than 10 years. Rheumatoid arthritis affects the forefoot more frequently than the hindfoot or midfoot, and any acquired adult forefoot disorder may occur in the rheumatoid arthritis patient. In the most common situation, numerous pathologic disorders are seen, including attenuation of capsular and ligamentous structures, contracture of the extensor tendons, subluxation of the interossei muscles, and subluxation of the metatarsal fat pad. These attributes of pathologic anatomy manifest themselves clinically as the various components of the rheumatoid forefoot, which include hallux valgus, metatarsus primus varus, and a prominent medial eminence. The lesser toes may be hammered or clawed with or without dislocation at the metatarsophalangeal joints (Fig. 1). Marked metatarsalgia occurs as a result of anterior subluxation of the fat pad. With time, articular degeneration occurs at the metatarsophalangeal and interphalangeal joints.

Nonoperative treatment includes the use of appropriate shoewear. Extra-depth shoes with a high, wide toe box may help accommodate the deformities. Molded Plastazote inserts are recommended to distribute weight-bearing pressure during the stance phase of gait. Range-of-motion exercises and other physical therapy modalities allow maintenance of the arc of motion of the involved articulations.

Surgical treatment must be tailored to each individual patient. Isolated deformities in the forefoot are treated in a way similar to that used for isolated forefoot deformities that occur in nonrheumatoid patients. Isolated hallux valgus without articular changes is treated with either a distal or proximal metatarsal osteotomy depending on the extent of the deformity. Isolated hallux valgus with articular changes at the metatarsophalangeal joint is treated with arthrodesis or a Keller resection arthroplasty. Isolated hammer or claw toe deformities without dislocation at the metatarsophalangeal joint are often treated with extensor tenotomy and dorsal capsulotomy with resection of the distal portion of the proximal phalanx. When a lesser toe deformity occurs in conjunction with dislocation at the metatarsophalangeal joint, resection of the base of the proximal phalanx is often necessary.

Late rheumatoid forefoot involvement with severe deformities, articular involvement, and plantar metatarsalgia often requires more complex forefoot reconstruction. In the younger, more active rheumatoid patient, the first ray is generally treated by means of an arthrodesis of the metatarsophalangeal joint; the older patient with a lower activity level may be best treated with a Keller resection arthroplasty. Reconstruction of the lesser toes often requires a Clayton-Hoffmann type procedure. This often includes manual osteoclasis at the interphalangeal joint combined with resection of the metatarsal heads. Resection of the proximal portion of the proximal phalanges is often required. With significant bony decompression, subtotal syndactylization of toe 2 to toe 3 and toe 4 to toe 5 often helps maintain alignment of the digits.

Patient Selection

Indications

1. The primary indication is severe rheumatoid involvement of the forefoot with hallux valgus, claw or hammer deformities of the lesser toes, articular degeneration at the metatarsophalangeal joints, and plantar metatarsalgia with hyperkeratotic lesions overlying the metatarsal heads (Fig. 1).
2. This major reconstructive procedure is best reserved for those patients who fail to achieve relief of symptoms with prescription shoewear and antiarthritic medications.

Contraindications

1. Elderly patients with other general medical conditions that preclude operative intervention may be better treated with prescription footwear.
2. Vascular evaluation is often obtained prior to surgery. Rheumatoid vascular involvement may lead to significant circulatory dysfunction that would interfere with wound healing.
3. Isolated forefoot deformities that occur early in the rheumatoid process may be better treated with simpler procedures similar to those utilized in nonrheumatoid patients. The patient should be informed that additional surgery will most likely be required in the future as the disease process progresses.

Surgical Procedure

Operative Technique: Correction of Hallux Valgus

1. In the older patient with a limited activity level, a Keller resection arthroplasty may be most appropriate (Fig. 2).
2. Younger rheumatoid patients who require a significant level of ambulation may do best with an arthrodesis of the first metatarsophalangeal joint. This helps provide a stable post that may allow a heel-to-toe gait.

Operative Technique: Clayton-Hoffmann Reconstruction

1. Manually manipulate the proximal interphalangeal joint to correct the hyperflexion deformity by means of osteoclasis (Fig. 3).
2. Mark the web incisions just plantar to the midline. The mark extends from the proximal interphalangeal joint to the center of the web on the lateral aspects of toes 2 and 4. Press adjacent toes together to transfer the mark (Fig. 4). This provides a guideline for syndactylization of toe 2 to toe 3 and toe 4 to toe 5.

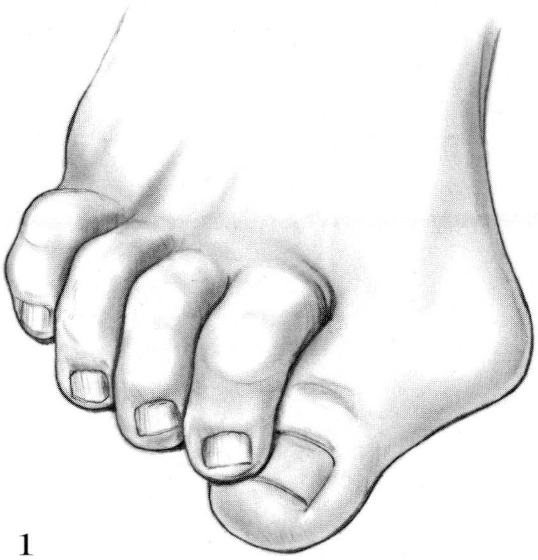

1

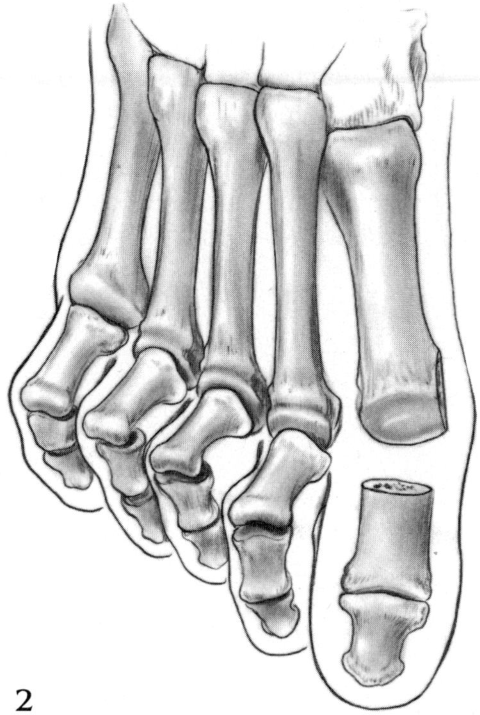

2

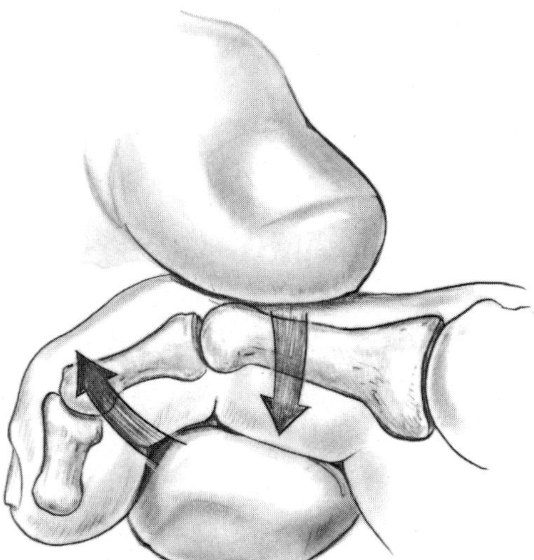

3

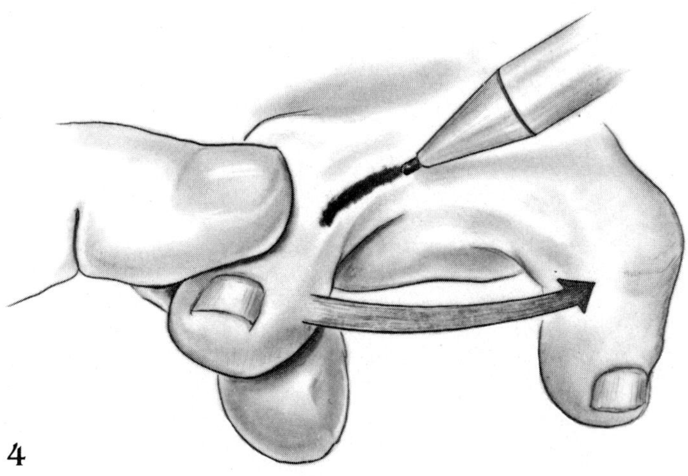

4

3. Extend the incision as a dorsal longitudinal incision from the base of the web proximally between metatarsals 2 and 3 and metatarsals 4 and 5 to end 2.5 cm proximal to the web (Fig. 5). Incise the skin along the mark (Fig. 6). Incise subcutaneous tissue along the line of the skin incision.

4. Reflect the skin and subcutaneous tissue medially and laterally to allow visualization of each metatarsal and proximal phalanx from a dorsal approach. Transect the extensor digitorum longus transversely. Incise the capsule and periosteum overlying the base of the proximal phalanx longitudinally and reflect subperiosteally (Fig. 7). Resect the base of the proximal phalanx with a power saw (Fig. 8). (Leave the base of the proximal phalanx of the fifth toe intact to provide a lateral post to prevent drift of the digits postoperatively.)

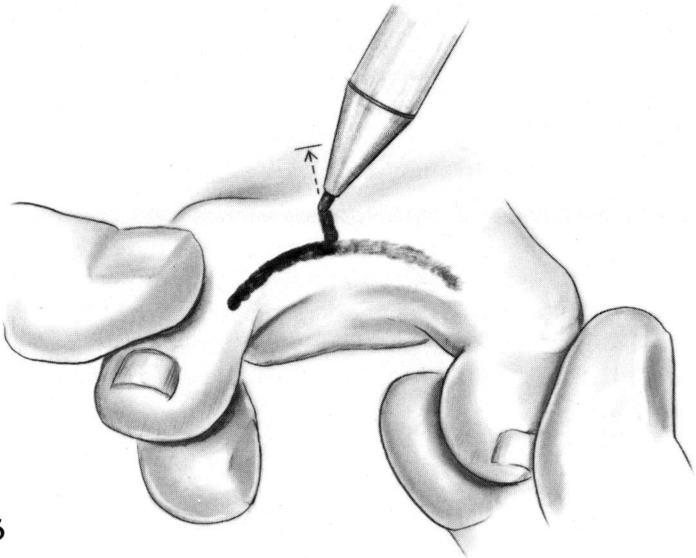

5

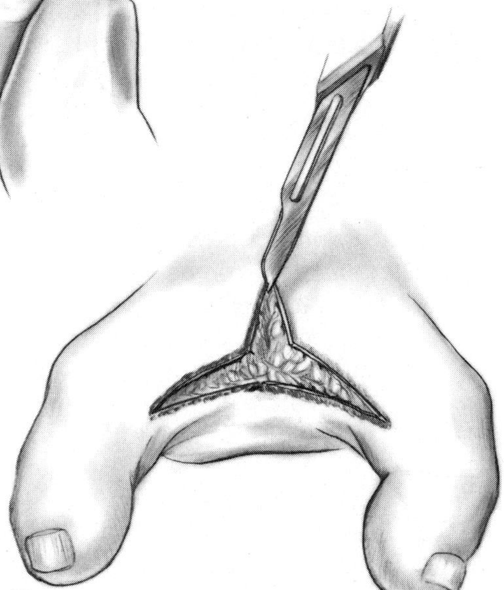

6

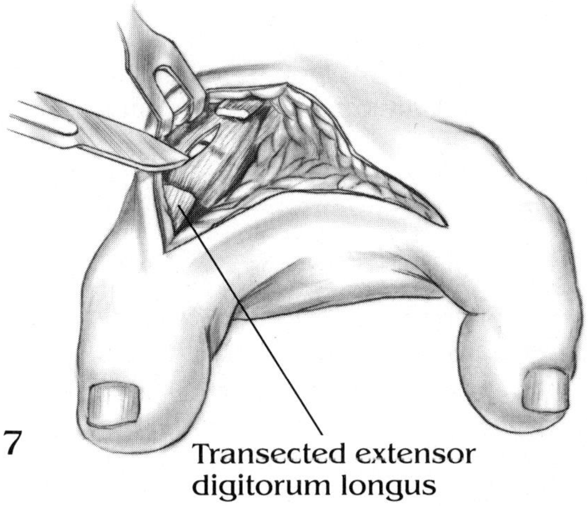

7

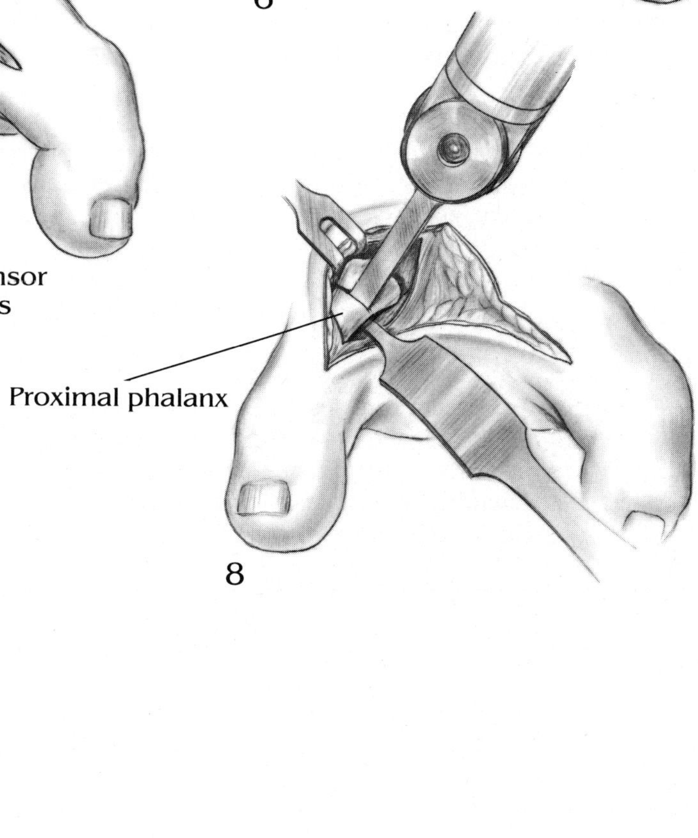

8

5. Incise the capsule and periosteum overlying the metatarsal head and neck. Reflect subperiosteally to expose the metatarsal head (Fig. 9). Resect the metatarsal head obliquely from dorsal distal to plantar proximal with a microsagittal saw (Fig. 10). Transect the metatarsal heads in such a way that the second metatarsal is level with the first metatarsal and metatarsals 3, 4, and 5 are each sequentially shorter than the metatarsal medial to it to form a smooth, tapering arc (Fig. 11).
6. Excise redundant skin in the form of a plantar triangular flap from the web incisions as needed. Close the web incisions with interrupted simple buried 3-0 chromic sutures from plantar to dorsal to syndactylize toe 2 to toe 3 and toe 4 to toe 5 (Figs. 12a and 12b). Close the dorsal longitudinal portion of the incisions that lie proximal to the web with vertical mattress 4-0 nylon sutures (Fig. 13).

Postoperative Care
1. A sterile dressing is applied.
2. A Robert Jones compression dressing is applied.
3. The initial postoperative dressings are changed weekly to observe wound healing and maintenance of alignment of the digits.
4. Sutures are removed at 3 weeks after surgery.
5. Heel walking in a stiff-soled postoperative shoe is allowed.

Technical Pitfalls
1. Insufficient removal of bone may lead to recurrence of symptoms as the stump of the metatarsal impinges against the remnant of the proximal phalanx.
2. Excessive bony decompression without syndactyly may lead to instability of the digits, resulting in various deformities.

Potential Complications
1. Delayed wound healing may occur in rheumatoid patients, particularly those receiving steroids or other rheumatologic medications. Consultation with the patient's rheumatologist may lead to discontinuation of medications prior to surgery.
2. Delayed wound healing at the syndactyly should be treated with local wound care. Antiseptic soaks and dressing changes are performed until wound healing occurs.
3. The rheumatoid process progresses despite surgical intervention, and recurrence of deformities is possible. Patients should be informed that additional surgery may be required in the future.
4. Symptoms may recur, particularly if inappropriate shoewear is worn. The patient should be informed that appropriate prescription shoewear is required after surgery.

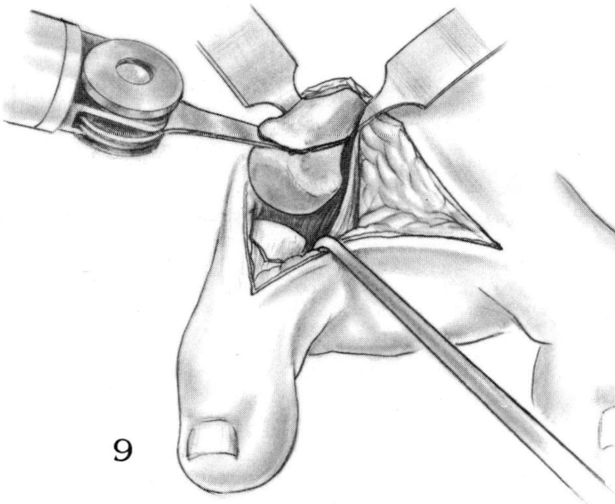
9

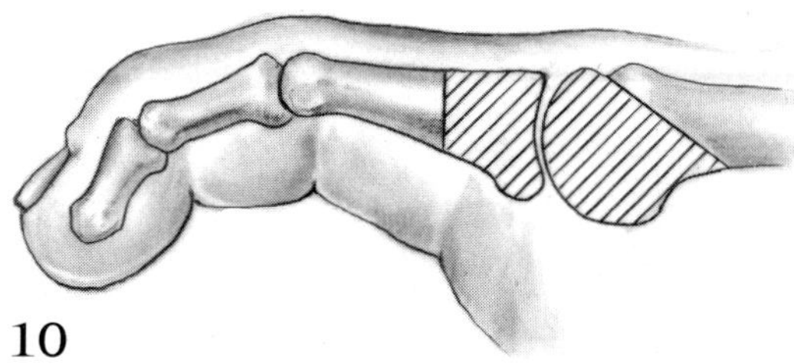
10

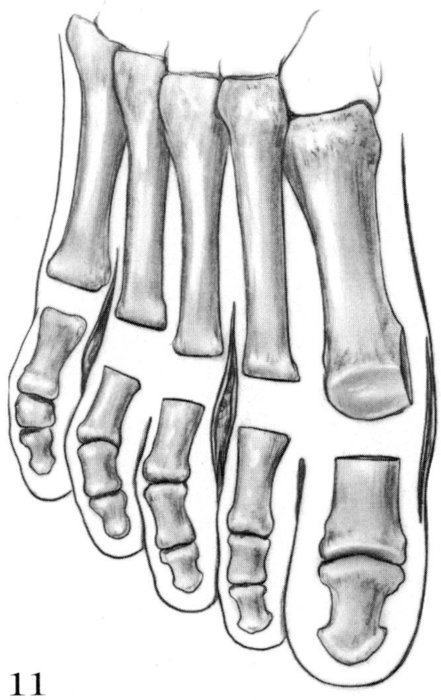
11

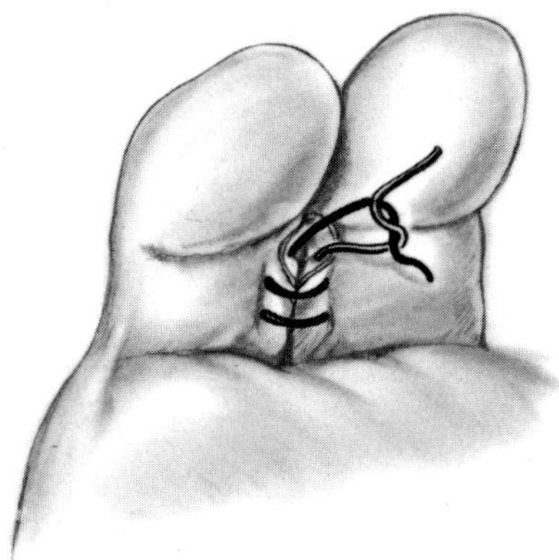
12a

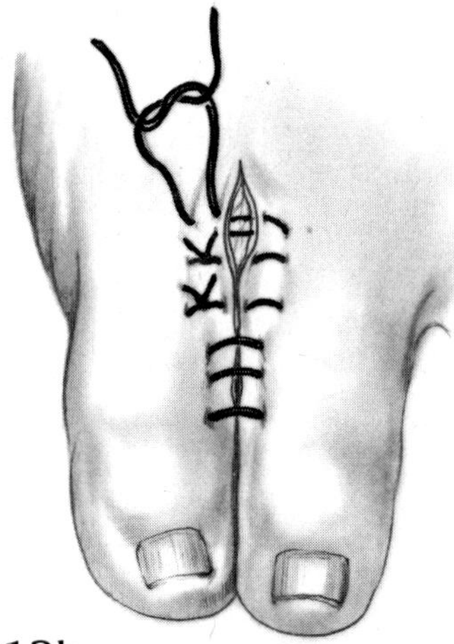
12b

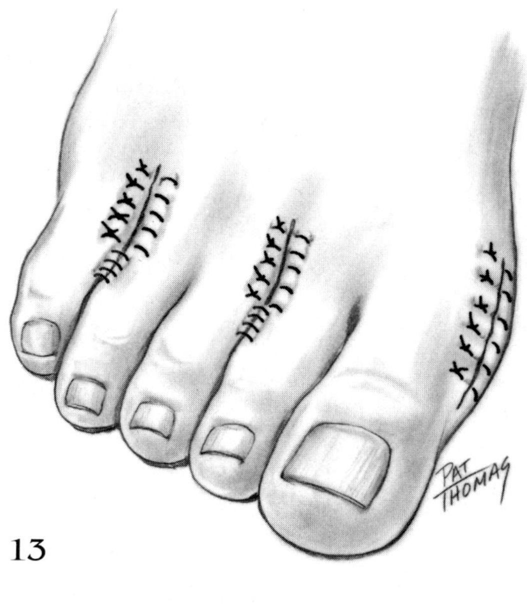

13

SECTION 3

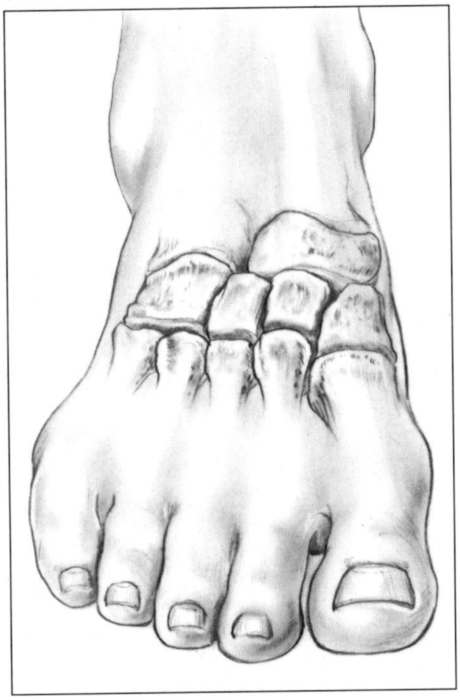

Midfoot

PART 12

Tarsometatarsal Arthrodesis

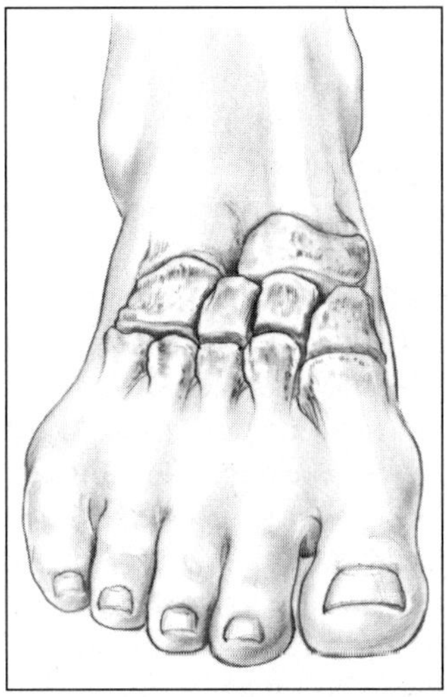

ARTHRODESIS OF THE TARSOMETATARSAL AND ASSOCIATED JOINTS

General Considerations

Arthritis of the tarsometatarsal joints is most often a consequence of a Lisfranc fracture-dislocation. This injury is likely to be associated with multiple intraarticular fractures, as well as significant injury to the articular cartilage and interosseous ligaments. The tarsometatarsal joints may also be the site of involvement of systemic inflammatory and metabolic disorders.

Patients present with pain and swelling about the dorsal and plantar aspect of the foot in the region of the involved joints. Pain is most often increased with weight-bearing activities. Physical examination reveals localized tenderness and swelling about the involved joints, and passive motion of the individual metatarsals may reproduce the patient's pain. These patients often walk with an antalgic gait.

Treatment is instituted with a medial longitudinal arch support and a shoe with a reinforced midfoot last. If symptoms persist, consideration can be given to arthrodesis of the involved joints.

Extensive preoperative planning is most important. Identification of the specific joints involved requires meticulous clinical evaluation to elicit localized areas of tenderness and pain. Anteroposterior tomograms of the midfoot are helpful to identify which articulations require arthrodesis. Most often the first, second, and third tarsometatarsal joints are involved; involvement of the fourth and fifth tarsometatarsal joints may require an additional incision to approach these articulations. The intercuneiform joints may also be involved in the arthritic process and should be included in the fusion if necessary. Residual deformity associated with a Lisfranc fracture-dislocation that has healed in an abnormal position may require correction either by mobilization and repositioning of the osseous structures or by combined osteotomy and arthrodesis of the tarsometatarsal joints.

Patient Selection

Indications

1. Traumatic arthritis secondary to Lisfranc fracture-dislocation
2. Arthritis in the tarsometatarsal and associated joints secondary to systemic inflammatory arthritis or metabolic disorders
3. Degenerative arthritis involving the midfoot

Contraindications

1. General medical conditions that preclude anesthesia and surgery
2. Neuropathic and vascular disorders that may lead to a marked increased risk for wound healing problems and other complications

Surgical Procedure

Operative Technique

1. A dorsal longitudinal incision 6 cm long is made, centered over the first tarsometatarsal joint. The incision is placed just medial to the extensor hallucis longus tendon (Fig. 1). Subcutaneous tissues are incised along the line of the skin incision. The joint capsules and periosteum overlying the first tarsometatarsal joint and, if necessary, the first intercuneiform joint are incised longitudinally and reflected subperiosteally to expose the involved articulations (Fig. 2).
2. A second dorsal longitudinal incision 6 cm long is made, centered over the tarsometatarsal joints. This incision is positioned between the bases of metatarsals 2 and 3 and slightly closer to the third metatarsal (Fig. 1). The subcutaneous tissue is incised along the line of the skin incision. The joint capsule and periosteum are incised longitudinally and reflected subperiosteally to expose the second and third tarsometatarsal joints, as well as the joint between the second and third cuneiforms, if exposure of these joints is required (Fig. 2).
3. A third dorsal longitudinal incision 6 cm long is made, centered over the tarsometatarsal joints. This incision is positioned between metatarsals 4 and 5 just medial to the base of the fifth metatarsal (Fig. 1). Subcutaneous tissue is incised along the line of the skin incision. The periosteum and capsule are incised longitudinally and reflected subperiosteally to expose the fourth and fifth tarsometatarsal joints.
4. Excise the articular surfaces between the involved joint surfaces with small osteotomes or a microsagittal saw (Figs. 2 and 3).
5. The fusion sites are fixed with multiple 0.062-inch (1.5-mm) Kirschner wires (Fig. 4). These wires are bent and buried beneath the skin.
6. Cancellous iliac bone graft is inserted in all of the fusion sites (Fig. 4).
7. The subcutaneous tissue is closed with interrupted simple 3-0 Vicryl sutures. Close the skin with vertical mattress 4-0 nylon sutures.

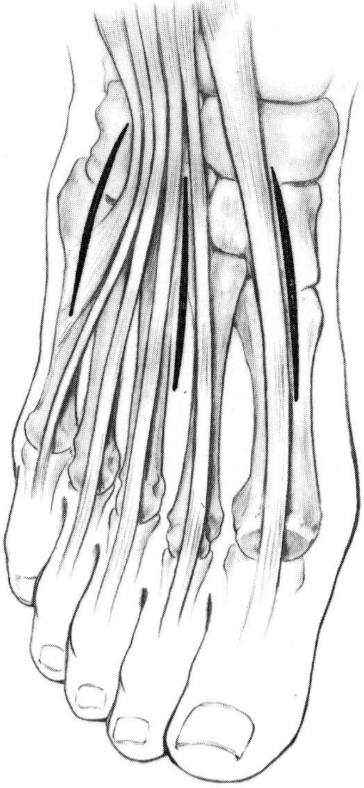

1

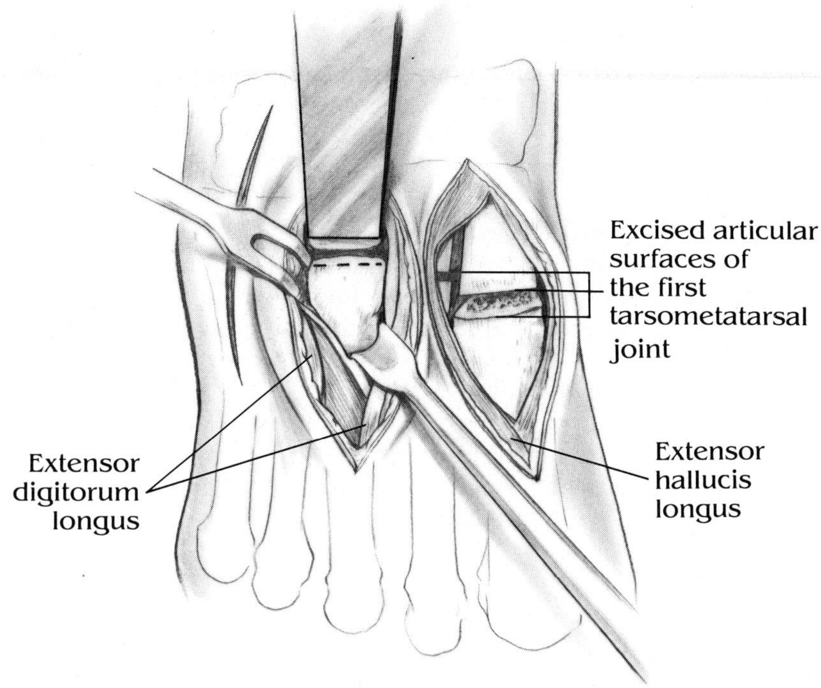

Excised articular surfaces of the first tarsometatarsal joint
Extensor digitorum longus
Extensor hallucis longus

2

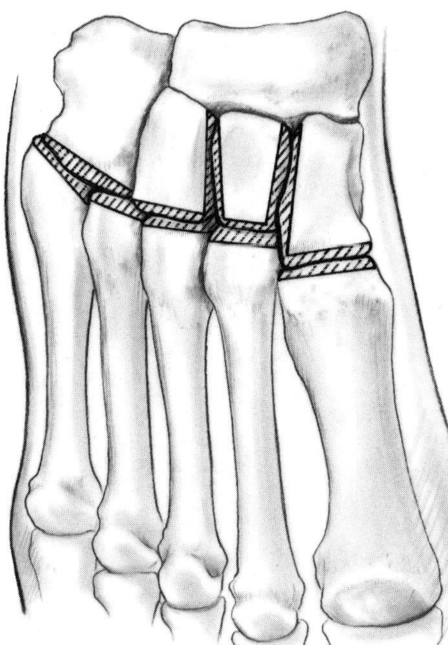

3

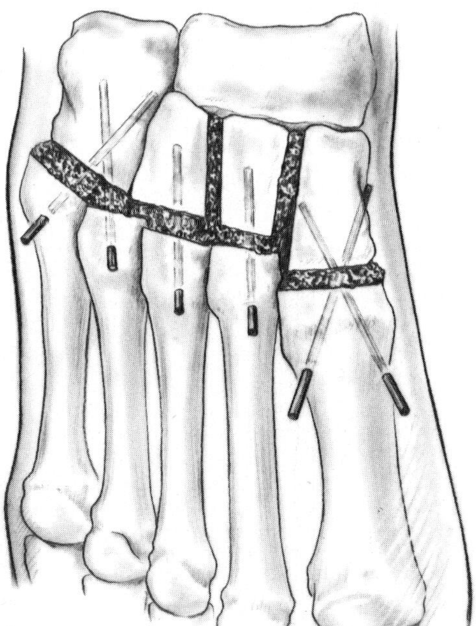

4

Postoperative Care

1. A Robert Jones compression dressing is applied for the the first 48 hours.
2. A short-leg cast is applied and the patient is kept non–weight bearing on crutches for 6 to 8 weeks until radiographs display progressive osseous union.
3. The cast is changed and sutures removed 3 weeks after surgery.
4. Pins are removed approximately 8 weeks after surgery.
5. The patient is allowed a slow, gradual, progressive return to weight-bearing activities within the limits of discomfort once the pins are removed.

Technical Pitfalls

1. Failure to correct any pre-existing deformity may lead to osseous prominences that can cause impingement against the shoe.
2. Extensive iliac bone graft is required to optimize osseous union.

Potential Complications

1. Delayed union and nonunion of the arthrodesis may occur.
2. Arthritis may occur at articulations distal and proximal to the fusion site secondary to the increased stresses applied to these joints with weight bearing after fusion.

PART 13

Arthrodesis Talonavicular Joint

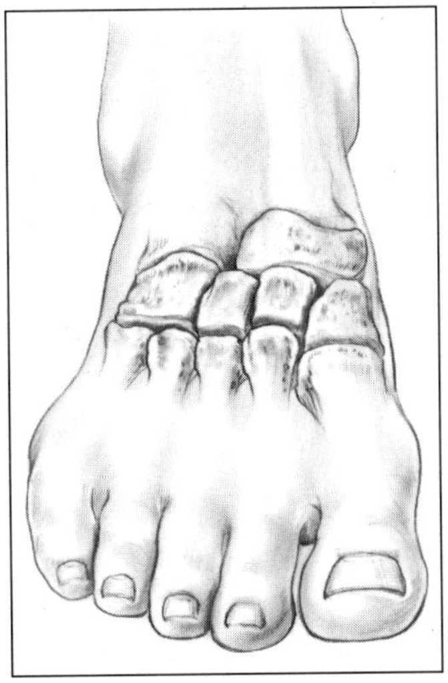

ISOLATED TALONAVICULAR ARTHRODESIS

General Considerations

Various systemic disorders manifest themselves at the talonavicular joint. This articulation may be the site of any of several arthritic conditions. Arthritis of the talonavicular joint may occur as a sequela to fracture or dislocation in the midfoot. Rheumatoid arthritis and other forms of systemic inflammatory arthropathy may affect this articulation. Long-standing subluxation of the talonavicular joint, such as that seen in rupture of the posterior tibial tendon or other disorders, may result in articular degeneration with loss of articular cartilage, narrowing of the joint space, and formation of periarticular osteophytes. Avascular necrosis of the tarsal navicular may lead to collapse of the bone. Deformation of the osseous structure leads to articular incongruity, which often results in degenerative arthritis at the talonavicular and/or the naviculocuneiform joint.

Patients with localized arthritis at the talonavicular joint present with pain and swelling at the medial aspect of the midfoot; this pain is increased with weight bearing and ambulation. Conservative modalities of treatment include the use of a medial longitudinal arch support, as well as a shoe with a reinforced midfoot last. These may provide relative immobilization of the damaged joint. Antiarthritic medications and other symptomatic treatments may also be helpful. If nonoperative treatment fails to provide relief of symptoms, consideration can be given to operative intervention. Arthrodesis of the talonavicular joint serves to eliminate the painful grinding of the incongruous articular surfaces. The technique described utilizes iliac bone graft and compression screw fixation.

Patient Selection

Indications

1. Degenerative arthritis or other forms of inflammatory arthropathy that affect the talonavicular joint
2. Traumatic arthritis of the talonavicular joint resulting from fracture or dislocation in the midfoot
3. Arthrosis secondary to avascular necrosis of the tarsal navicular
4. Metabolic or infectious arthritis involving the talonavicular articulation

Contraindications

1. The talonavicular joint is often involved in arthritic processes that occur more diffusely in the region of the hindfoot. Isolated talonavicular fusion is only effective if this joint alone is involved in the pathologic process. Involvement of the subtalar and calcaneocuboid joint, in addition to the talonavicular joint, requires triple arthrodesis, in which all involved joints are fused.
2. General medical conditions that preclude general anesthesia and surgery are a contraindication.
3. Neurologic or vascular dysfunction may increase the risk of complications associated with surgery on the distal peripheral extremity.

Surgical Procedure

Operative Technique

1. A dorsomedial incision 8 cm long is made. The incision is positioned between the tibialis anterior tendon and the extensor hallucis longus tendon and extends from the level of the ankle joint to end at the level of the medial cuneiform (Fig. 1). Incise the subcutaneous tissue along the line of the skin incision. Incise the retinaculum longitudinally.
2. Retract the tibialis anterior tendon medially and the extensor hallucis longus tendon laterally. This allows visualization of the talonavicular joint.
3. Incise the capsule and periosteum longitudinally and reflect subperiosteally to expose the talonavicular joint (Fig. 2).
4. Excise the articular surface of the talonavicular joint with an osteotome (Fig. 3).

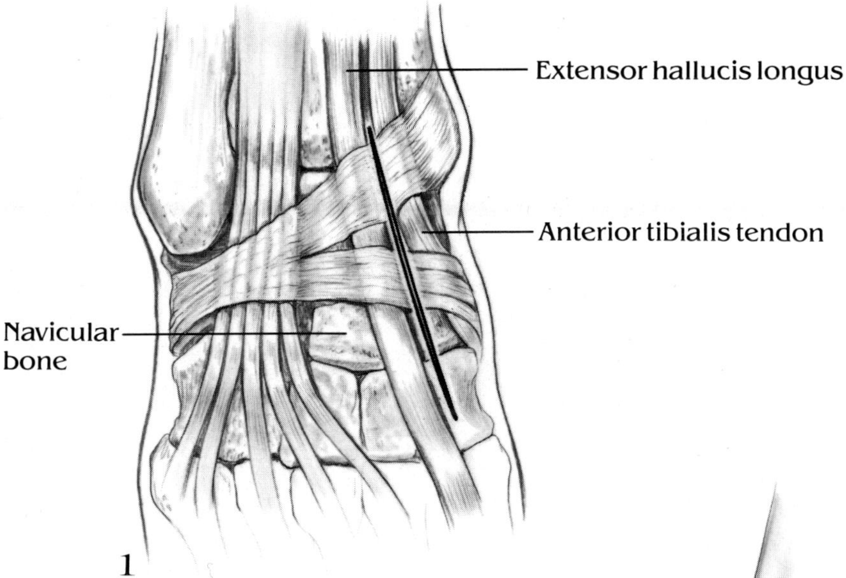
Extensor hallucis longus
Anterior tibialis tendon
Navicular bone
1

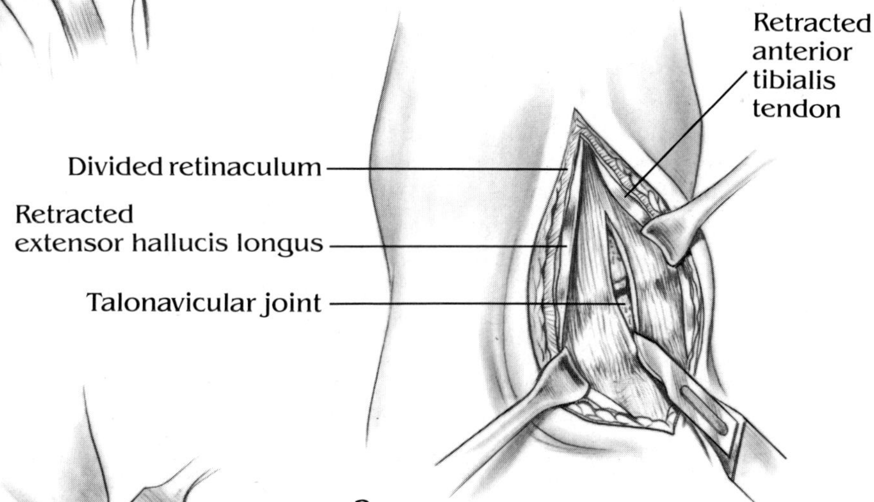
Retracted anterior tibialis tendon
Divided retinaculum
Retracted extensor hallucis longus
Talonavicular joint
2

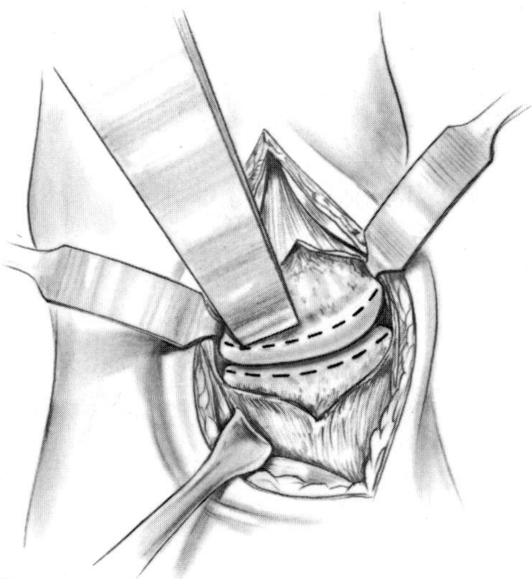
3

5. Fix the arthrodesis with a 4.0-mm cancellous screw inserted from the distal medial aspect of the navicular tuberosity into the head and neck of the talus (Fig. 4).
6. Create a trough 5 mm wide and 1½ cm long across the talonavicular joint with a microsagittal saw (Fig. 5).
7. Deepened the trough with a curet. Pack the arthrodesis site with cancellous iliac graft. Pack the trough with corticocancellous iliac graft (Fig. 6).
8. Close the retinaculum with interrupted figure-of-eight 2-0 Vicryl sutures. Close the subcutaneous tissue with interrupted simple 3-0 Vicryl sutures. Close the skin with interrupted vertical mattress 3-0 nylon sutures.

Postoperative Care

1. A well-padded short-leg cast is applied with the foot in neutral position at the ankle.
2. The cast is changed and the sutures removed 2 to 3 weeks after surgery.
3. The patient is maintained non–weight bearing on crutches for 6 weeks after surgery.
4. The cast is removed at 6 weeks, and the patient is begun on a slow, gradual return to weight-bearing activities within the limits of discomfort.
5. The patient is allowed to bear weight in a rubber-soled shoe containing a soft, flexible insert with a medial longitudinal arch support.

Technical Pitfalls

1. Complete decortication of the talonavicular joint is required, as inadequate preparation of the fusion surfaces may result in pseudarthrosis. The use of cancellous bone graft, as well as inlaid bone graft, may minimize the risk of delayed union and nonunion.
2. Adequate compression fixation may help ensure osseous union.

Potential Complications

1. Delayed union and pseudarthrosis of the arthrodesis may occur.
2. Arthrodesis of the talonavicular joint may increase the stress on the articulations proximal and distal to the fusion site. The patient should be forewarned of the possibility of further progression of arthritis in the distal peripheral extremity.

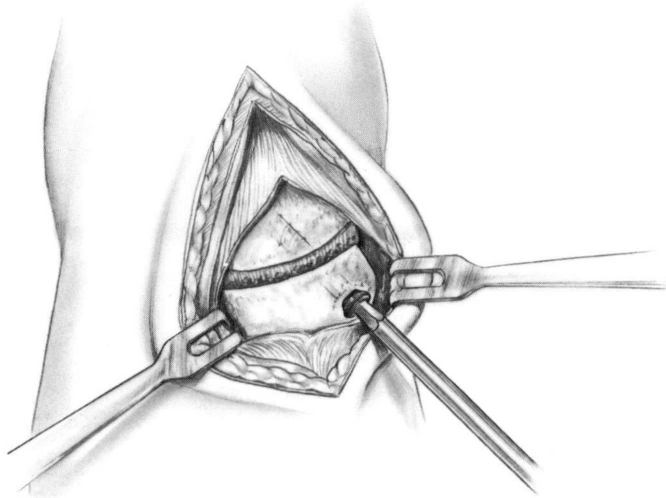

4

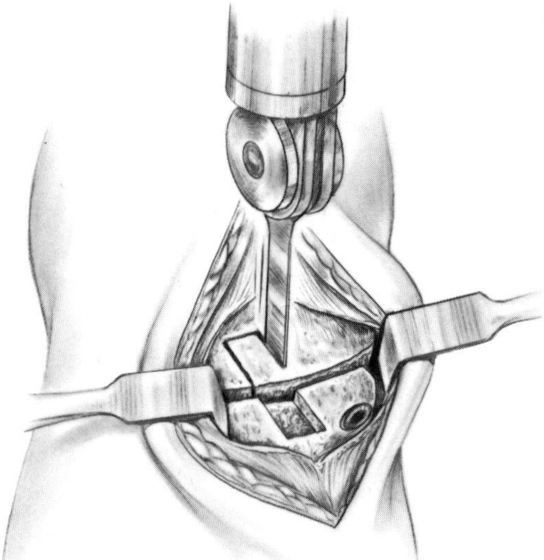

5

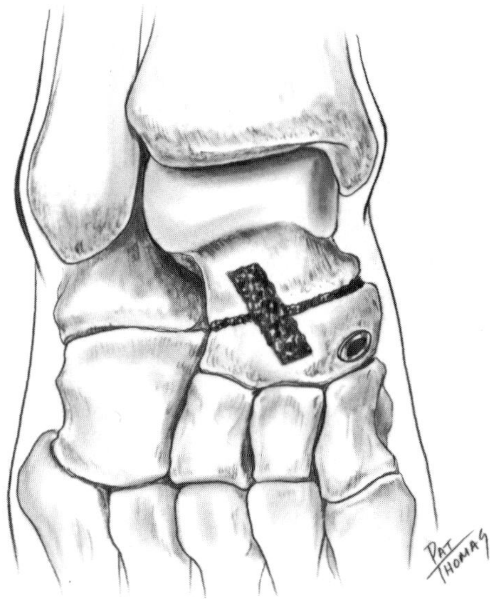

6

PART 14

Operations for Dorsal Bossing Midfoot

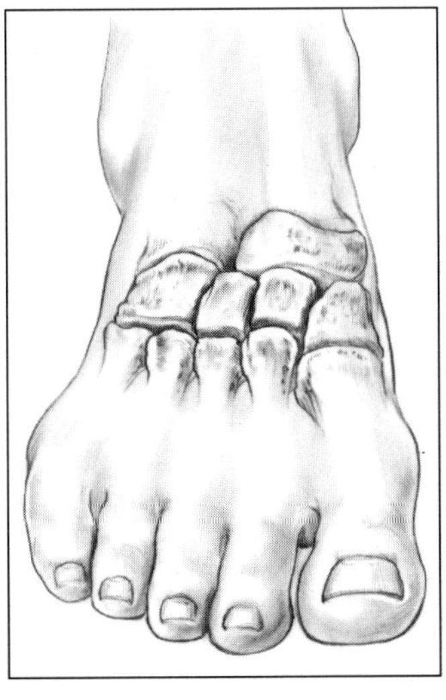

EXCISION DORSAL BOSSING FIRST TARSOMETATARSAL JOINT

General Considerations

Dorsal bossing of the first tarsometatarsal joint is a common acquired disorder of the foot. Formation of a hypertrophic osteophyte in this region may be the first manifestation of osteoarthritis or traumatic arthritis of this articulation.

Patients present with a prominent dorsal eminence in the region of the first tarsometatarsal joint, and mechanical impingement from the tongue of the shoe may cause pain. Physical examination may reveal localized tenderness at the tarsometatarsal articulation, as well as erythema of the skin overlying the bony prominence. Padding of the tongue of the shoe, in addition to various types of float pads applied to the foot, may help alleviate mechanical impingement from shoewear.

Surgical intervention requires bony decompression of the region. Evaluation of a lateral radiograph of the foot will allow identification of the bony eminence. Most often resection of the dorsal aspect of the base of the first metatarsal, as well as the dorsal aspect of the articulating portion of the medial cuneiform, is required.

Patient Selection

Indications. The primary indication is a dorsal bossing of the first tarsometatarsal joint that is not responsive to conservative measures.

Contraindications

1. Hypertrophic spurring in this region may be associated with more diffuse arthrosis at the tarsometatarsal joint. If clinical evaluation and radiographs indicate degenerative changes throughout the tarsometatarsal joint, excision of the bony eminences will not be sufficient. Arthrodesis of the first tarsometatarsal joint is often necessary in addition to bony decompression.
2. Neurologic, vascular, or other medical disorders may lead to increased risk of infection or wound healing problems.

Surgical Procedure

Operative Technique

1. A dorsal longitudinal incision approximately 4 cm long is made. The incision is centered over the exostosis and placed medial to the extensor hallucis longus tendon (Fig. 1). Subcutaneous tissue is divided along the line of the skin incision. The exostosis is exposed subperiosteally. The dorsalis pedis artery and the deep perforating artery in the first web space are to be avoided.
2. The exostosis is excised flush with the dorsum of the foot using a microsagittal saw or hand osteotome. The osteophyte is excised from the base of the metatarsal, as well as from the distal portion of the medial cuneiform (Fig. 2).
3. The cut surface is smoothed with a rasp (Fig. 3).
4. The subcutaneous tissue is closed with interrupted simple 3-0 Vicryl sutures. The skin is closed with interrupted vertical mattress sutures of 4-0 nylon.

Postoperative Care

1. A sterile compression dressing is applied.
2. Limitation of weight-bearing activities is recommended.
3. Sutures are removed 2 to 3 weeks after surgery.
4. The patient is allowed a slow, gradual return to weight-bearing activities and shoewear within the limits of discomfort.

Technical Pitfalls

1. Inadequate resection of bone may lead to persistent symptoms after surgery.
2. Care must be taken to avoid damage to the vascular structures that lie at the proximal aspect of the first web space.

Potential Complications. Recurrence of the bony eminence is possible.

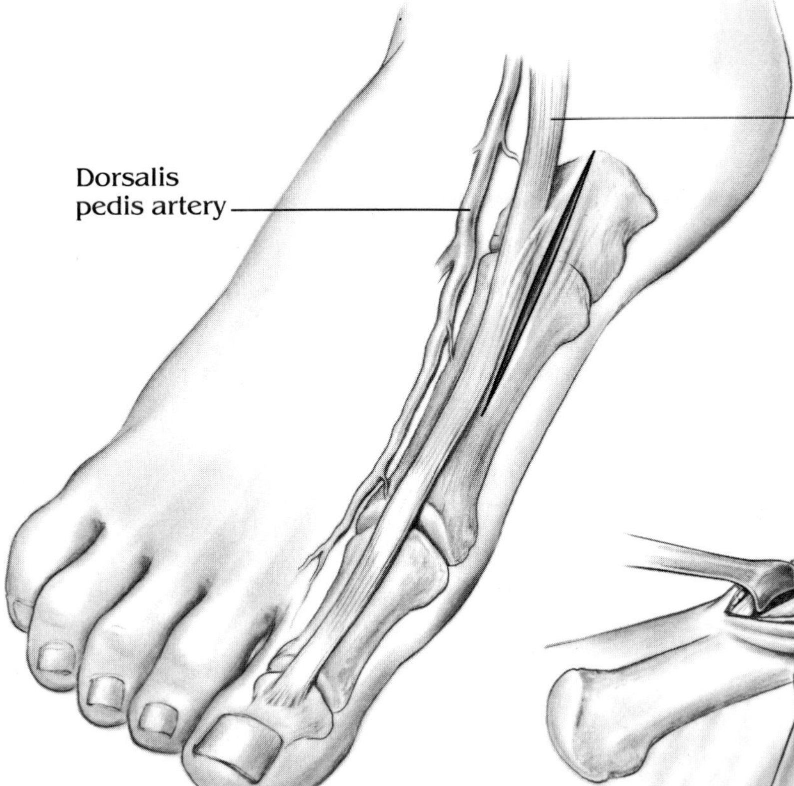

1

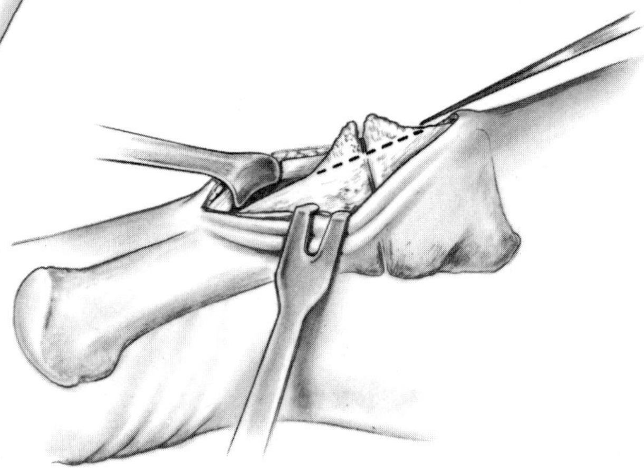

2

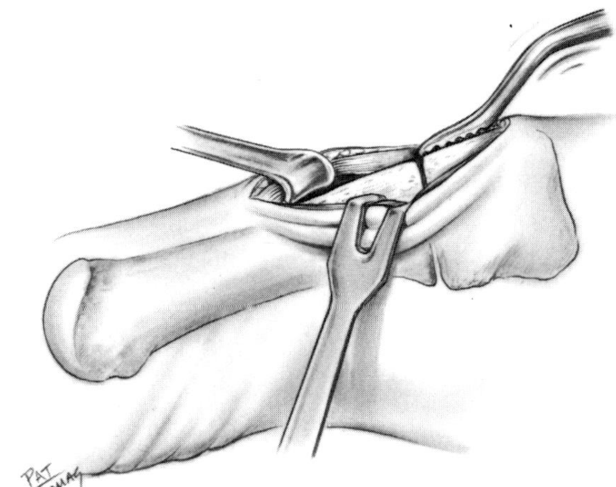

3

PART 15

Operations for Painful Accessory Navicular

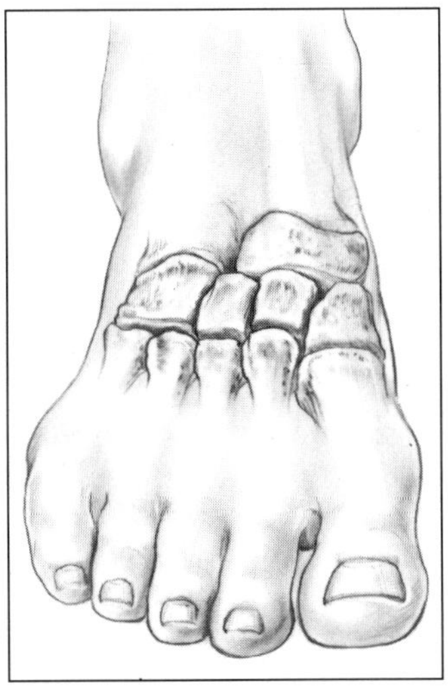

EXCISION ACCESSORY NAVICULAR

General Considerations

An accessory navicular is a congenital abnormality in which a navicular tuberosity develops from a second center of ossification. Typically, the accessory bone is separated from the navicular by a synchondrosis. It is thought to occur in 5% to 15% of the population.

Although the condition is most often asymptomatic, pain may occur as a result of mechanical pressure of the prominent accessory bone against the midfoot last of the shoe. Some patients describe a twisting injury that initiates the onset of symptoms. It has been hypothesized that sudden contraction of the posterior tibial tendon may lead to a partial or complete tear of the synchondrosis. It may be difficult to distinguish this process from a fracture of the navicular tuberosity.

Patients note localized pain in the region of the navicular tuberosity. Physical examination may identify localized tenderness and erythema of the skin overlying the bony prominence. Patients with separation of the synchondrosis may note reproduction of pain with active contraction of the posterior tibial tendon against resistance, as this tendon inserts on the navicular tuberosity and may in part insert on the accessory bone.

Treatment includes the use of a soft, flexible, medial longitudinal arch support to roll the bony prominence away from the irritating portion of the midfoot last. Posting the insert medially may also help alleviate symptoms. These modalities may also serve to decrease excursion of the posterior tibial tendon during the stance phase of gait, which may contribute to improvement in symptoms. Symptomatic measures, including limitation of weight-bearing activities and anti-inflammatory medications, may be helpful. If conservative measures fail, excision of the accessory navicular may be appropriate. If a significant portion of the posterior tibial tendon inserts on the accessory bone, reimplantation of that tendon into the navicular through drill holes may be required.

Patient Selection

Indications

1. Pain caused by impingement of the bony prominence against the midfoot last of the shoe
2. Failure of conservative measures

Contraindications. Young patients with symptomatic accessory naviculars may note improvement of symptoms with time. Fusion of the accessory bone with the body of the navicular has been reported to occur and often leads to resolution of symptoms.

Surgical Procedure

Operative Technique

1. A medial longitudinal skin incision 4 cm long is made. The incision is centered over the accessory navicular and runs along the course of the posterior tibial tendon. Subcutaneous tissue is incised along the line of the skin incision (Fig. 1).
2. The skin and subcutaneous tissue are reflected to expose the posterior tibial tendon. The accessory bone is identified by development of the distal aspect of the posterior tibial tendon and its insertion at the navicular tuberosity by means of sharp and blunt dissection along the superior border of the tendon (Fig. 2).
3. If the posterior tibial tendon appears to insert on the navicular, the accessory bone may be exposed by splitting the posterior tibial tendon longitudinally. The fibers are retracted, allowing visualization of the accessory navicular (Fig. 3).

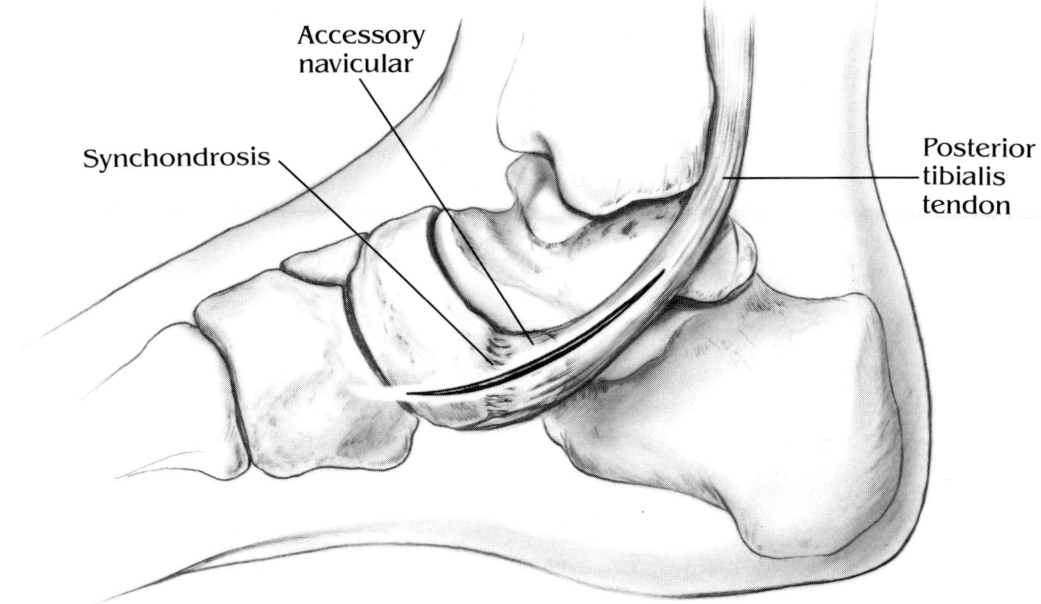
Accessory
navicular
Synchondrosis
Posterior
tibialis
tendon

1

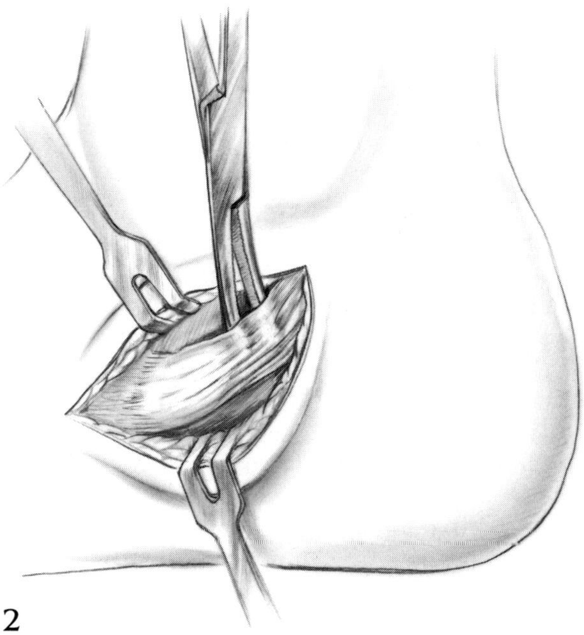

2

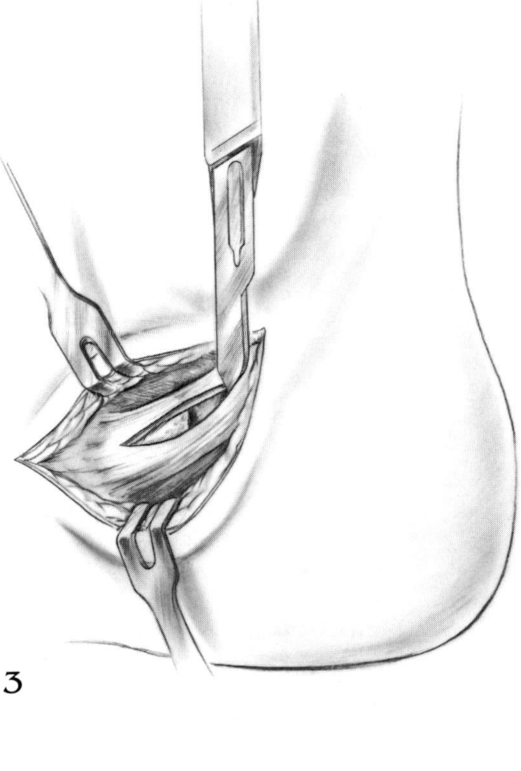

3

4. The accessory bone is grasped with a towel clamp, and traction is applied to demonstrate the junction of the accessory bone with the navicular. The accessory navicular is enucleated by means of excision at the synchondrosis (Fig. 4).
5. If the remaining medial tuberosity of the navicular is prominent or roughened, it may be excised with a small osteotome. The cut surface is smoothed with a rasp.
6. The tendon is repaired with interrupted simple buried 2-0 Dexon sutures (Fig. 5).
7. If the posterior tibial tendon finds extensive insertion on the accessory navicular, excision of the accessory navicular may require detachment of the tendon insertion (Fig. 6). If this is necessary, the tendon is reinserted into the medial aspect of the navicular through drill holes. The medial surface of the bone is roughened to provide a satisfactory bed for insertion of the tendon. Two drill holes are then made from the cut surface through the cortical bone at the medial aspect of the navicular. A modified Kessler box suture of 1-0 nylon is passed through the distal end of the stump of the posterior tibial tendon. The ends of the suture are passed through the drill holes and tied over cortical bone while holding the foot in inversion and plantarflexion.
8. The skin is closed with interrupted vertical mattress 3-0 nylon sutures.

Postoperative Care

1. Simple excision of the accessory navicular requires a compression dressing. Sutures are removed at 3 weeks postoperatively, and the patient is allowed a slow, gradual return to weight-bearing activity within the limits of discomfort. Shoes with a medial longitudinal arch support are recommended.
2. If advancement of the tibialis posterior tendon is required, cast immobilization with the foot in inversion and plantarflexion is necessary until adequate anchoring of the tendon stump has occurred. This requires 6 weeks of immobilization and the use of crutches non–weight bearing. Once the cast is removed, a progressive return to weight-bearing activities is allowed. A medial longitudinal arch support is utilized in rubber-soled shoes to decrease excursion of the tendon during the stance phase of gait.

Technical Pitfalls

1. Failure to excise a prominent medial tuberosity of the navicular may lead to residual symptoms after surgery.
2. If a significant portion of the posterior tibial insertion must be detached to excise the accessory navicular, reattachment through drill holes is required to maintain the integrity of the muscle tendon unit.

Potential Complications. Weakening of the insertion of the posterior tibial tendon may lead to tendon dysfunction with time.

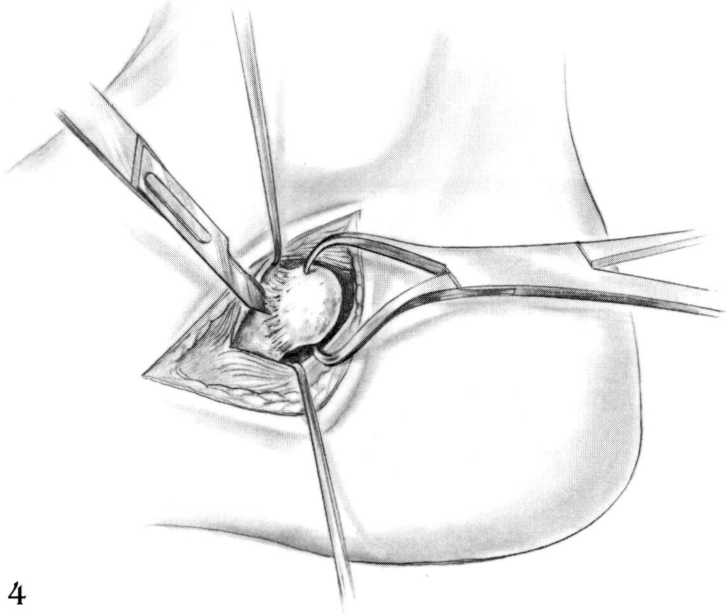

4

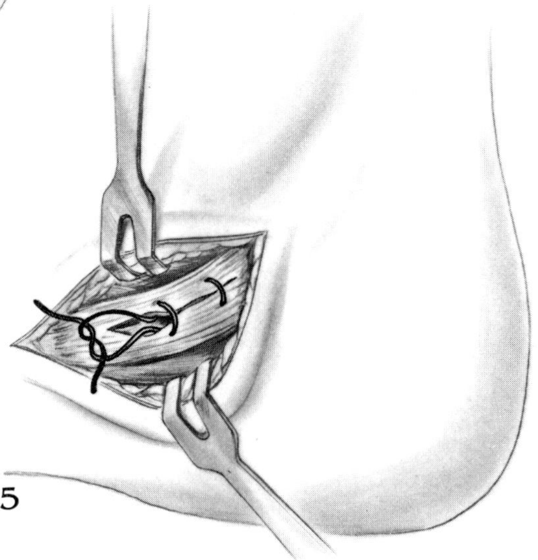

5

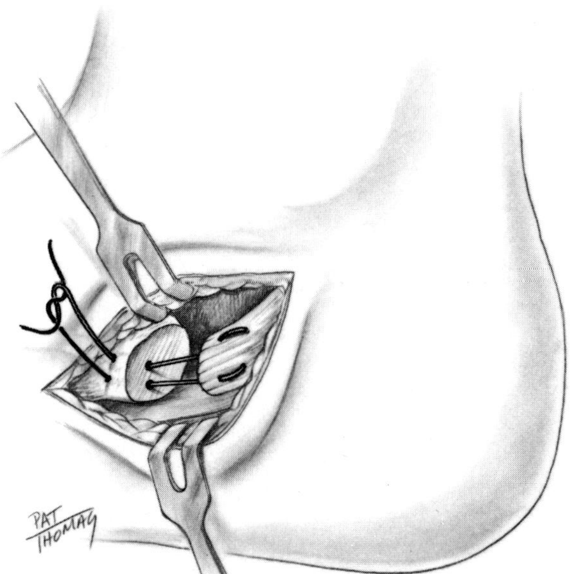

6

SECTION 4

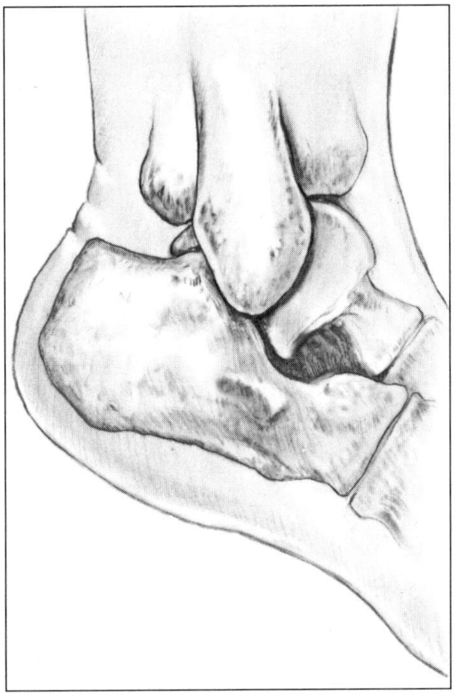

Hindfoot

PART 16

Arthrodesis Subtalar Joint

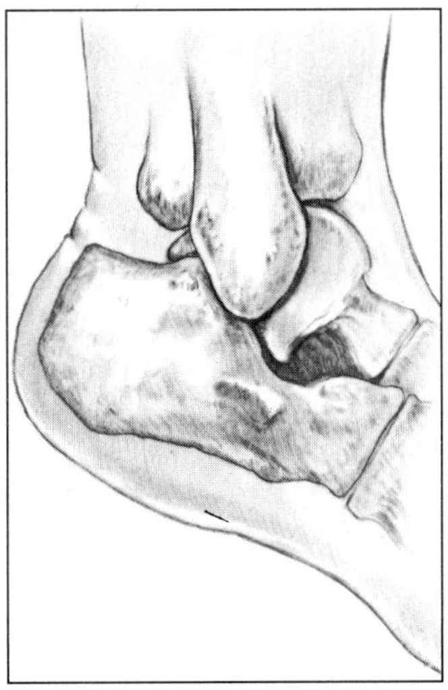

ISOLATED SUBTALAR ARTHRODESIS

General Considerations

Isolated subtalar arthrodesis provides for surgical stabilization of the deformed or arthritic hindfoot. It allows for correction of a varus or valgus deformity, as well as the elimination of the painful grinding of incongruous talocalcaneal articular surfaces during motion, weight bearing, and ambulation. The operative technique uses a moldable bone graft first described by K. A. Johnson and is a relatively simple and effective method of achieving fusion of the subtalar joint and alleviating the symptoms associated with pathologic disorders of this articulation.

Isolated Moldable Subtalar Arthrodesis Compared With Other Hindfoot Fusions

Advantages

1. Preservation of the talonavicular and calcaneocuboid articulations
2. Minimal shortening of the height of the hindfoot
3. Adequate fixation (using pin or screw)
4. Increased stability
5. Rapid healing (using bone graft)
6. High incidence of union
7. Single incision

Disadvantages

1. Can correct only varus and valgus deformity
2. Can be used to relieve localized symptoms originating from the subtalar joint alone

Patient Selection

Indications

1. Traumatic, degenerative, or inflammatory arthritis of the subtalar joint
2. Metabolic disorders (e.g., gout)
3. Neoplastic disorders leading to localized destruction of the subtalar joint
4. Localized arthritis secondary to malalignment of the talocalcaneal joint
5. Talocalcaneal coalition with secondary subtalar arthritis
6. Varus or valgus deformity of the hindfoot secondary to congenital anomalies, neurologic disorders, or acquired disorders

Contraindications

1. Advanced age
2. Vascular insufficiency
3. Diabetes mellitus
4. Neuropathic disorders of the foot
5. Active local or systemic infections
6. Presence of pathologic disorders involving the ankle, Chopart joint, or midfoot that require more extensive fusion
7. Presence of deformities of the foot not amenable to correction at the subtalar joint alone

Surgical Procedure

Operative Technique

1. An oblique skin incision is made, centered over the sinus tarsi from 1 cm distal and posterior to the tip of the lateral malleolus and extending anteriorly and distally to the region of the second cuneiform (Fig. 1). Incise subcutaneous tissue along the line of the skin incision.
2. Incise the extensor retinaculum longitudinally and retract the extensor tendons superiorly (Fig. 2).
3. Incise the origin of the extensor digitorum brevis muscle and reflect distally to expose the sinus tarsi (Fig. 3). Excise fat from the sinus tarsi. Using subperiosteal dissection, retract the peroneal tendons posteriorly to expose the posterior subtalar joint (Fig. 3).
4. Incise the joint capsule and insert a lamina spreader in the sinus tarsi to expose the entire articulation (Fig. 4).

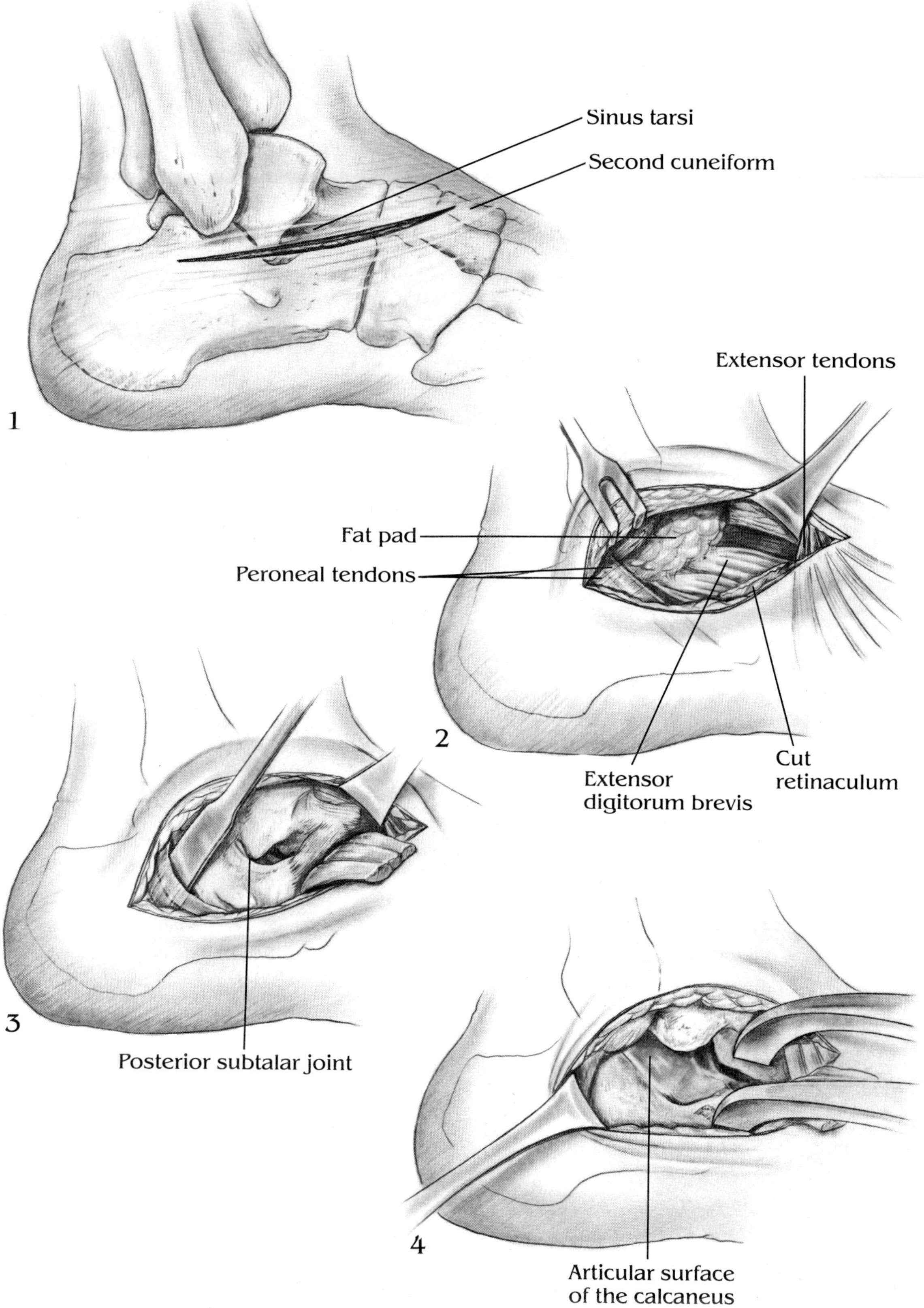
Sinus tarsi
Second cuneiform
1
Extensor tendons
Fat pad
Peroneal tendons
2
Extensor digitorum brevis
Cut retinaculum
3
Posterior subtalar joint
4
Articular surface of the calcaneus

5. Excise articular cartilage and subchondral bone from the subtalar joint, including the anterior, middle and posterior facets, with an osteotome (Fig. 5). Decorticate all surfaces of the sinus tarsi (Fig. 6).
6. Hold the ankle joint and the calcaneus in neutral position and insert a smooth Steinmann pin medial to the anterior tibial tendon from the neck of the talus into the calcaneus (Fig. 7). Cut the pin off under the skin.
7. Fill in the fusion site with cancellous iliac graft (Fig. 7).
8. Reattach the flap of the extensor digitorum brevis muscle with interrupted figure-of-eight 2-0 Vicryl sutures. Close the subcutaneous tissue with interrupted simple 3-0 Vicryl sutures. Close the skin with interrupted vertical mattress 3-0 nylon sutures (Fig. 8).

Postoperative Care

1. A soft compression dressing is applied for 48 hours.
2. A short-leg cast is applied.
3. The cast is changed and sutures removed at 3 weeks.
4. The patient is kept non–weight bearing on crutches for 6 weeks.
5. The pin is removed and a short-leg walking cast applied at 6 weeks.
6. The short-leg walking cast is removed at 12 weeks.

Technical Pitfalls

1. Excessive removal of subchondral bone
2. Improper positioning of the subtalar joint (correct position: 7 to 10 degrees of valgus)
3. Excessive soft tissue handling

Potential Complications

1. Delayed union
2. Nonunion
3. Wound necrosis
4. Infection
5. Malalignment leading to a nonplantigrade foot

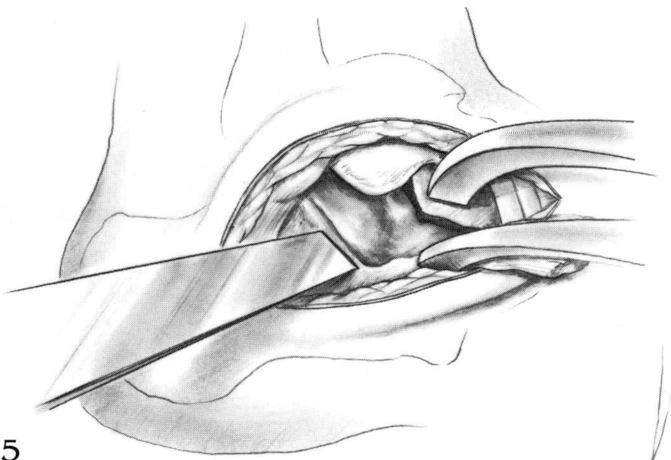

5

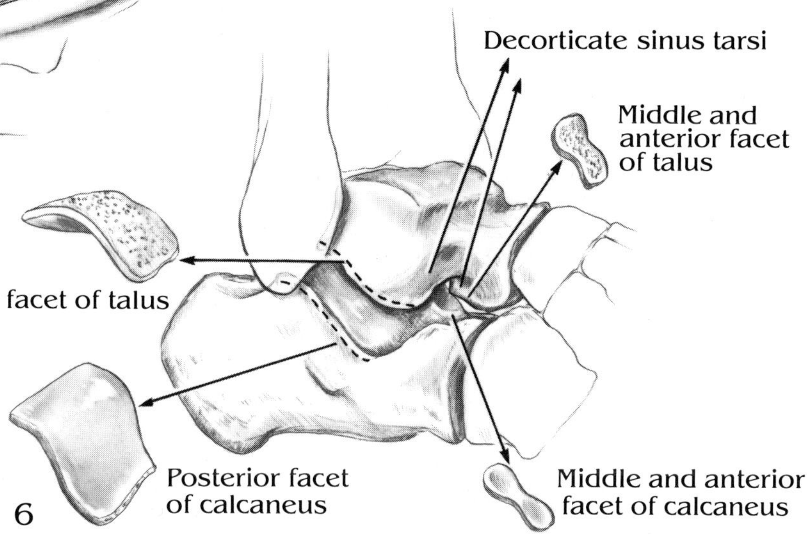
Decorticate sinus tarsi
Middle and anterior facet of talus
Posterior facet of talus
Posterior facet of calcaneus
Middle and anterior facet of calcaneus

6

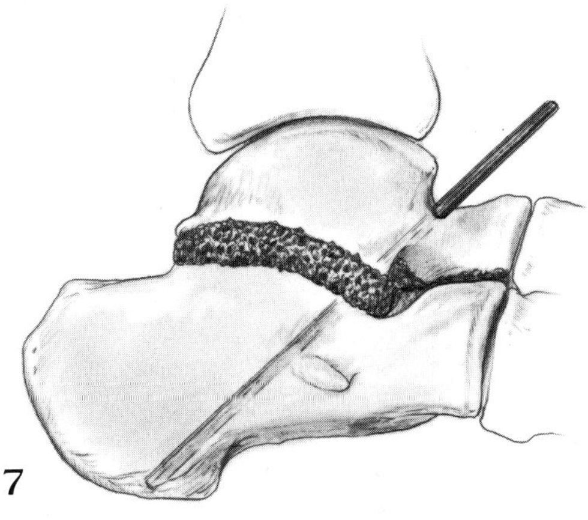

7

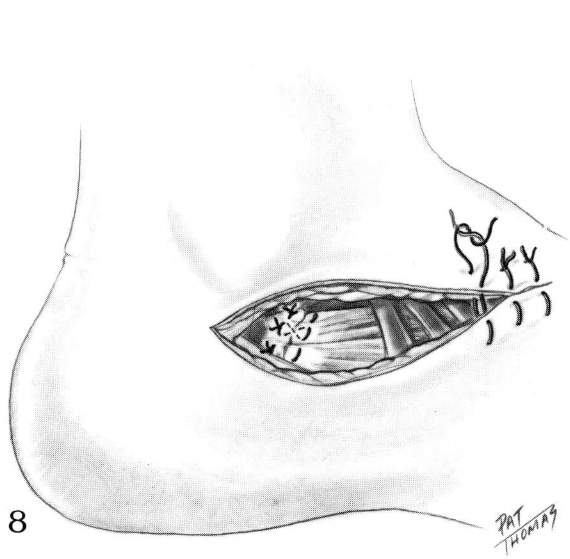
PAT THOMAS

8

PART 17

Triple Arthrodesis

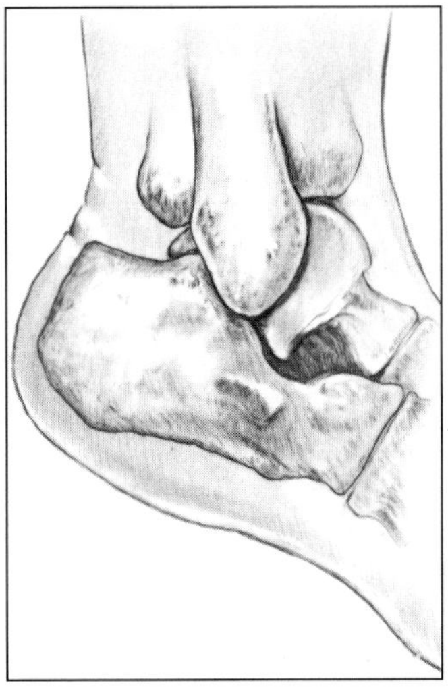

TRIPLE (QUADRUPLE) ARTHRODESES

General Considerations

The triple arthrodesis is a further extension of the technique described for isolated subtalar arthrodesis. This procedure enables correction of a deformity at Chopart's joint, as well as the talocalcaneal joint. It also serves to eliminate painful motion of incongruous arthritic joints of the hindfoot. Fusion of the subtalar, calcaneocuboid, and talonavicular joints is performed using pin fixation and iliac bone graft. In addition, a fourth articulation between the navicular and cuboid bone has been reported. It is believed that this interface may also be involved in hindfoot arthritis. This joint surface is also fused in the quadruple arthrodesis.

Exposure of the articular surfaces to be arthrodesed requires extensive exposure at the dorsolateral aspect of the hindfoot. Although in most cases the talonavicular joint can be well exposed with a dorsolateral incision, occasionally a second medial incision is made.

Patient Selection

Indications

1. Traumatic, degenerative, or inflammatory arthritis of the hindfoot involving the talonavicular and calcaneocuboid joint in addition to the subtalar joint
2. Deformity of the hindfoot that includes malalignment at Chopart's joint

Contraindications

1. If the subtalar joint only is involved in the disease process, an isolated subtalar fusion is preferable.
2. If the ankle joint is also arthritic, it may be necessary to incorporate that articulation in the form of a pantalar arthrodesis.
3. Vascular insufficiency may lead to increased risk of infection and wound healing.
4. Neuropathic conditions may increase the risk of nonunion and delayed wound healing.
5. Advanced age or general medical conditions that prohibit extensive hindfoot reconstruction or anesthesia are contraindications.

Surgical Procedure

Operative Technique

1. An oblique skin incision centered over the sinus tarsi is made, similar to that described for isolated subtalar arthrodesis. This is a longitudinal incision beginning 1 cm posterior and distal to the tip of the lateral malleolus and extending anteriorly and distally to the level of the middle cuneiform (Fig. 1). The dorsalis pedis artery lies in close proximity to the distal aspect of the incision. It is generally advisable to palpate and mark the dorsalis pedis pulse before the tourniquet is inflated to avoid injury to this important structure. Subcutaneous tissue is incised along the line of the skin incision.
2. The extensor retinaculum is incised longitudinally, and the extensor tendons are retracted superiorly. The origin of the extensor digitorum brevis muscle is incised sharply and reflected distally to expose the sinus tarsi (Fig. 2). Excise the adipose contents of the sinus tarsi. The peroneal tendons are retracted posteriorly by subperiosteal dissection to expose the posterior subtalar joint.
3. The capsule and periosteum overlying the subtalar, calcaneocuboid, and talonavicular joints are incised and reflected subperiosteally to expose those articulations in their entirety (Fig. 3). The capsule and periosteum overlying the articulation between the navicular and cuboid bones are also incised and reflected subperiosteally.

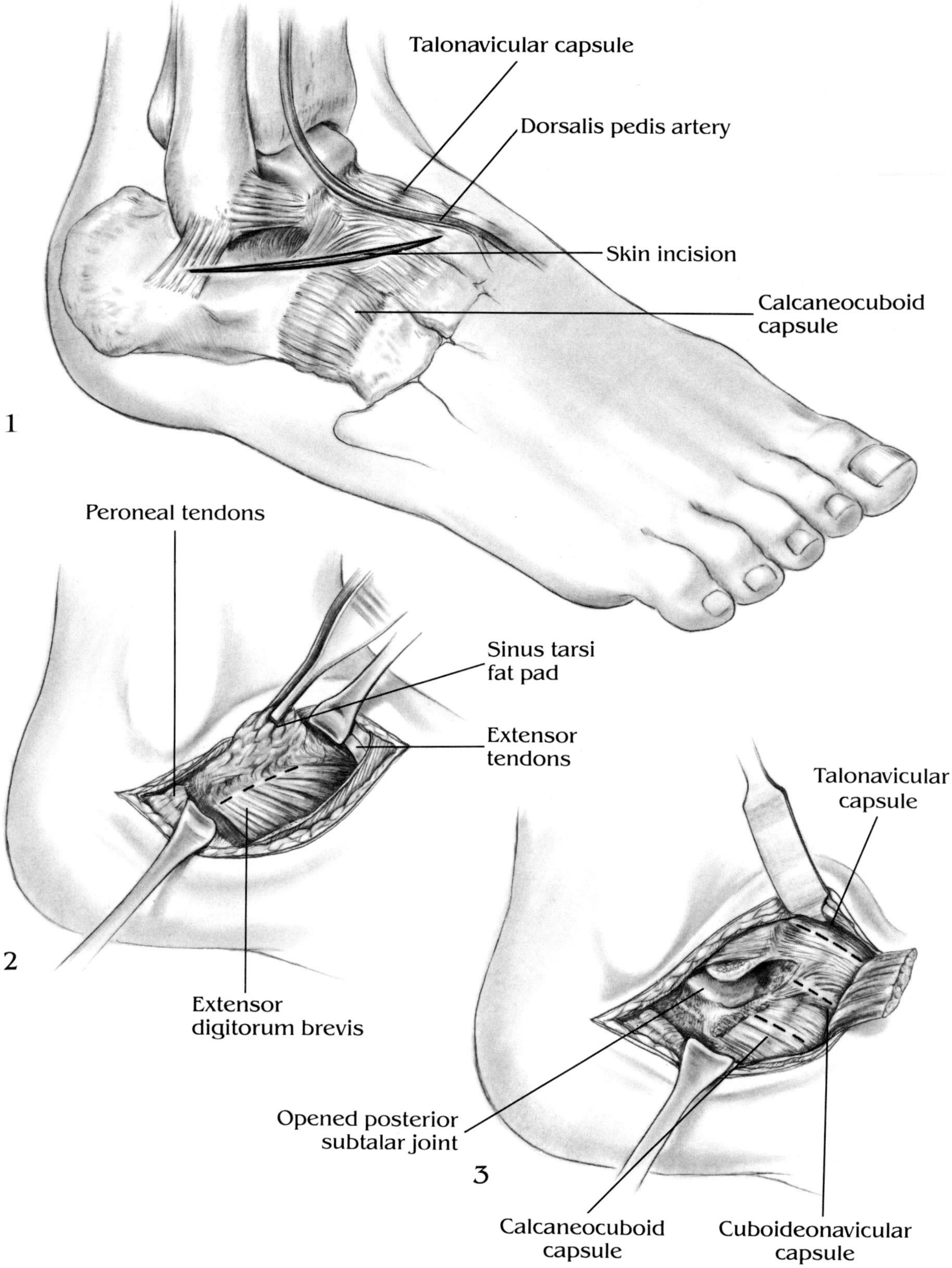
Talonavicular capsule
Dorsalis pedis artery
Skin incision
Calcaneocuboid capsule
1
Peroneal tendons
Sinus tarsi fat pad
Extensor tendons
2
Extensor digitorum brevis
Talonavicular capsule
Opened posterior subtalar joint
3
Calcaneocuboid capsule
Cuboideonavicular capsule

4. If the medialmost aspect of the talonavicular joint is not visible, a second medial incision may be utilized. Make a medial longitudinal skin incision 5 cm long and centered over the talonavicular joint. The incision is placed between the anterior tibial tendon and posterior tibial tendon (Fig. 4). Subcutaneous tissue is divided along the line of the skin incision. The anterior tibial tendon is identified, mobilized, and protected throughout the remainder of the procedure. The capsule and periosteum overlying the talonavicular joint are incised longitudinally and reflected subperiosteally. This should allow exposure of the talonavicular articulation in its entirety (Fig. 5).
5. Excise articular cartilage and subchondral bone from the subtalar joint with an osteotome as described in "Isolated Subtalar Arthrodesis" (Fig. 6). This excision includes the anterior, middle, and posterior facets. Decorticate all surfaces of the sinus tarsi. A small lamina spreader is utilized to expose the entire articulation.

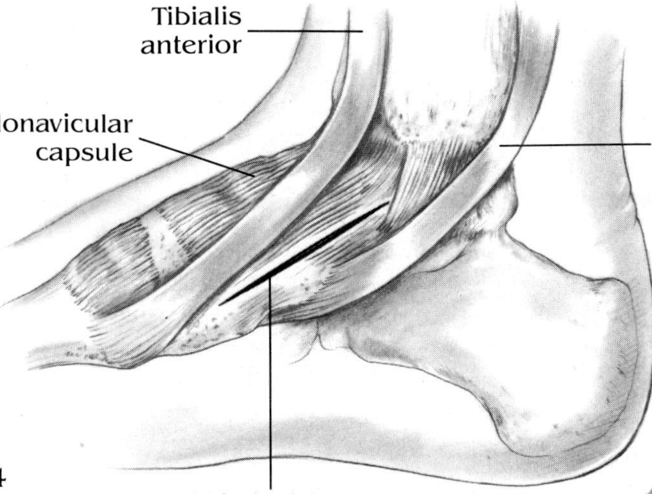
Tibialis anterior
Talonavicular capsule
Tibialis posterior
Skin incision

4

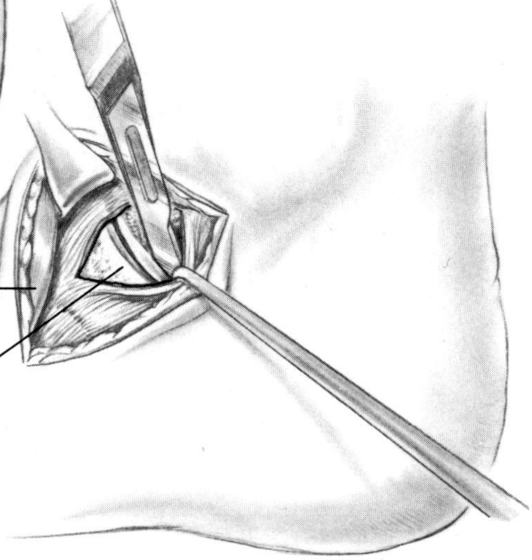
Tibialis anterior
Talonavicular joint

5

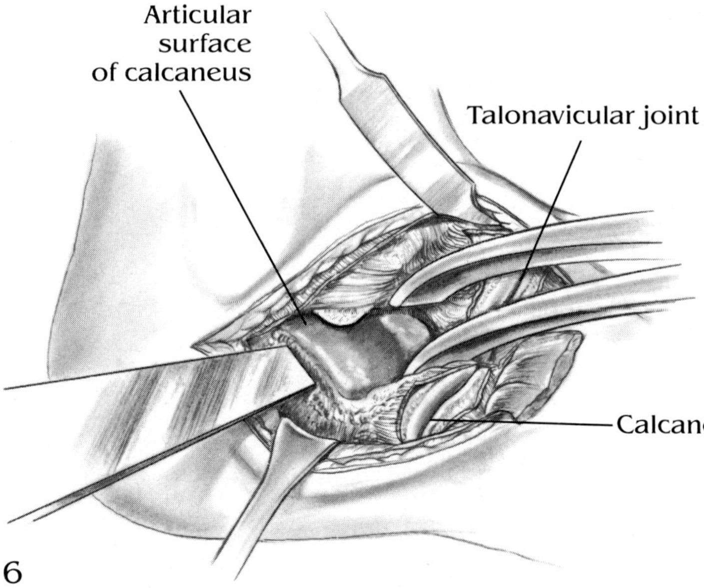
Articular surface of calcaneus
Talonavicular joint
Calcaneocuboid joint

6

6. Excise articular cartilage from the calcaneocuboid and talonavicular joints with hand osteotomes (Fig. 7). The articulation between the navicular and the cuboid is also decorticated.
7. With the ankle and calcaneus in neutral position, a smooth Steinmann pin is inserted medial to the anterior tibial tendon from the neck of the talus into the calcaneus to fix the subtalar joint as previously described (Fig. 8a).
8. The midfoot is then held in neutral position in relation to the hindfoot. A smooth Steinmann pin is inserted percutaneously to transfix the calcaneocuboid joint. The pin is inserted through a 1-cm incision at the dorsolateral aspect of the foot at the lateral margin of the cuboid. It is inserted longitudinally to engage the cancellous bone in the neck of the calcaneus (Fig. 8b).
9. An additional pin is inserted from the distal medial aspect of the navicular in the region of the navicular tuberosity into the neck of the talus (Fig. 8b).
10. Fusion sites are packed with cancellous iliac graft.
11. Closure is performed in a manner similar to that used in isolated subtalar arthrodesis. The flap of the extensor digitorum brevis muscle is reattached. The subcutaneous tissue and skin are closed in layers.

Postoperative Care
1. A soft compression dressing is applied for 48 hours.
2. A short-leg cast is then applied.
3. The patient is maintained non–weight bearing on crutches for 6 weeks.
4. The cast is changed and sutures removed at 3 weeks.
5. At 6 weeks the pins are removed, and a short-leg walking cast is applied.
6. The short-leg walking cast is removed at 12 weeks after surgery.

Technical Pitfalls
1. Care is taken to avoid injury to the dorsalis pedis artery, as noted previously.
2. Excessive retraction of soft tissue may lead to a localized area of wound necrosis.

Potential Complications
1. Delayed union
2. Nonunion
3. Wound necrosis
4. Infection

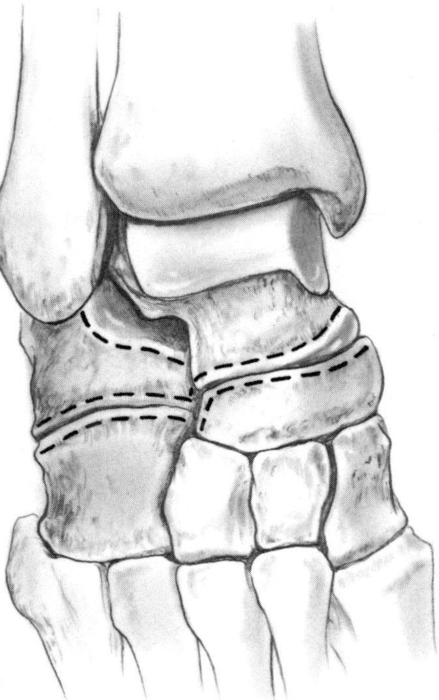

7

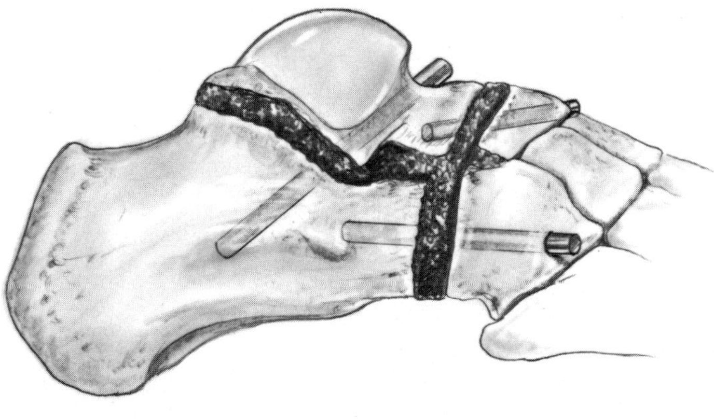

8a

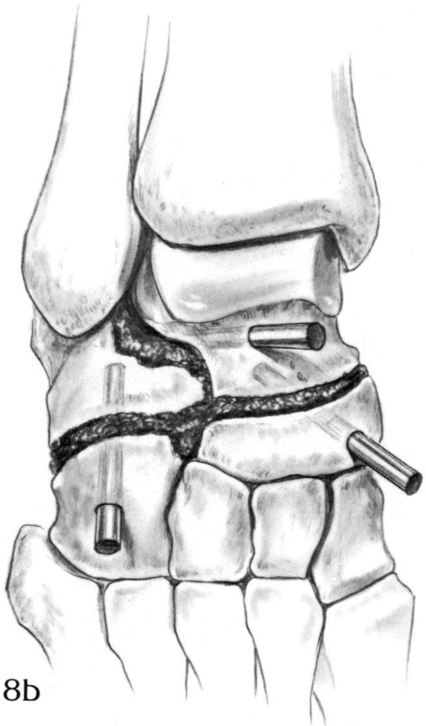

8b

PART 18

Operations for Os Trigonum Syndrome

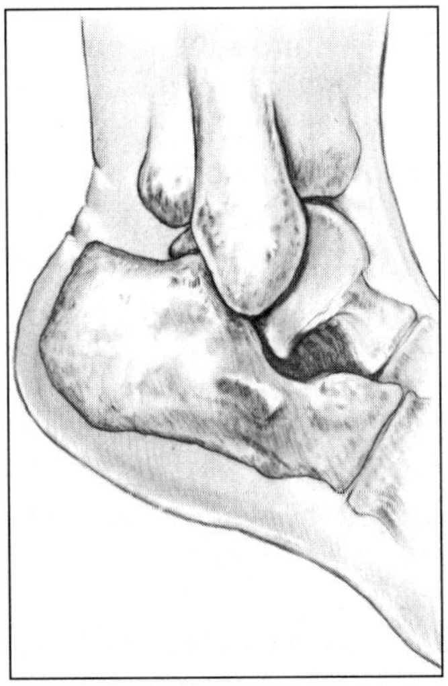

EXCISION OS TRIGONUM

General Considerations

The os trigonum is an accessory bone that lies at the posterior process of the talus. It is thought to arise from a separate ossification center that appears between 8 and 11 years of age. Most often this osseous structure proceeds to unite with the parent bone within 1 year of its appearance, at which time it goes on to form the lateral tubercle of the posterior process of the talus. In approximately 7% of the population it does not unite with the talus and goes on to form an os trigonum. The os trigonum may cause pain in the retrocalcaneal space that is increased with weight-bearing activities and plantarflexion of the foot.

It is often difficult and may be impossible to differentiate a symptomatic os trigonum from a fracture of the lateral tubercle of the posterior process of the talus. This fracture is caused by forced plantarflexion of the foot, which leads to impingement of the posterior tibial plafond on the posterolateral process of the talus. A second mechanism that has been proposed is that of excessive dorsiflexion of the ankle, which may lead to fracture of the lateral tubercle of the posterior process by means of avulsion of the posterior talofibular ligament.

Pain in the retrocalcaneal region may be associated with either a fracture of the lateral tubercle of the posterior process of the talus or a rupture of the synchondrosis that attaches a true os trigonum to the talus. The physical examination reveals localized tenderness at the lateral aspect of the retrocalcaneal space just anterior to the Achilles tendon. Passive plantarflexion of the foot may reproduce the symptoms. A lateral radiograph of the foot often enables identification of the osseous fragment, but if overlap of osseous structures makes visualization difficult, tomograms or a computed tomographic scan of the ankle may be helpful.

Retrocalcaneal pain associated with a fracture fragment or os trigonum is treated in a similar fashion. Acute symptoms may be treated with cast immobilization, followed by a slow, gradual return to weight-bearing activities within the limits of discomfort. Rubber-soled shoes may help decrease impact loading during the stance phase of gait. Other symptomatic measures include the use of anti-inflammatory medications. Persistent pain associated with an os trigonum or an ununited fracture fragment may require surgical excision to alleviate symptoms.

Patient Selection

Indications

1. Chronic pain at the posterior aspect of the ankle after fracture of the lateral tubercle of the posterior process of the talus
2. Symptomatic os trigonum that fails to respond to conservative treatment

Contraindications

1. Older or inactive patients with mild episodic symptoms
2. Patients whose general medical condition makes them susceptible to increased risks of surgery and general anesthesia

Surgical Procedure

Operative Technique

1. A posterolateral incision 10 cm long is made. The incision is positioned 1 cm lateral to the Achilles tendon and ends distally at the insertion of the tendon on the os calcis (Fig. 1). Incise subcutaneous tissue along the line of the skin incision. Identify the sural nerve and retract it laterally. The Achilles tendon is retracted medially.
2. Incise deep fascia longitudinally. Incise fat and areolar tissue to the posterior surface of the tibia between the flexor hallucis longus and peroneal tendons (Fig. 2).
3. Reflect the origin of the flexor hallucis longus muscle medially. Incise the periosteum over the tibia longitudinally. Incise the capsule and synovium of the ankle and subtalar joint longitudinally and reflect subperiosteally to expose the posterior process of the talus (Fig. 3).
4. Separate the osseous fragment from the talus by dividing its fibrous tissue junction with a scalpel. This allows excision of the os trigonum or fracture fragment (Fig. 4).
5. Examine the posterior subtalar joint. The inferior aspect of the os trigonum or the fracture fragment often contains an articular surface for the posterior talocalcaneal joint. Trauma or chronic inflammation in this area may lead to articular degeneration at that portion of the posterior subtalar joint that articulates with the osseous fragment. If this is the case, localized resection of arthritic articular surface or osteophytes at the superior surface of the calcaneus may be performed.
6. The wound is copiously irrigated with triple antibiotic solution. Deep fascia may be closed with interrupted simple 3-0 Vicryl sutures. The skin is closed with interrupted vertical mattress 3-0 nylon sutures.

Postoperative Care

1. A Robert Jones compression dressing is applied.
2. The dressing and sutures are removed 3 weeks after surgery.
3. A slow, gradual return to weight bearing is allowed within the limits of discomfort.
4. Range-of-motion exercises are instituted after removal of the sutures.

Technical Pitfalls

1. Care should be taken to avoid injury to the sural nerve.
2. Osteophytes at the portion of the posterior facet of the calcaneus that articulates with the os trigonum or fracture fragment should be resected to provide the optimum chance of alleviating symptoms.
3. Active range-of-motion exercises must be instituted quickly after the postoperative immobilization device has been removed.

Potential Complications

1. Sural nerve dysfunction
2. Limitation of motion as a result of scarring at posterior ankle and subtalar joints

---

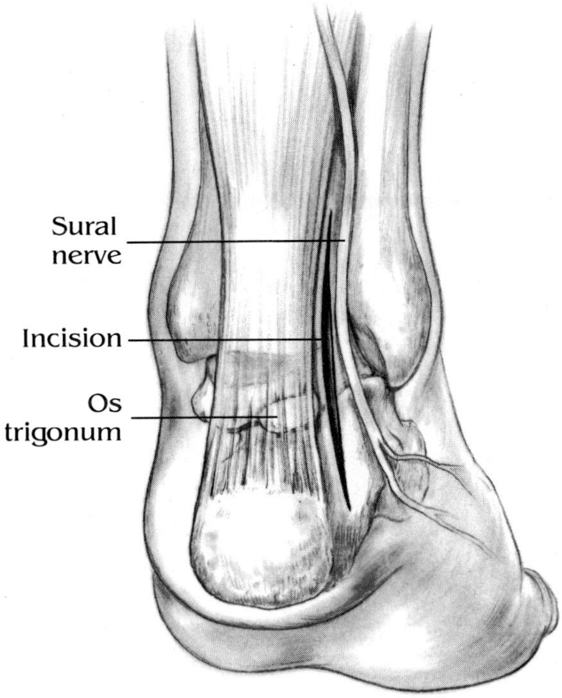

Sural nerve
Incision
Os trigonum

1

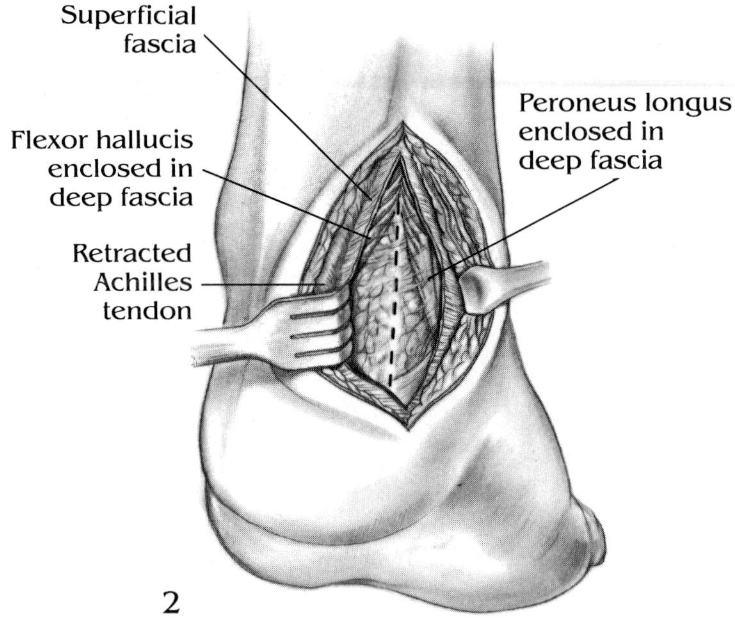

Superficial fascia
Flexor hallucis enclosed in deep fascia
Retracted Achilles tendon
Peroneus longus enclosed in deep fascia

2

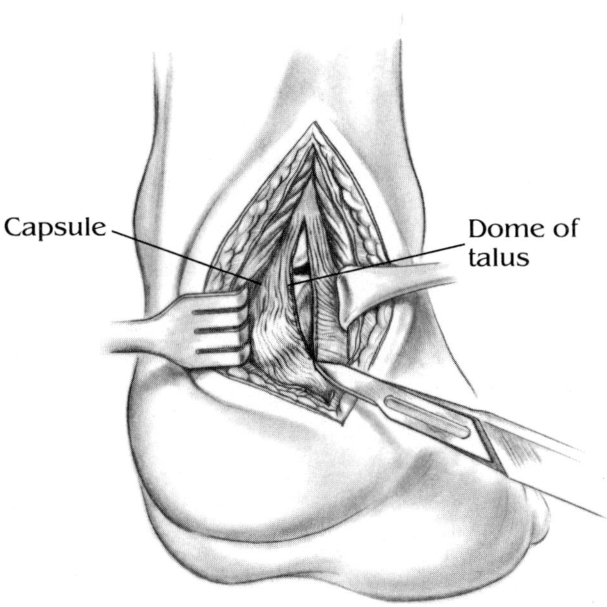

Capsule
Dome of talus

3

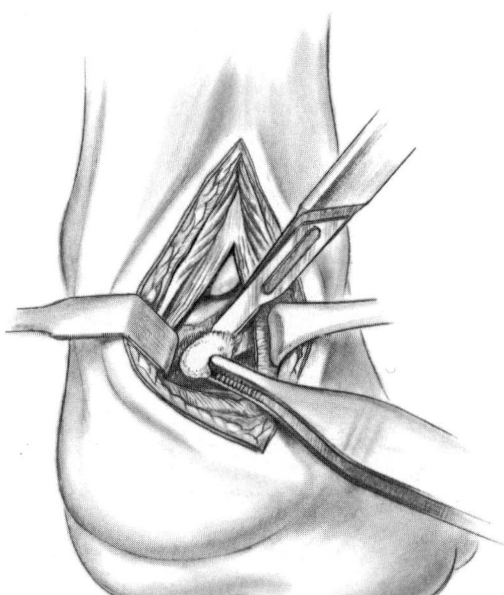

4

PART 19

Operations for Haglund Deformities

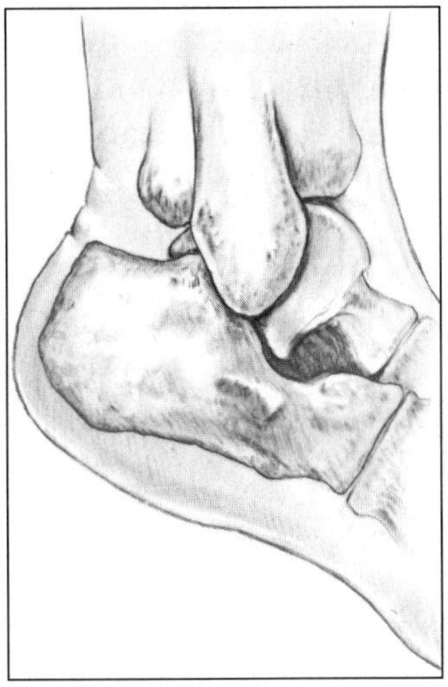

EXCISION HAGLUND'S EXOSTOSIS

General Considerations

It is believed that the structural configuration of the calcaneus is related to various pathologic disorders at the posterior aspect of the heel. Prominence of the posterosuperior tuberosity of the calcaneus has been implicated in the etiology of Achilles tendinitis, retrocalcaneal bursitis, precalcaneal bursitis, and "pump bumps." Prominence of the calcaneus in this region may cause impingement of the adjacent soft tissues between the heel counter of the shoe and the underlying bone, and repetitive mechanical pressure leads to inflammation of these soft tissue structures.

Patients describe localized pain and swelling in the region. Physical examination enables identification of the specific soft tissue structure(s) involved in the inflammatory process. Lateral radiographs of the foot reveal the prominent posterosuperior tuberosity of the calcaneus.

Conservative treatment includes soft rubber-soled shoes to decrease impact loading. The use of an open-heeled shoe or footwear with a soft, flexible heel counter may alleviate mechanical pressure. The use of a heel lift applied to the inner sole of the shoe may elevate the inflamed area above the heel counter. Anti-inflammatory medication and limitation of weight bearing are also useful. If conservative measures fail to provide relief, bony decompression of the posterosuperior tuberosity of the calcaneus may be helpful.

Patient Selection

Indications

1. Any of the following pathologic disorders affecting the posterior aspect of the heel thought to be secondary to a prominent posterosuperior tuberosity of the calcaneus:
   a. Achilles tendinitis
   b. Precalcaneal bursitis
   c. Retrocalcaneal bursitis
   d. Pump bump
2. Active individuals with previously noted posterior calcaneal problems who have failed to respond to a long trial of conservative treatment

Contraindications

1. Patients who present with acute symptoms of relatively recent onset are better treated with conservative methods, as persistent or recurrent symptoms are possible after surgery.
2. Elderly individuals with limited activity levels may be better treated with shoe modifications and appropriate medication.
3. Inadequate neurologic status or vascular supply to the distal peripheral extremity is a contraindication.

Surgical Procedure

Operative Technique

1. A longitudinal skin incision 5 cm long is made along the lateral border of the Achilles tendon (Fig. 1). The incision extends from 2½ cm proximal to the posterosuperior angle of the calcaneus to 2½ cm distal to this landmark. Incise subcutaneous tissue along the line of the skin incision. Identify and retract the sural nerve laterally.
2. Incise periosteum on the calcaneus and reflect subperiosteally to expose the posterosuperior eminence (Fig. 2). Plantarflex the ankle and insert a Hohmann retractor to retract and protect the Achilles tendon and its insertion.
3. Resect the posterosuperior tuberosity of the calcaneus with a cut oriented obliquely from anterosuperior to posteroinferior with an osteotome (Fig. 3). Include any prominent osseous ridge lateral to the tendon (pump bump) in the bony decompression.
4. Smooth the prominent medial and lateral borders of the cut surface of the calcaneus with a rasp (Fig. 4).
5. Close the subcutaneous tissue with interrupted simple 3-0 Vicryl sutures. Close the skin with interrupted vertical mattress 3-0 nylon sutures.

Postoperative Care

1. A Robert Jones compression dressing is applied.
2. The patient is maintained non–weight bearing on crutches for 3 weeks.
3. Sutures are removed at 3 weeks after surgery.
4. A slow, gradual return to weight-bearing activity is permitted. The patient is asked to wear shoes with a 1½-inch heel lift applied to the outer sole when standing or walking. The height of the lift is sequentially decreased over the course of 4 to 6 weeks.

Technical Pitfalls

1. Care should be taken to avoid injury to the sural nerve, which lies in the region of the incision.
2. Removal of too little bone may lead to residual prominence and persistent symptoms.
3. Removal of too much bone may weaken the insertion of the Achilles tendon.
4. Inadequate smoothing of the medial and lateral borders of the cut surface may lead to bony prominence at these sites.

Potential Complications

1. Recurrence of the bony prominence
2. Weakening of the Achilles tendon insertion and subsequent rupture
3. Inadequate removal of bone, resulting in persistent symptoms

---

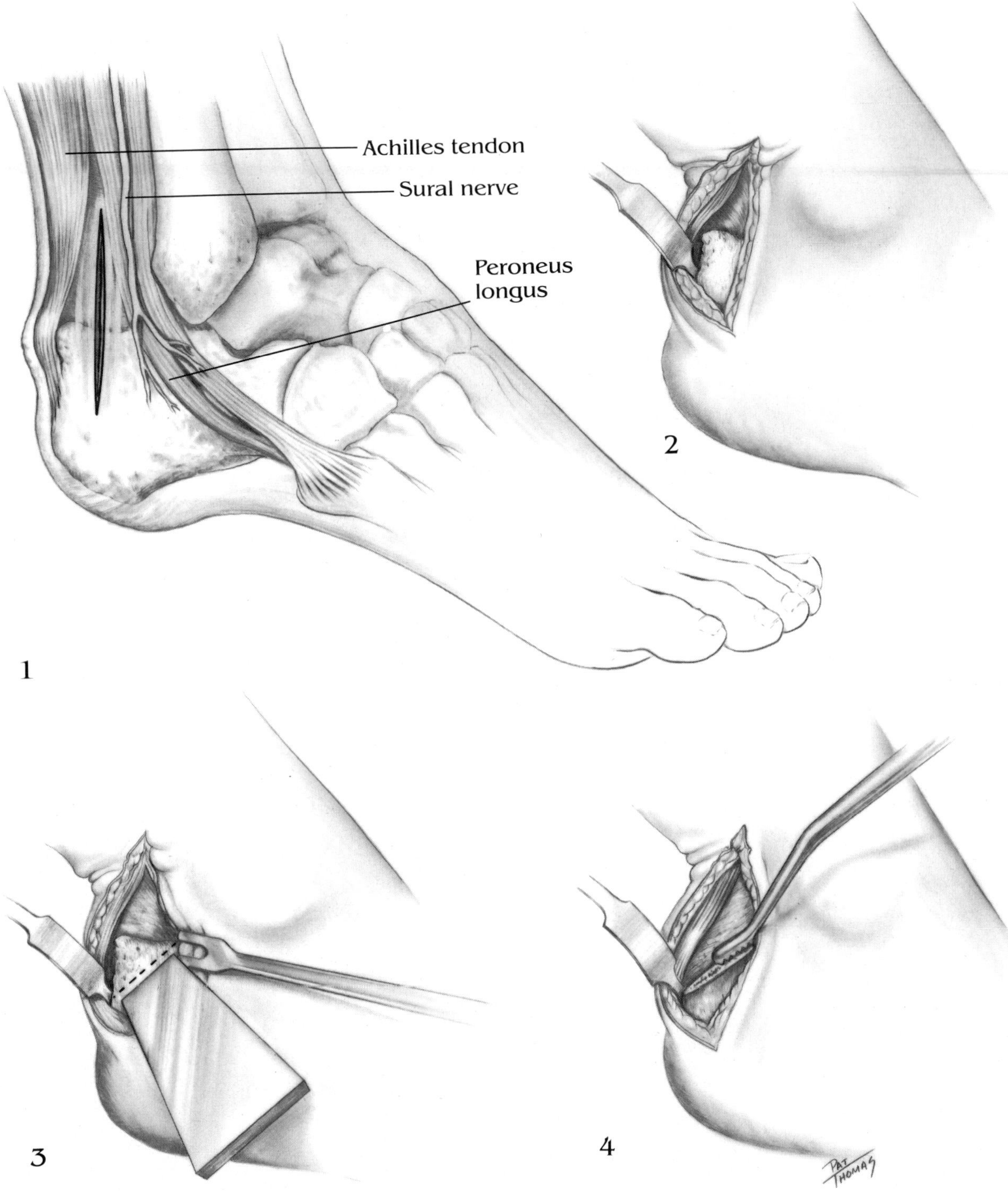
Achilles tendon
Sural nerve
Peroneus longus
1
2
3
4

SECTION 5

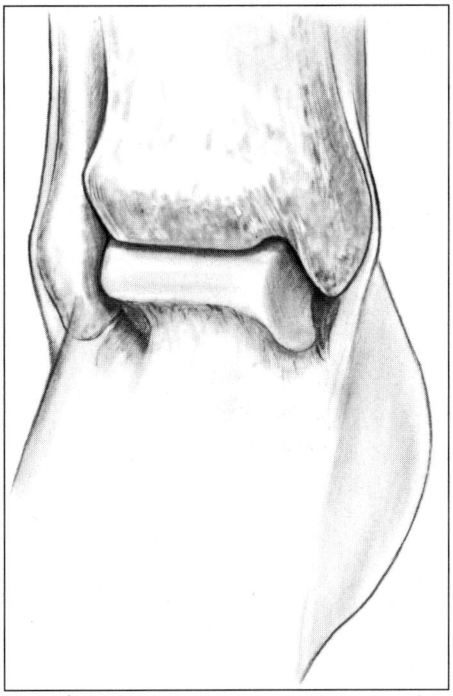

Ankle

PART 20

Ankle Arthroscopy

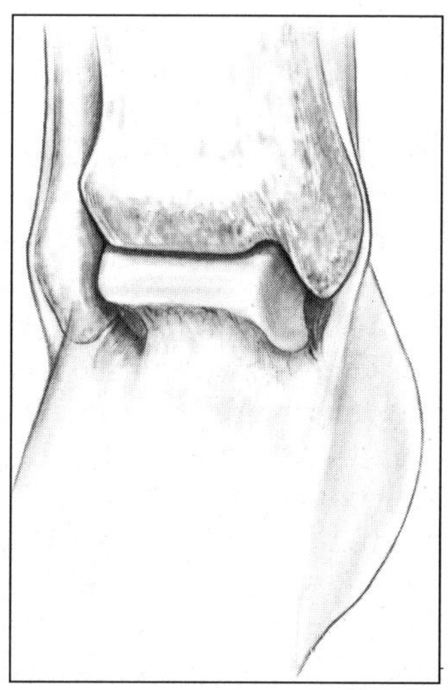

DIAGNOSTIC AND OPERATIVE ARTHROSCOPY OF THE ANKLE

General Considerations

Arthroscopy has proved to be a valuable tool for the diagnosis and treatment of disorders of the ankle. It has a significant diagnostic role in the evaluation of intra-articular pathology that eludes identification on radiographic analysis and other laboratory studies. Arthroscopy may help the clinician avoid unnecessary arthrotomy and may provide insight for planning treatment options.

A typical situation in which arthroscopy may be useful includes patients with chronic pain after an ankle sprain. Arthroscopic exploration of the ankle may provide valuable insight regarding the status of the articular cartilage and enable identification of various types of intra-articular disorders. Typical lesions that may be diagnosed by means of arthroscopy include synovitis, impingement syndrome, intra-articular adhesions, osteochondritis dissecans, loose bodies, and osteochondral fractures. Other diagnostic applications of ankle arthroscopy may include evaluation of disorders of the synovial lining, including synovitis resulting from inflammatory disorders and pigmented villonodular synovitis. Nontraumatic articular disorders such as degenerative joint disease, neoplastic lesions, and metabolic disorders may also be identified by means of this technique.

Operative arthroscopy may allow surgical treatment of various intra-articular disorders. Synovial biopsy or a more extensive synovectomy may be performed through the arthroscope under direct visualization. This may play a role in rheumatoid arthritis and other inflammatory arthropathies of the ankle joint. Removal of loose bodies, lysis of adhesions, and excision of intra-articular osteophytes may enable arthroscopic debridement arthroplasty of the arthritic ankle. Excision, curettage, and drilling of osteochondritic lesions may be done through the arthroscope. Operative arthroscopic techniques allow valuable surgical procedures to be performed with minimal morbidity and complications.

Patient Selection

Indications

1. Arthroscopy may be used to evaluate and treat persistent pain and limitation of motion after traumatic injury to the ankle joint.
2. Arthroscopy may also be used to evaluate articular damage after injury.
3. Synovial biopsy and synovectomy may be useful in the evaluation and treatment of disorders of the synovium.
4. Arthroscopy may be used in the evaluation of nontraumatic articular disorders such as degenerative arthritis, neoplastic lesions, and metabolic disorders.

Contraindications

1. Diagnosis of the majority of intra-articular disorders may be achieved by means of noninvasive radiographic examinations.
2. Identification of soft tissue abnormality involving periarticular structures is not possible by means of the arthroscope. These disorders may be more easily identified by means of magnetic resonance imaging and other diagnostic modalities.

Surgical Procedure

Preparation for Surgery

1. The procedure is carried out in an operating room under strict asceptic conditions.
2. Copies of the patient's medical records and radiographic tests should be available during the procedure.
3. A tourniquet is applied but not inflated. It may be used to obtain hemostasis during the procedure.
4. General anesthesia or regional blocks may be utilized depending on the age, medical condition, and preference of the patient.
5. The patient is placed in the supine position. A knee holder or bolster may be utilized to improve the position of the limb for arthroscopic evaluation. Tilting the limb obliquely by means of a sandbag placed under the hip may allow easy access to the posterolateral portal, if required.
6. The use of invasive or noninvasive distraction devices may be helpful in providing easy access to all areas of the articulation.
7. The 4.0-mm scope used for evaluation of larger joints may provide optimum visualization of the ankle joint. In situations in which distraction is difficult, smaller arthroscopes may be required. Small, angled arthroscopes such as the 2.7-mm oblique arthroscope may be helpful. Small scopes with wide-angle lenses may provide visualization equal to that obtainable with larger scopes.

Operative Technique

1. Palpate and identify the dorsalis pedis pulse, the anterior tibial tendon, and the extensor digitorum longus tendons.
2. Dorsiflex and plantarflex the ankle to identify the ankle joint.
3. Insert a 14-gauge needle lateral to the extensor digitorum longus tendon (Fig. 1). Aspirate the joint and then inject 10 to 15 mm of irrigation fluid. The needle is connected to plastic tubing, which allows egress of irrigation fluid.
4. A small incision is made through the skin at the level of the joint medial to the anterior tibial tendon. Care should be taken to avoid injury to the great saphenous vein, which is anterior to the medial malleolus (Fig. 1). A sharp trocar in its sleeve is inserted and passed through the joint capsule. The sharp obturator is exchanged for a blunt obturator, which is inserted through the synovium into the ankle joint (Fig. 2).
5. The obturator is removed, and the endoscope inserted into the sleeve. A piece of plastic tubing is connected to the valve of the trocar sleeve, which allows inflow of continuous irrigation fluid (Fig. 2).

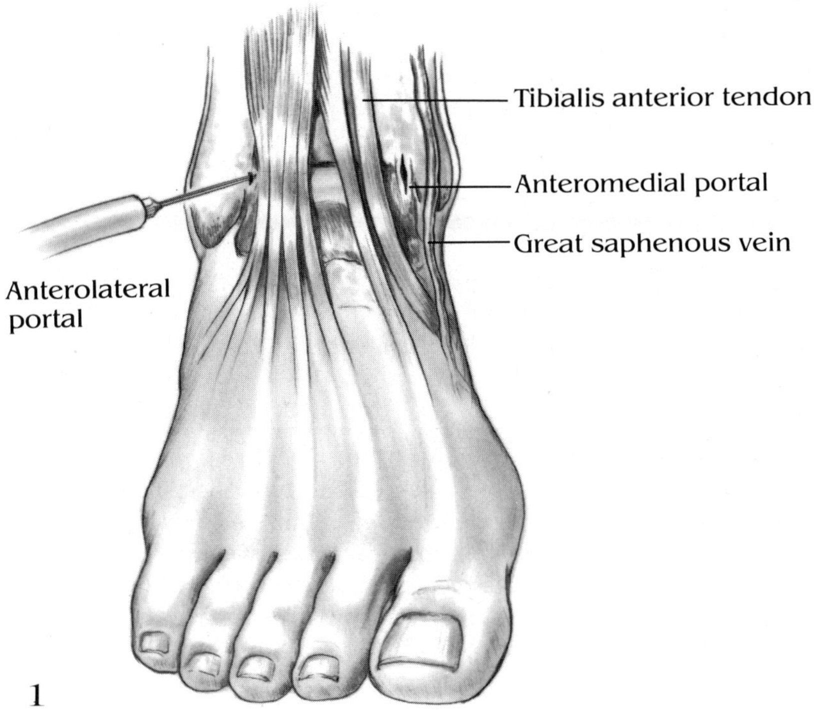
Tibialis anterior tendon
Anteromedial portal
Great saphenous vein
Anterolateral portal

1

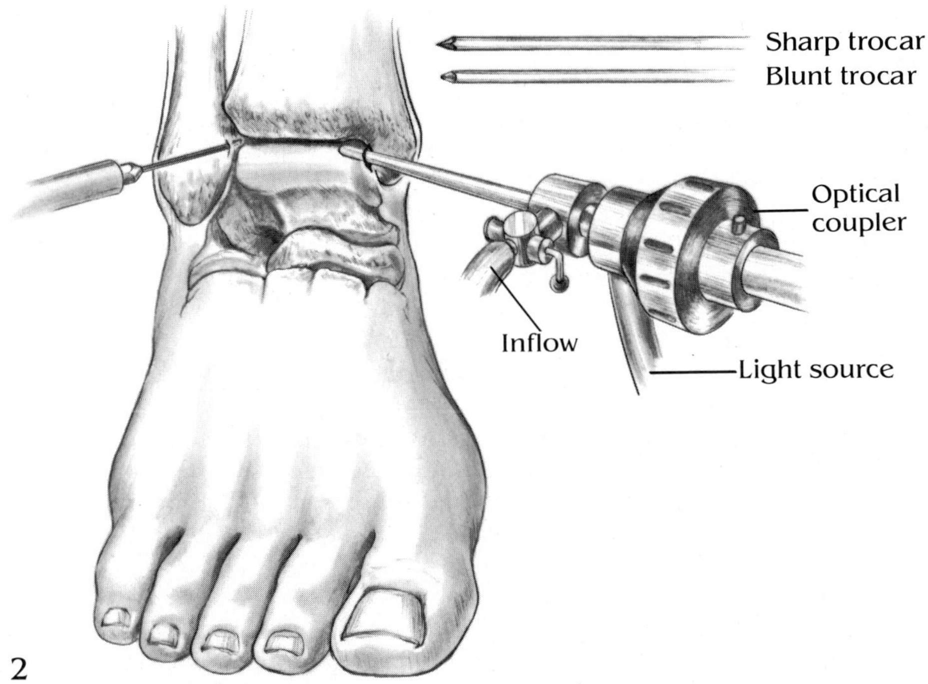
Sharp trocar
Blunt trocar
Optical coupler
Inflow
Light source

2

6. A systematic examination of the joint is performed (Fig. 3). Manipulation by eversion, inversion, plantarflexion, dorsiflexion, and application of traction allows for evaluation of the articulation. Structures to be examined from medial to lateral include the fibers of the deep deltoid ligament (Fig. 3a), the medial malleolus, the medial talomalleolar articulation (Fig. 3b), the anterior tibiotalor joint (Fig. 3c), the distal tibiofibular articulation (Fig. 3d), the lateral talomalleolar articulation (Fig. 3e), the lateral synovial wall, and the anterior talofibular ligament (Fig. 3f).
7. A posterolateral portal is often required. An incision is made lateral to the Achilles tendon. The sharp trocar, followed by a blunt trocar, is inserted through the capsule and into the joint. Care is taken to avoid injury to the sural nerve and short saphenous vein (Fig. 4).
8. Various instruments, including forceps, probes, rongeurs, burrs and articular shavers, may be inserted through any of the three portals (Fig. 4). Generally, surgical instruments are inserted through the portal in proximity to the pathologic entity. The arthroscope is inserted through a second alternate portal. Possible arthroscopic surgical procedures include excision and curettage of osteochondritis dissecans lesions, removal of loose bodies, and lysis of adhesions. Synovial biopsy and more extensive synovectomy may be performed through the arthroscope. Resection of osteophytes may enable debridement of an arthritic joint.
9. The skin edges are approximated with one or two simple sutures of 3-0 nylon.

Postoperative Care

1. A sterile dressing and a Robert Jones compression dressing with a U-shaped plaster splint are applied.
2. The patient is kept on crutches non–weight bearing.
3. The dressing and sutures are removed and weight bearing allowed in a slow, progressive manner within the limits of discomfort.

Technical Pitfalls

1. The branches of the superficial peroneal nerve in the area of the anterolateral portal should be avoided.
2. The great saphenous vein at the anteromedial portal should be avoided.
3. Care should be taken to avoid the sural nerve and short saphenous vein during insertion of the instruments at the posterolateral portal.
4. Articular damage should be avoided by using a blunt obturator in a well-distended capsule.

Potential Complications

1. Injury to the neurovascular structures that lie in proximity to the portals
2. Bending or breaking of the optics or instruments inside the joint cavity
3. Infection

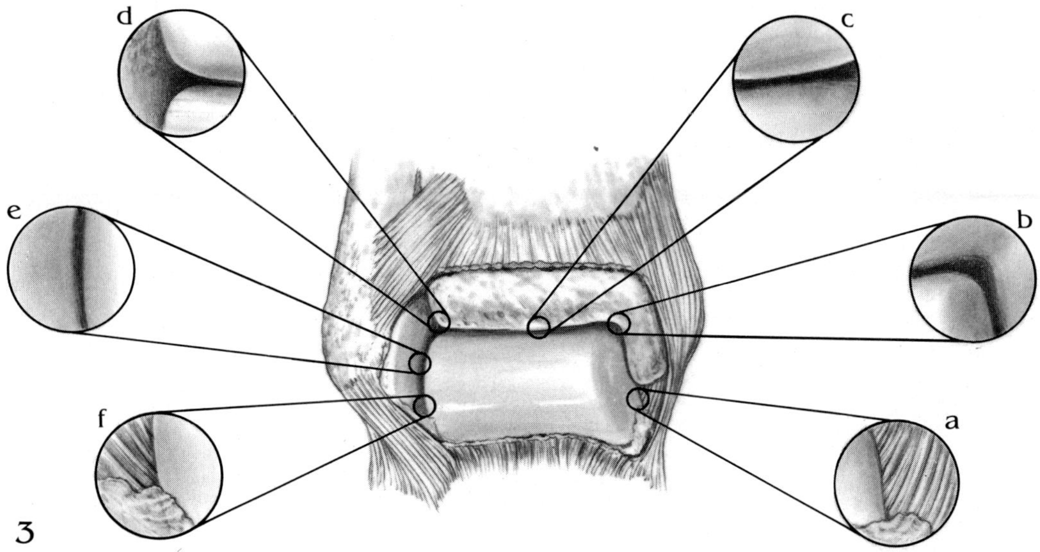

3

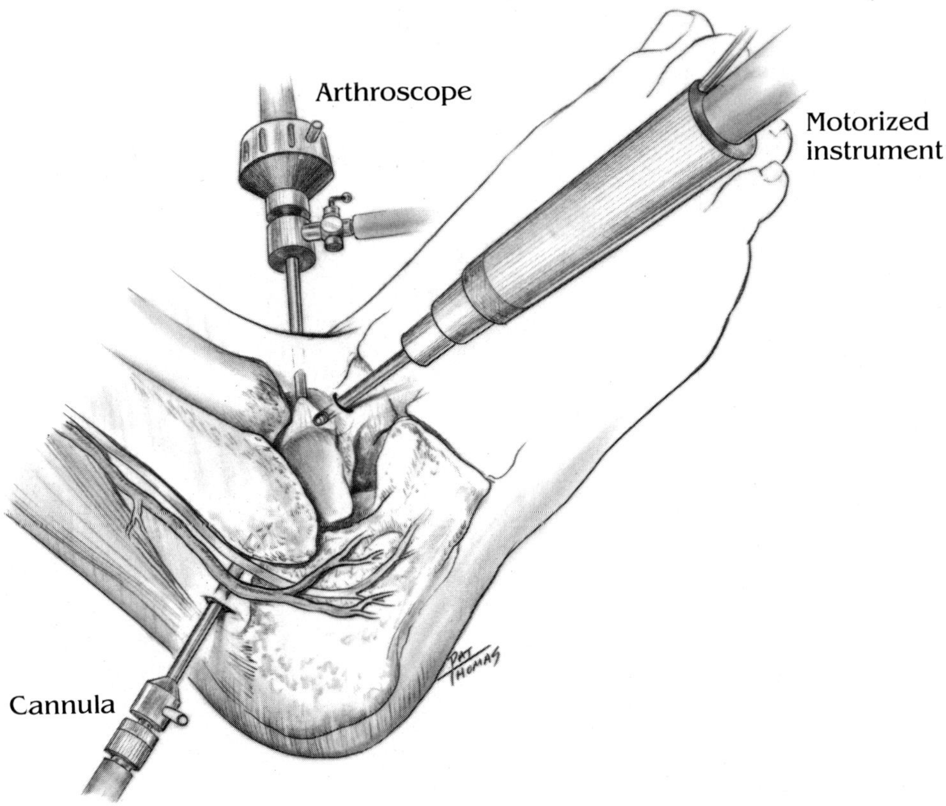

4

PART 21

Anterior Arthrotomy of the Ankle Joint for Removal of Loose Bodies; Synovectomy; and Debridement Arthroplasty

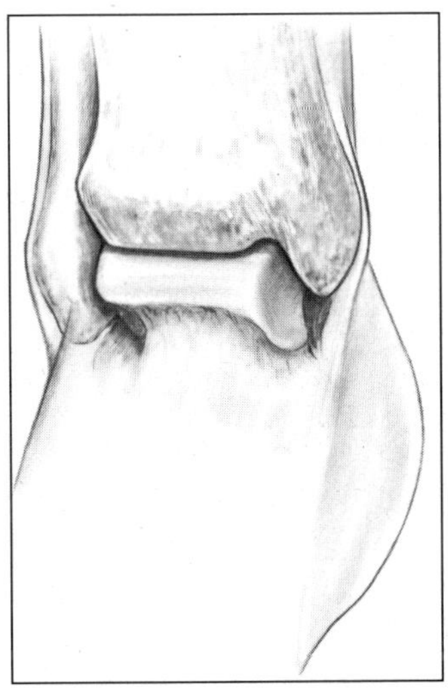

ANTERIOR ARTHROTOMY OF THE ANKLE JOINT FOR REMOVAL OF LOOSE BODIES; SYNOVECTOMY; AND DEBRIDEMENT ARTHROPLASTY

General Considerations

Various intra-articular disorders of the ankle can occur as a result of traumatic injury. Pathologic entities including synovitis, osteochondritis dissecans, osteochondral fractures, and articular osteophytes are commonly seen. Any of these problems may lead to pain, swelling, clicking, locking, and sensations of "giving way" in the region of the ankle joint. Identification of the specific abnormality may require radiographs, tomograms, arthrograms, or computed tomographic scans.

Nonoperative management may be successful in many patients. Treatment modalities include external bracing, anti-inflammatory medications, and physical therapy. If patients describe persistent symptoms despite conservative measures, consideration can be given to surgical intervention. Many of these pathologic entities may be amenable to arthroscopic surgery as described in the previous chapter. Some situations may require arthrotomy of the ankle joint.

In general, the surgical approach used for arthrotomy about the ankle joint most often depends on the location of the specific intra-articular pathology. The posterolateral approach, most often used for pathologic disorders affecting the posterior aspect of the ankle joint, is well delineated in the chapter, "Excision Os Trigonum." Various anterior approaches may be used to gain access to the anterior portion of the articulation. The most common incision utilized in approaching the ankle joint is the anterior utility incision between the tibialis anterior and the extensor hallucis longus tendons. Less commonly, an anteromedial or anterolateral approach may be used.

Patient Selection

Indications

1. Chondral and osteochondral fractures of the ankle
2. Osteochondritis dissecans
3. Loose bodies
4. Intra-articular adhesions
5. Synovitis of the ankle joint
6. Traumatic or degenerative joint disease

Contraindications. Many intra-articular lesions of the ankle joint are amenable to arthroscopic evaluation and treatment, which may be associated with less morbidity and more rapid rehabilitation in some cases.

Surgical Procedure: Operative Approaches

Operative Technique: Arthrotomy—Anterior Utility Incision

1. A longitudinal incision 8 cm long is made from 3 cm proximal to the ankle joint to 5 cm distal to this articulation (Fig. 1). The incision is placed between the anterior tibial and extensor hallucis longus tendons. Subcutaneous tissue is divided along the line of the skin incision.
2. Divide the transverse and oblique extensor retinaculum. Deepen the incision in the interval between the anterior tibial tendon medially and the extensor hallucis longus tendon laterally (Fig. 2). Retract the anterior tibial tendon medially. Retract the extensor hallucis longus tendon and neurovascular bundle laterally.
3. Divide the joint capsule and synovium longitudinally. Expose the ankle joint and talar neck subperiosteally (Fig. 3).

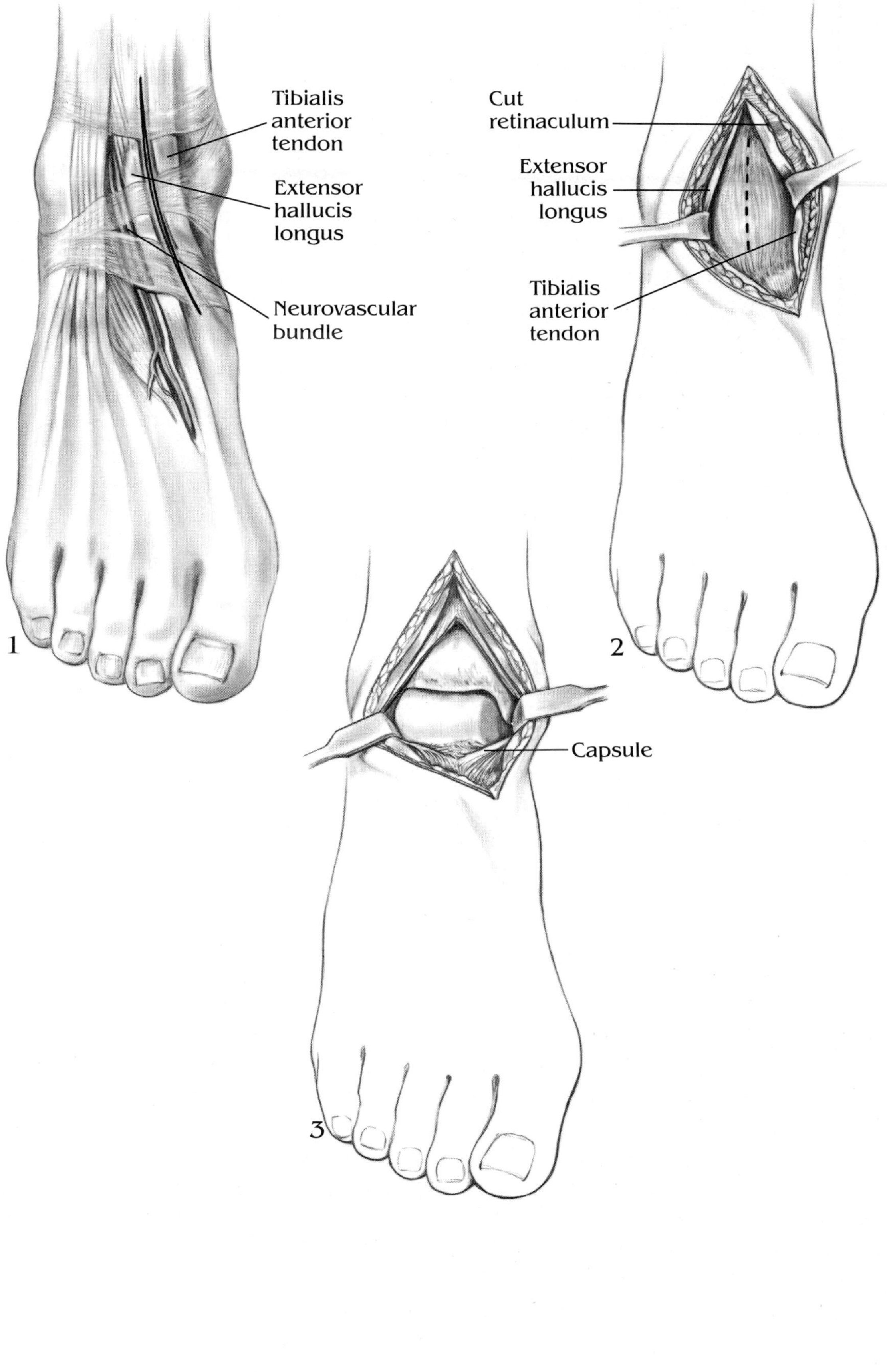
Tibialis anterior tendon
Extensor hallucis longus
Neurovascular bundle
1
Cut retinaculum
Extensor hallucis longus
Tibialis anterior tendon
2
Capsule
3

Operative Technique: Arthrotomy—Anterolateral Incision

1. An anterolateral longitudinal incision 8 cm long is made. The incision is placed 1 cm medial to the anterior margin of the fibula and lateral to the extensor tendons (Fig. 1). The incision extends from 4 cm proximal to the ankle joint to 4 cm distal to that articulation at about the level of the base of the fourth metatarsal. Incise subcutaneous tissue along the line of the skin incision.
2. Identify, mobilize, and protect the branches of the superficial peroneal nerve.
3. Incise deep fascia as well as the superior and inferior retinaculum longitudinally. Retract the extensor tendons and peroneus tertius tendon medially (Fig. 2).
4. Incise the periosteum over the tibia and the capsule over the ankle joint longitudinally (Fig. 2). Reflect the capsule and periosteum subperiosteally to expose the anterior tibia, the neck of the talus, and the ankle joint. Reflect the capsule and periosteum laterally to expose the lateral gutter of the ankle joint, as well as the fibular malleolus (Fig. 3).

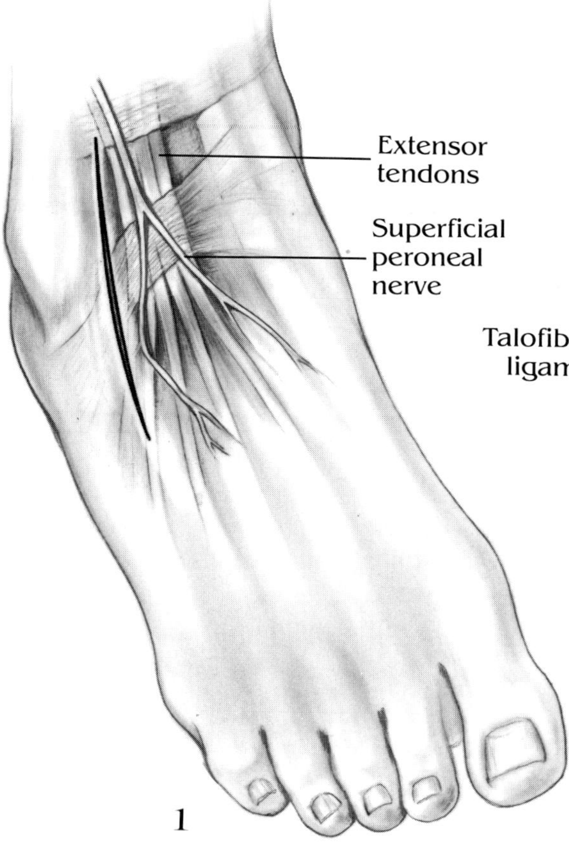
Extensor
tendons
Superficial
peroneal
nerve

1

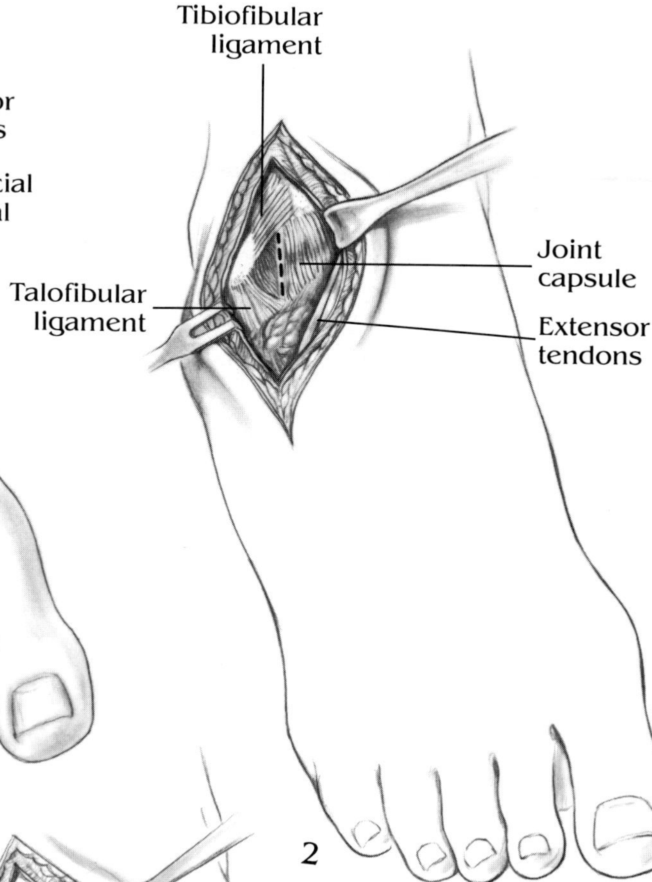
Tibiofibular
ligament
Joint
capsule
Talofibular
ligament
Extensor
tendons

2

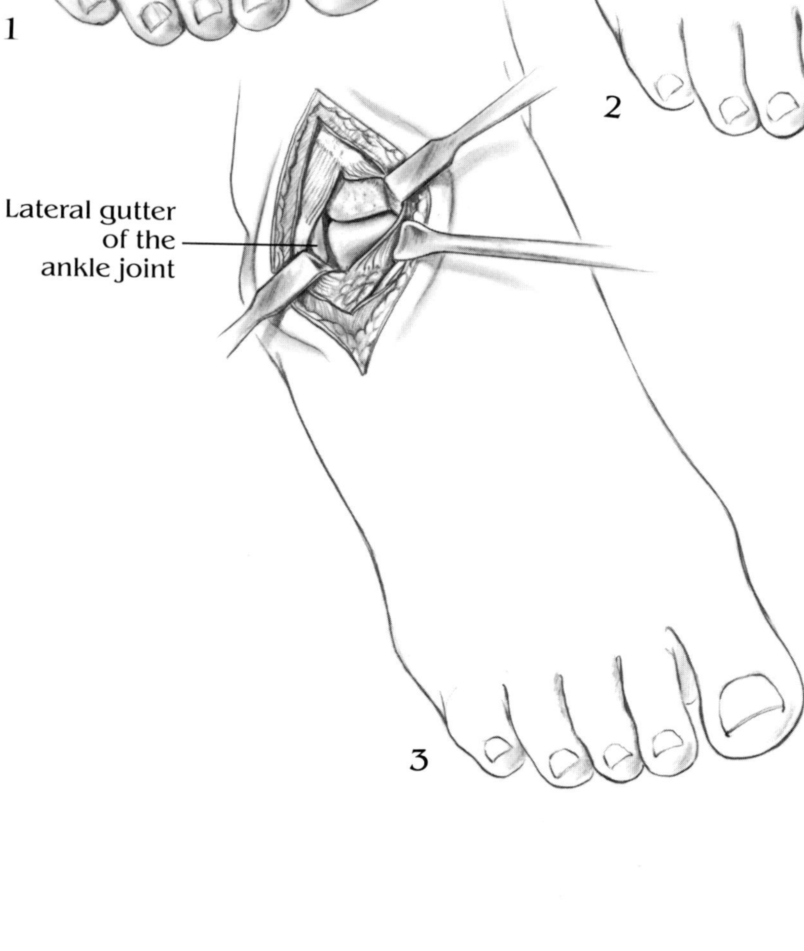
Lateral gutter
of the
ankle joint

3

Operative Technique: Arthrotomy—Anteromedial Incision

1. An anteromedial longitudinal incision 8 cm long is made, beginning 3 cm proximal to the ankle joint. The incision is placed medial to and paralleling the anterior tibial tendon (Fig. 1). Curve the incision gently posteriorly, following the anterior margin of the medial malleolus to end 3 cm distal to the malleolus. Incise subcutaneous tissue along the line of the skin incision.
2. It may be necessary to divide the saphenous vein below the ankle joint. Divide the dorsal retinacular ligament longitudinally (Fig. 2).
3. Divide the joint capsule longitudinally and reflect subperiosteally to expose the lower end of the tibia and the dome of the talus (Fig. 3).

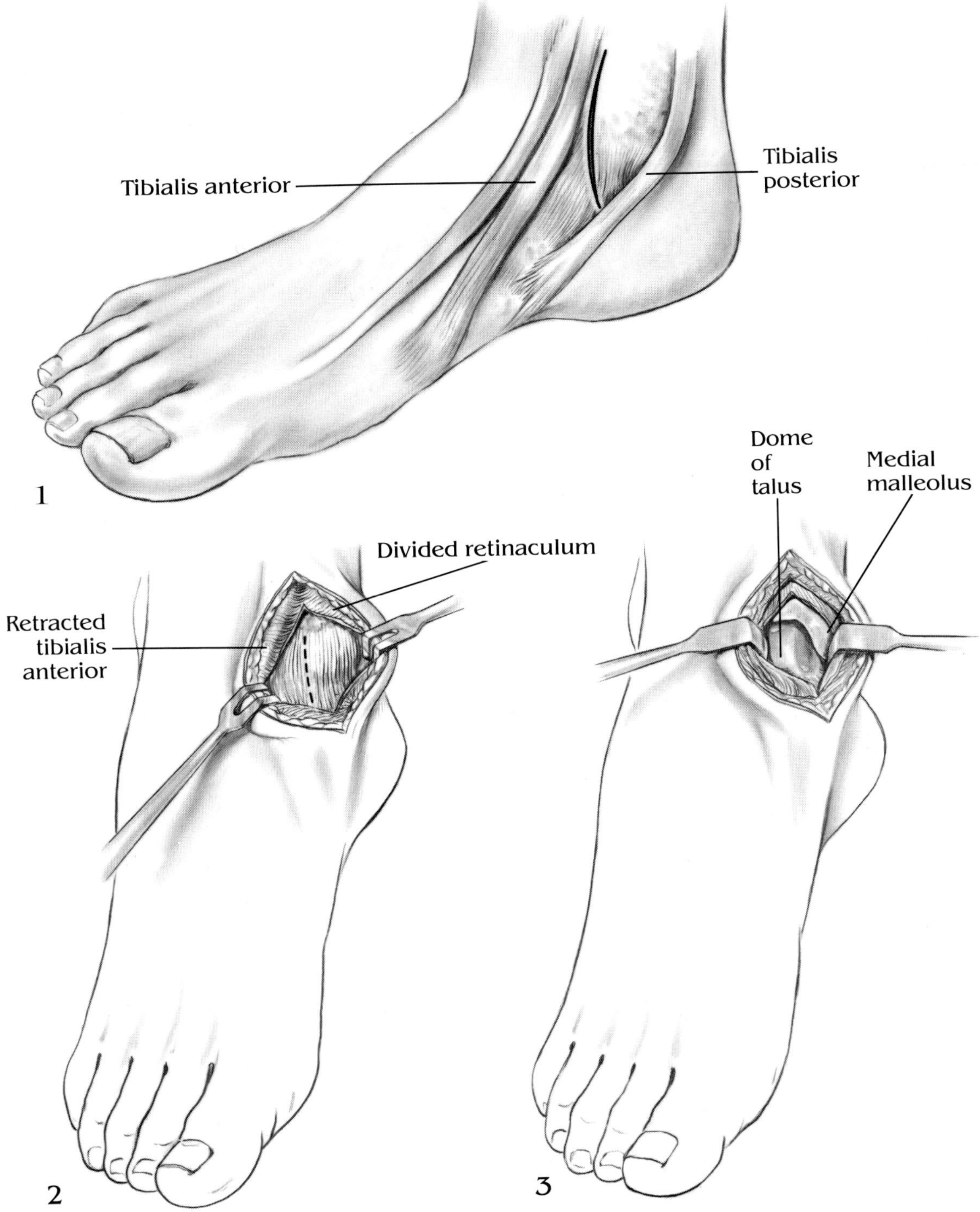
Tibialis anterior
Tibialis posterior
1
Retracted tibialis anterior
Divided retinaculum
2
Dome of talus
Medial malleolus
3

Surgical Procedure: Operative Intervention Addressing Intra-articular Disorders

Operative Technique: Synovectomy Ankle Joint

1. Identify the plane between the synovium and capsule. With dissecting scissors, separate the synovium from the capsule (Fig. 1).
2. Excise hypertrophic synovium in the regions accessible through the incision.
3. Curet areas of abnormal synovium that are difficult to reach (Fig. 2).
4. Close the capsule with interrupted figure-of-eight 2-0 Vicryl sutures. Reapproximate the retinaculum with interrupted figure-of-eight 2-0 Vicryl sutures. Reapproximate subcutaneous tissue with interrupted simple 3-0 Vicryl sutures. Close the skin with interrupted vertical mattress 3-0 nylon sutures.

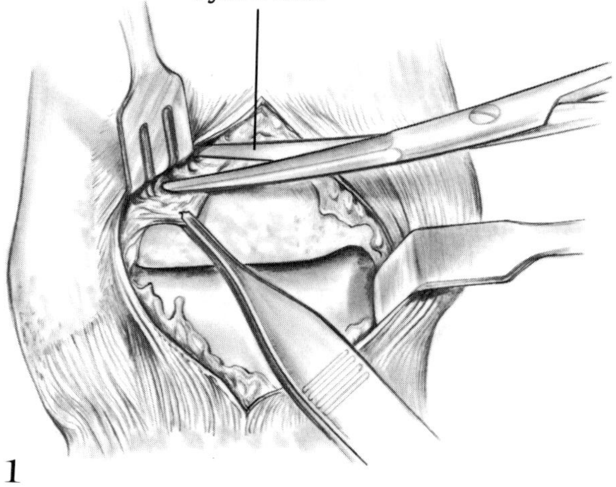

1

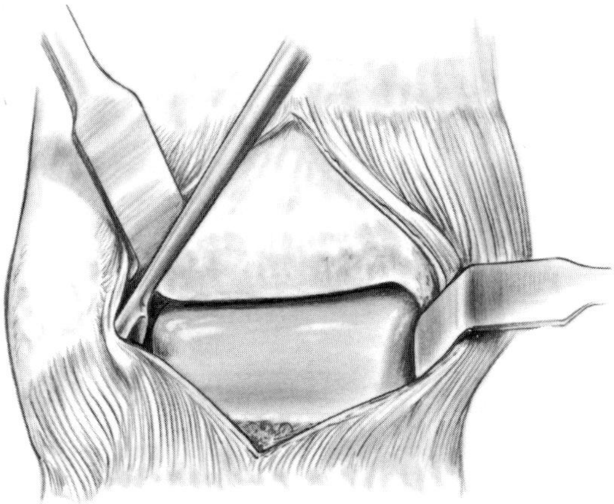

2

Operative Technique: Debridement Arthroplasty Ankle Joint

1. Meticulously examine the ankle joint in a systematic fashion.
2. Remove loose bodies that are visible (Fig. 1).
3. Excise areas of osteophyte at the anterior margin of the tibia and the dorsal aspect of the talar neck with an osteotome (Fig. 2). Decompress other areas of osteophytes that are identified. Smooth the cut surface with a rasp.
4. Plantarflex the foot maximally. Identify and address any areas of osteochondral defect or other abnormalities.
5. Close the capsule with interrupted figure-of-eight 2-0 Vicryl sutures. Reapproximate the retinaculum with interrupted figure-of-eight 2-0 Vicryl sutures. Reapproximate subcutaneous tissue with interrupted simple 3-0 Vicryl sutures. Close skin with interrupted vertical mattress 3-0 nylon sutures.

Postoperative Care

1. A sterile dressing is applied.
2. A Robert Jones compression dressing incorporating a U-shaped sugar-tong type plaster splint is applied to provide protected mobilization.
3. The patient is kept non–weight bearing on crutches for 3 weeks following surgery.
4. Sutures are removed at 3 weeks.
5. A slow, gradual return to weight-bearing activity is permitted. Range-of-motion exercises are instituted.

Technical Pitfalls

1. Identification and ligation of the saphenous vein below the ankle are often required when using the anteromedial approach.
2. Identification and protection of the branch of the superficial peroneal nerve is necessary when using the anterolateral approach.
3. Failure to adequately close the dorsal retinaculum may lead to abnormal mobility of the extensor tendons.

Potential Complications

1. Inflammation, scarring, or injury to the branches of the superficial peroneal nerve at the anterior aspect of the ankle joint may lead to neurologic symptoms.
2. All portions of the ankle joint are not accessible through an isolated anterior approach, and thus complete synovectomy is not feasible. Residual hypertrophic synovium may lead to persistent symptoms after surgery.
3. Debridement arthroplasty of the ankle is thought to provide partial and temporary relief of traumatic arthritis of that articulation. Residual symptoms should be expected.

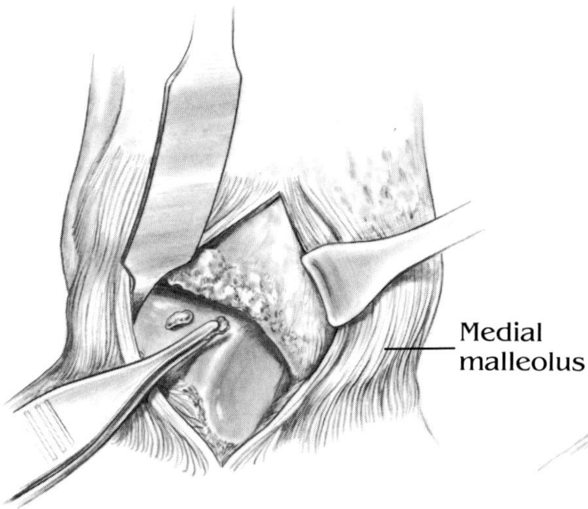
Medial
malleolus

1

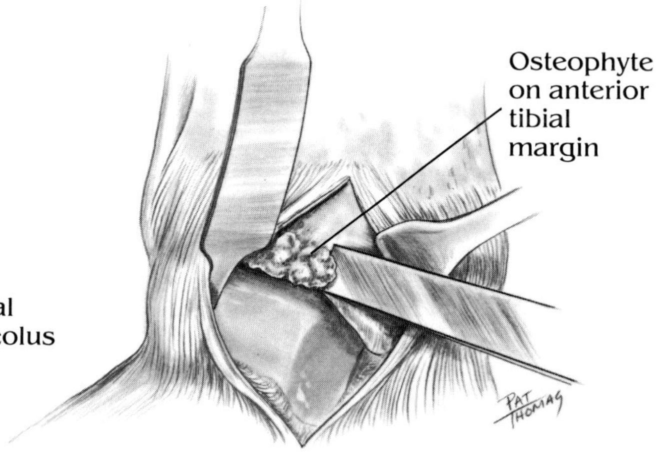
Osteophyte
on anterior
tibial
margin
PAT
THOMAS

2

PART 22

Operations for Osteochondritis Dissecans of the Talus

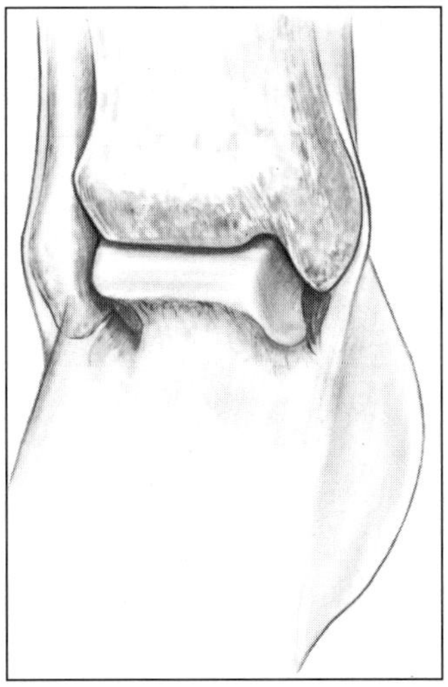

EXCISION, CURETTAGE, AND DRILLING OSTEOCHONDRITIS DISSECANS OF THE TALUS

General Considerations

The term *osteochondritis dissecans* refers to osteochondral fractures of the talus caused by trauma. An inversion injury produces a force that is transmitted across the ankle joint through the articular cartilage of the talus and into subchondral bone. The osteochondral fragment is devoid of a blood supply, and avascular necrosis of the fracture fragment often occurs.

Patients typically present with pain and swelling at the ankle joint after inversion injury. Physical examination allows identification of localized tenderness at the talar dome. These lesions most often occur at the anterolateral or posteromedial aspect of the talar dome. Radiographic evaluation may include plain radiographs, an arthrogram/tomogram of the ankle, a computed tomographic scan, or a magnetic resonance imaging scan. The purpose of radiographic evaluation is to localize the injury and to discern whether the overlying articular cartilage is intact.

Treatment depends on whether the overlying articular cartilage is intact and on the extent of detachment of the osteochondral fragment from the remainder of the talar dome. Conservative management for lesions that are minimally displaced may include use of a non–weight-bearing short-leg cast. Those lesions that do not heal may lead to persistent symptoms necessitating surgical excision of the fracture fragment. Lesions that are significantly displaced also require removal of the fragment. Complete treatment for fragments that require extirpation includes removal of the fragment, curettage of the base of the lesion, and drilling of the bed to stimulate vascularization and encourage healing.

Excision, curettage, and drilling can be accomplished by numerous techniques. Some osteochondritic lesions are amenable to arthroscopic surgery, whereas other lesions may require arthrotomy of the ankle joint. The specific surgical approach depends on the exact location of the lesion as determined by preoperative radiographic evaluation. Surgical exposures utilized include the anterior utility incision, the anteromedial approach, the anterolateral approach, and the posterolateral approach. These approaches are described in "Anterior Arthrotomy of the Ankle Joint for Removal of Loose Bodies; Synovectomy; and Debridement Arthroplasty."

Osteochondritic lesions located on the central or posterior aspect of the medial margin of the talar dome may be inaccessible from standard anterior approaches to the ankle joint. Lateral radiographs of the ankle with the foot held in maximum dorsiflexion and plantarflexion may be helpful to identify those lesions that require medial malleolar osteotomy.

Surgical Procedure: Excision, Curettage, and Drilling Osteochondritis Dissecans of the Talus by Means of an Anteromedial Approach Incorporating a Medial Malleolar Osteotomy

Operative Technique

1. An anteromedial incision 8 cm long is made, beginning 3 cm proximal to the ankle joint (Fig. 1). The incision is placed medial and parallel to the anterior tibial tendon. Curve the incision gently posteriorly, following the anterior margin of the medial malleolus to end 3 cm distal to the malleolus. Incise subcutaneous tissue along the line of the skin incision.
2. Reflect the skin and subcutaneous tissue to expose the anterior ankle joint capsule and medial malleolus (Fig. 2). Divide the dorsal retinacular ligaments longitudinally. Divide the anterior ankle joint capsule longitudinally and reflect subperiosteally to expose the dome of the talus (Fig. 3).

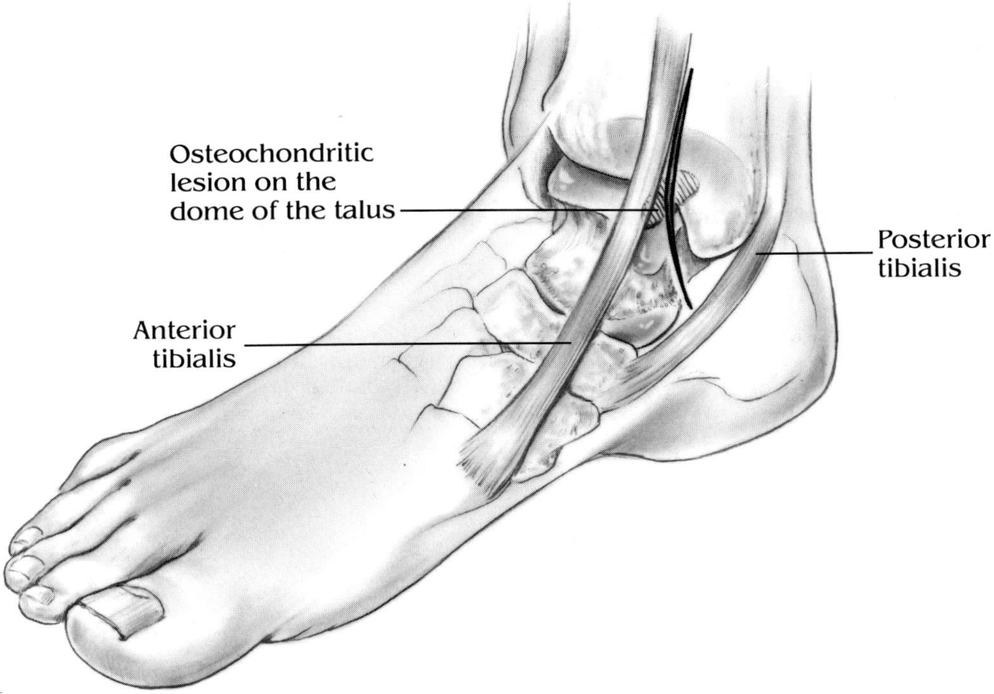
Osteochondritic
lesion on the
dome of the talus
Posterior
tibialis
Anterior
tibialis

1

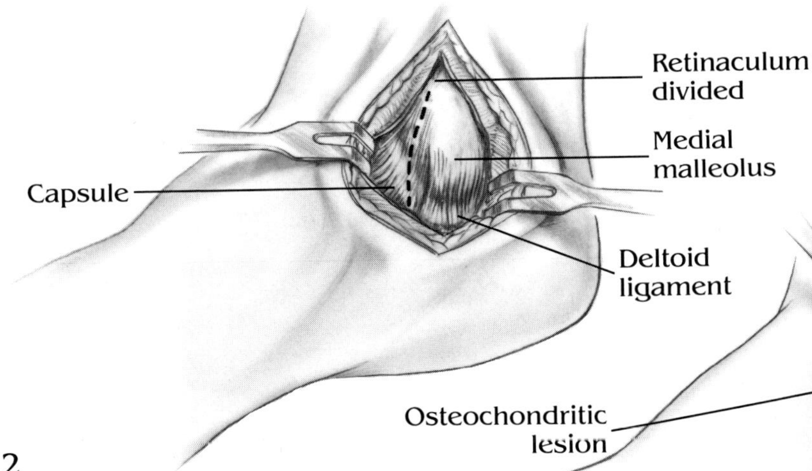
Retinaculum
divided
Medial
malleolus
Capsule
Deltoid
ligament

2

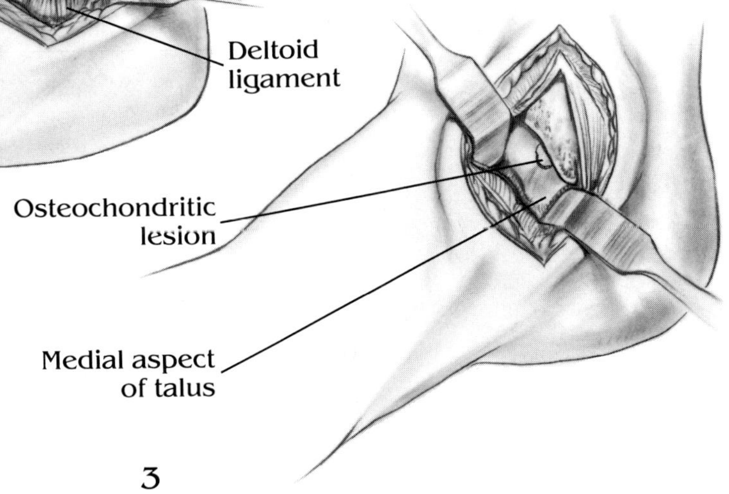
Osteochondritic
lesion
Medial aspect
of talus

3

3. If the osteochondritic lesion is not accessible via the anterior medial approach, consideration may be given to osteotomy of the medial malleolus.

4. Incise the posterior tibial tendon sheath and the flexor retinaculum and retract the tendon posteriorly to expose the posterior margin of the medial malleolus (Fig. 4). Drill one or two holes from the tip of the malleolus into the metaphysis of the tibia with a 2.5-mm drill bit (Fig. 5). Measure the length of the drill hole made with a depth gauge. Insert a 4-mm cancellous screw through each channel in the usual fashion. The screws are then removed from the medial malleolus.

5. Osteotomize the medial malleolus obliquely from proximal medial to distal lateral to enter the ankle joint at the level of the junction of the medial malleolus with the tibial plafond (Fig. 6).

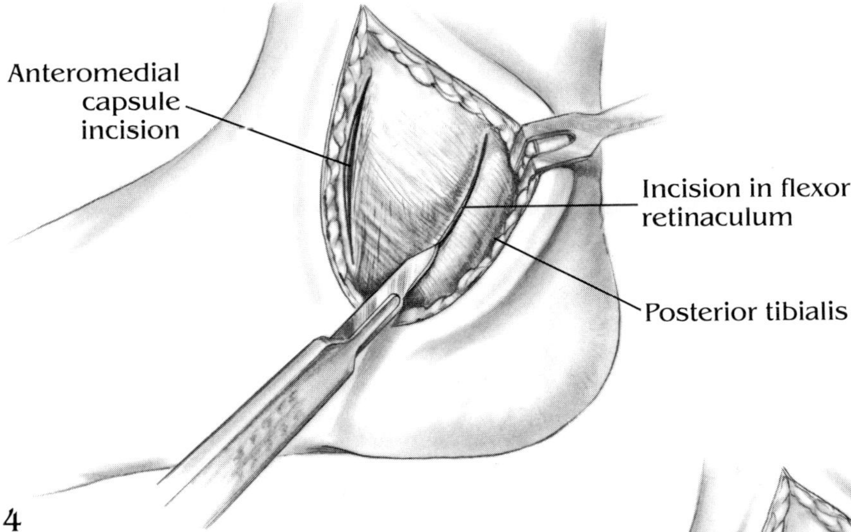
Anteromedial capsule incision
Incision in flexor retinaculum
Posterior tibialis

4

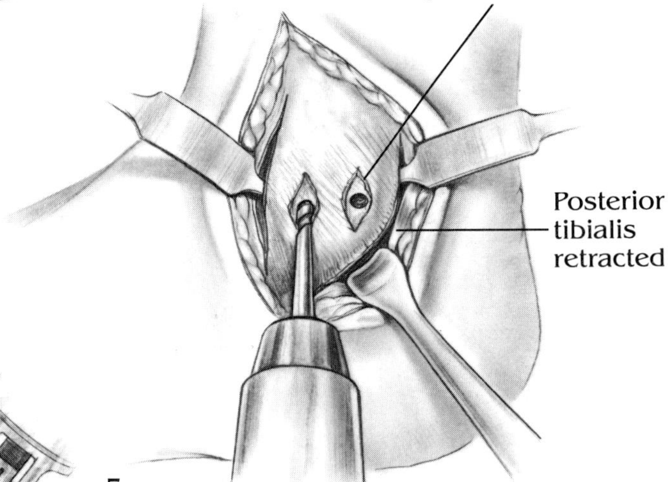
Opened periosteum
Posterior tibialis retracted

5

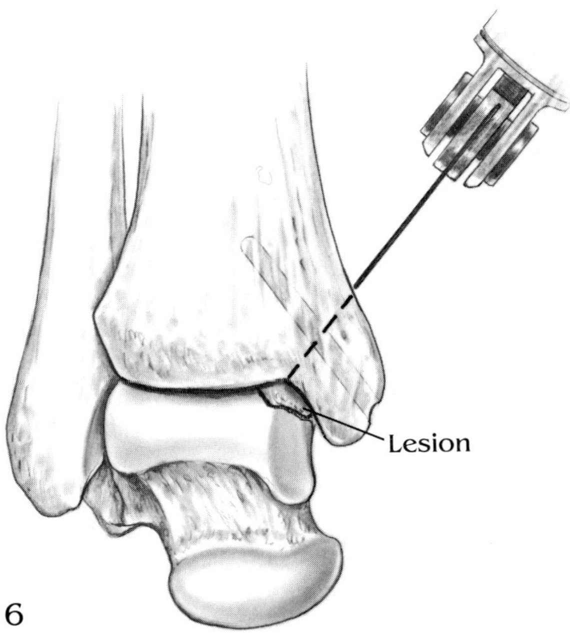
Lesion

6

6. Retract the medial malleolus distally. Evert the ankle to allow exposure of the osteochondral fragment (Fig. 7).
7. Inspect the joint in a systematic fashion. Identify the softened cartilage overlying the osteochondritic lesion, as well as the osteochondral fragment. Remove the fragment by incising the overlying cartilage perpendicular to the subchondral bone (Fig. 8).
8. Curet the osseous bed of the lesion (Fig. 9).
9. Drill 8 to 12 drill holes with a small drill bit or a Kirschner wire in the base of the lesion, deep enough to permit exudation of blood (Fig. 10).
10. Copiously lavage the joint.
11. Reduce the medial malleolus and reinsert the cancellous screws (Fig. 11).
12. Close the ankle joint capsule and dorsal retinaculum with interrupted figure-of-eight 2-0 Vicryl sutures. Close the flexor retinaculum with interrupted figure-of-eight 2-0 Vicryl sutures. Reapproximate subcutaneous tissue with interrupted simple 3-0 Vicryl sutures. Close the skin with interrupted vertical mattress 3-0 nylon sutures.

Postoperative Care

1. A sterile dressing is applied.
2. A Robert Jones compression dressing incorporating a U-shaped plaster splint is applied. An alternative form of immobilization is a well-padded short-leg cast.
3. The patient is maintained non–weight bearing on crutches for 6 weeks or until radiographs reveal union of the medial malleolar osteotomy.
4. A slow, gradual return to weight-bearing activities and normal shoewear is then permitted.

Technical Pitfalls

1. Medial malleolar osteotomy may not be required. Preoperative lateral radiographs with the foot in maximum dorsiflexion and plantarflexion may help in the preoperative planning for the surgical procedure.
2. Care should be taken to position the medial malleolar osteotomy so that the joint is entered at the junction of the malleolus and the tibial plafond. If the osteotomy enters the joint too far distally, osseous overlap may make exposure of the osteochondritis dissecans lesion difficult.
3. The posterior tibial tendon should be identified and retracted to avoid injury during the osteotomy.

Potential Complications

1. Delayed union or nonunion of the medial malleolar osteotomy
2. Progression of arthritis in the ankle joint as a result of chondral damage sustained at the time of the original injury

---

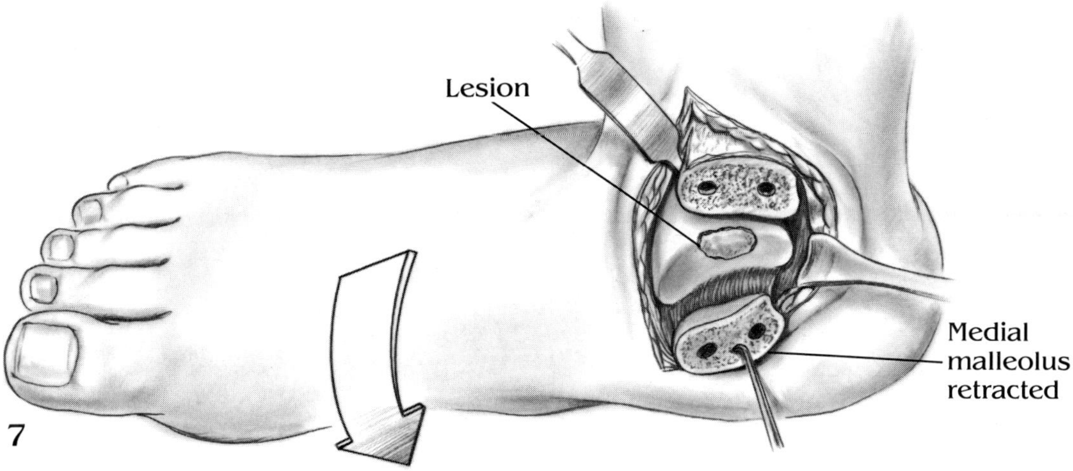

7

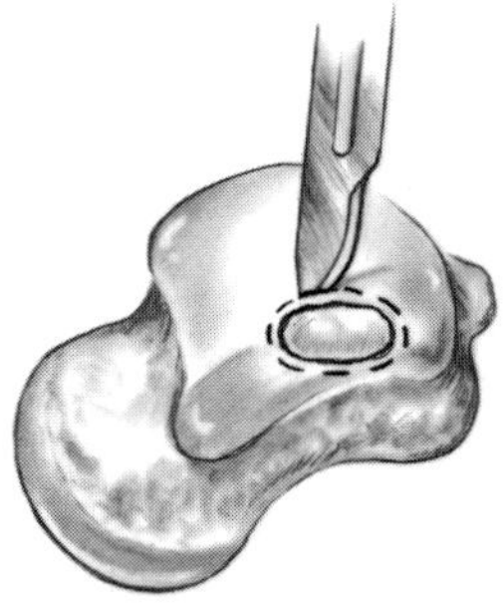

8

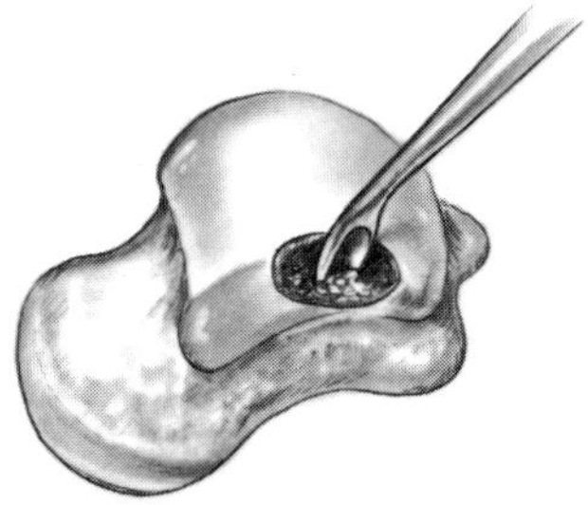

9

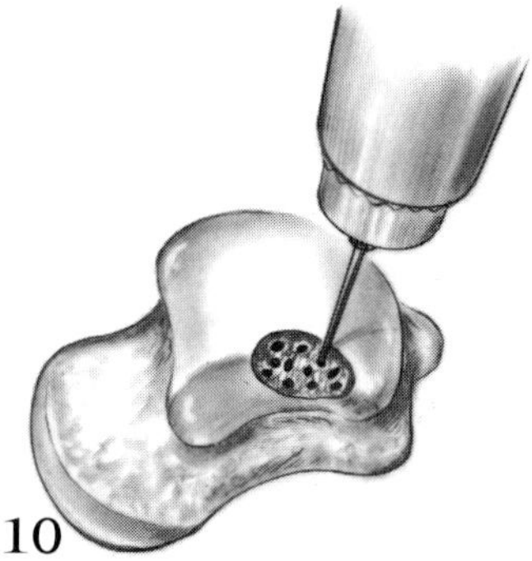

10

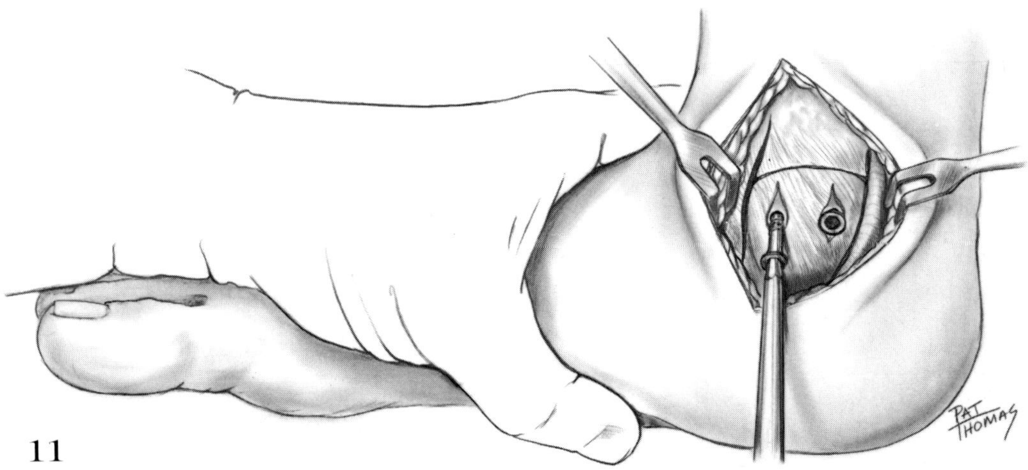

11

PART 23

Operations for Ankle Instability

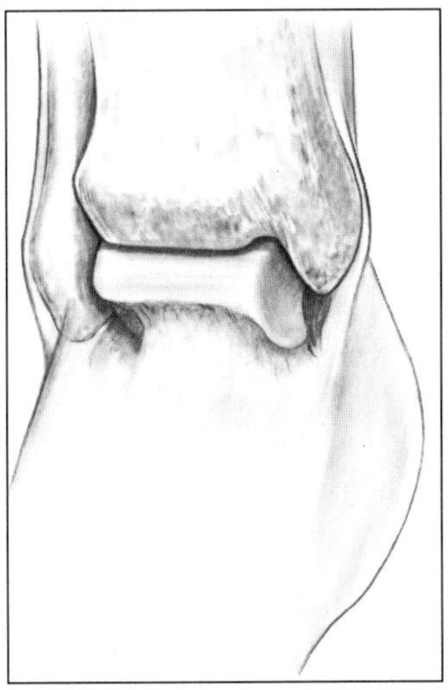

CHRISMAN-SNOOK PROCEDURE

General Considerations

The Chrisman-Snook procedure is utilized for reconstruction of the lateral collateral ligament complex of the ankle. It is an effective technique for patients who present with chronic recurrent instability of the ankle resulting from a severe ankle sprain.

This technique utilizes one half of the peroneus brevis tendon as a substitute for the ruptured anterior talofibular ligament and calcaneofibular ligament. The tendon is routed through drill holes in the fibula and calcaneus and anchored with multiple interrupted absorbable sutures. The distal end of the transplanted tendon graft may be directed to the fibula to reinforce the reconstruction or to the neck of the talus to reconstruct the interosseous talocalcaneal ligament and thus alleviate subtalar instability. This procedure is particularly appropriate in heavy patients who engage in rigorous ambulation and other athletic endeavors. It is most useful in cases in which remnants of the original lateral collateral ligaments are inadequate to allow satisfactory reconstruction by means of a direct repair.

Comparison of the Chrisman-Snook Procedure With Other Reconstruction Techniques

Advantages

1. This procedure provides sturdy reconstruction using local autogenous material.
2. Orientation of the distal end of the tendon graft toward the talar neck may correct concomitant subtalar instability.

Disadvantage. Sacrifice of a portion of the peroneus brevis tendon is required.

Patient Selection

Indications

1. Chronic recurrent instability following inversion twisting injuries after failure of conservative treatment with bracing and physical therapy
2. Young, active patients who engage in rigorous athletic endeavors
3. Combined ankle and subtalar instability

Contraindications

1. The same inversion injury that caused rupture of the lateral collateral ligament complex may result in dislocation of the peroneal tendons with injury to the peroneus longus and brevis. If the peroneus brevis tendon is damaged, alternative techniques of reconstruction may be considered.
2. Older patients with lower activity levels may be better treated with nonoperative methods.
3. The procedure is contraindicated in patients with medical conditions that preclude major reconstructive surgery and general anesthesia.

Surgical Procedure

Operative Technique

1. A lateral longitudinal incision 18 cm long is made. The incision begins 12 cm proximal to the tip of the fibula and extends distally along the posterior margin of the fibula. The incision is curved anteriorly and distally around the tip of the malleolus and extended along the course of the peroneus brevis tendon to end at the level of the insertion of that tendon on the base of the fifth metatarsal (Fig. 1). Subcutaneous tissue is divided along the line of the skin incision. The sural nerve is identified, mobilized, and protected throughout the remainder of the procedure.
2. The skin and subcutaneous tissues are reflected over the anterior aspect of the fibula and the ankle joint. The anterior joint capsule and anterior talofibular ligament are identified (Fig. 1).
3. The peroneal tendon sheath is incised. The peroneus longus tendon is retracted to expose the peroneus brevis tendon. The peroneus brevis tendon is split in half longitudinally as far proximal as possible. It is divided from its insertion on the base of the fifth metatarsal to its musculotendinous junction (Fig. 2). The longest half is transected proximally. Muscle is reflected from the cut end of the tendon stump. The distal end of the tendon graft is left attached at the base of the metatarsal. A stay suture of 1-0 nylon is applied to the proximal end. If the tendon is small, the entire tendon may be utilized and the muscle belly sutured to that of the peroneus longus.

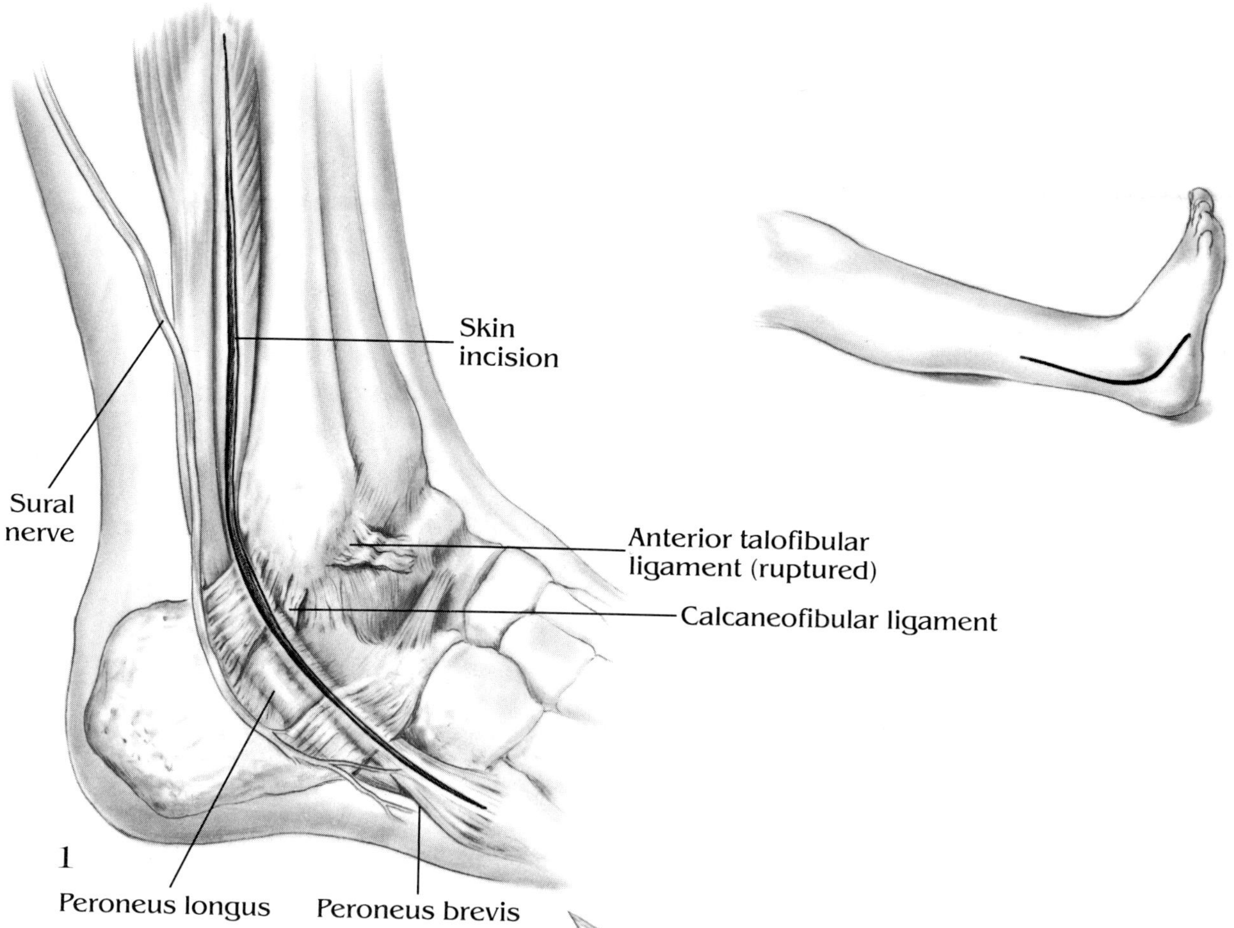
Skin
incision
Sural
nerve
Anterior talofibular
ligament (ruptured)
Calcaneofibular ligament
Peroneus longus
Peroneus brevis

1

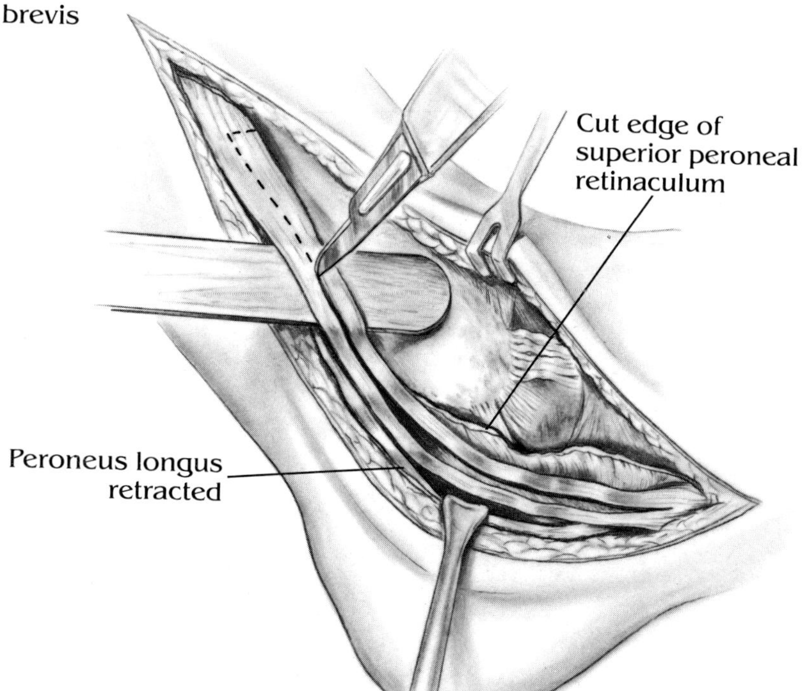
Cut edge of
superior peroneal
retinaculum
Peroneus longus
retracted

2

4. A hole is drilled from anterior to posterior through the fibula at or just proximal to the tibiotalar joint. The hole generally is located approximately 2½ cm proximal to the tip of the fibula. The hole is drilled obliquely from anteroproximal to posterodistal (Fig. 3). The hole is made with a 3.5-mm drill bit and then enlarged with drill bits up to 6 mm in diameter and curets. The tendon graft is passed through the hole in the fibula from anterior to posterior.
5. The lateral aspect of the calcaneus is exposed subperiosteally in the region of attachment of the calcaneofibular ligament. Two oblique drill holes are made 2 cm apart in the calcaneus to create a horizontal tunnel. The drill holes are connected with curets (Fig. 4).

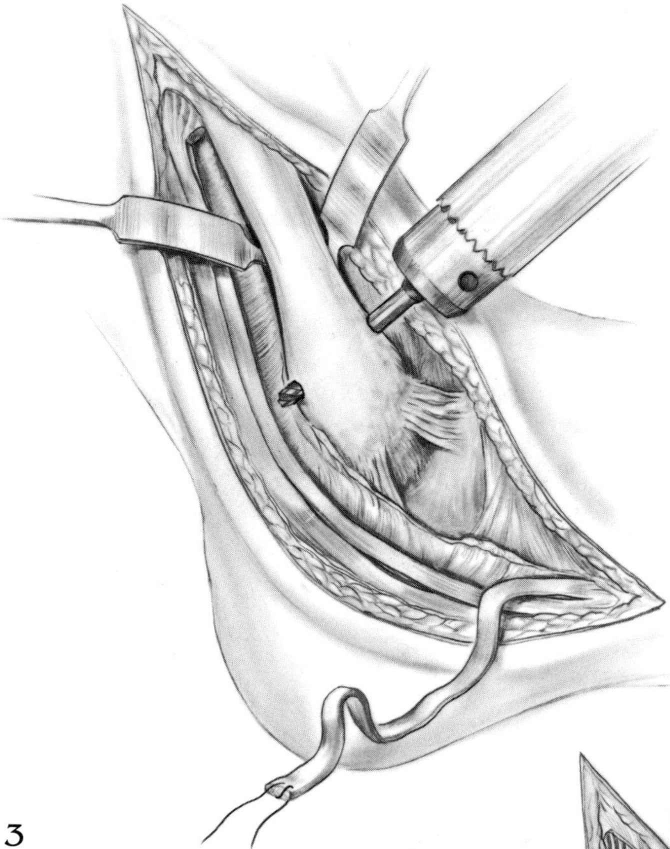

3

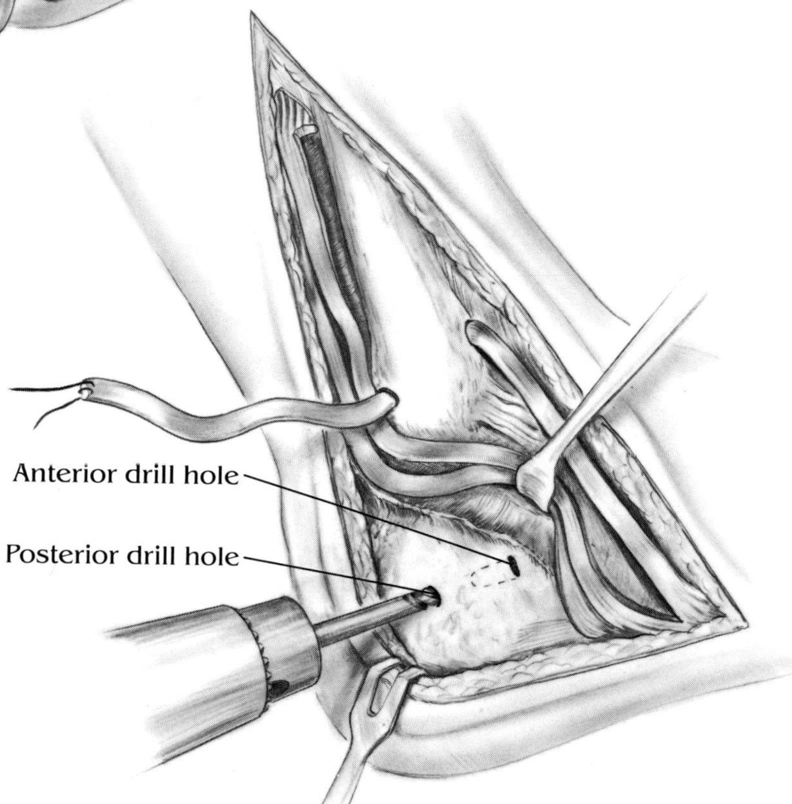

4

6. With the foot held in neutral plantarflexion-dorsiflexion and moderate eversion and the graft held taut, the graft is sutured to the remnant of the anterior talofibular ligament and adjacent periosteum at the talus with interrupted figure-of-eight 1-0 Dexon sutures. The graft is then sutured to the periosteum surrounding the anterior and posterior drill holes in the fibula with interrupted figure-of-eight 1-0 Dexon sutures (Fig. 5).
7. The peroneal tendons are returned to the fibular groove. The tendon graft is passed through the horizontal tunnel in the calcaneus from posterior to anterior, superficial to the peroneal tendons. The graft is pulled taut and sutured to the periosteum at the ends of the tunnel with interrupted figure-of-eight 1-0 Dexon sutures (Fig. 6).
8. The remaining graft may be passed back to the anterior portion of the graft at the anterior end of the fibular tunnel to reinforce reconstruction of the calcaneofibular ligament (Fig. 7). If subtalar instability is suspected, the remaining graft may be passed back to the neck of the talus and sutured to the periosteum overlying this region with interrupted figure-of-eight 1-0 Dexon sutures.
9. Hemostasis is obtained. The peroneal sheath is closed with interrupted figure-of-eight 2-0 Vicryl sutures. Subcutaneous tissue is reapproximated with interrupted simple 3-0 Vicryl sutures. The skin is closed with interrupted vertical mattress 3-0 nylon sutures.

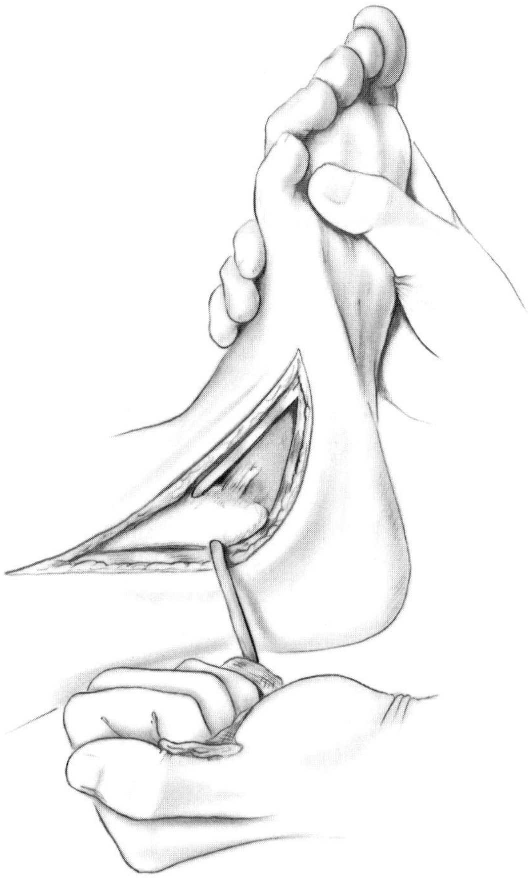

5

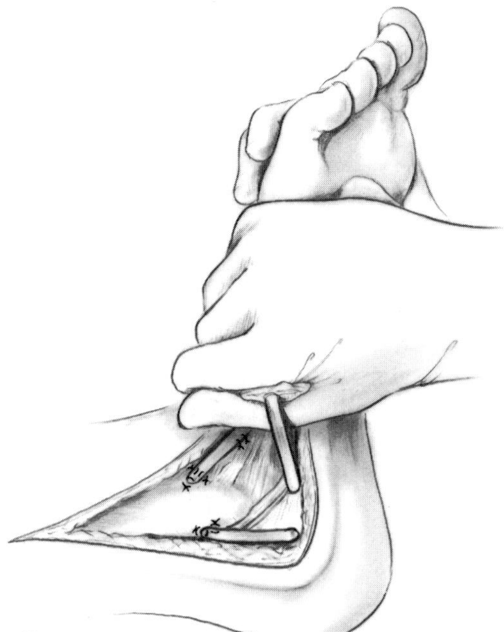

6

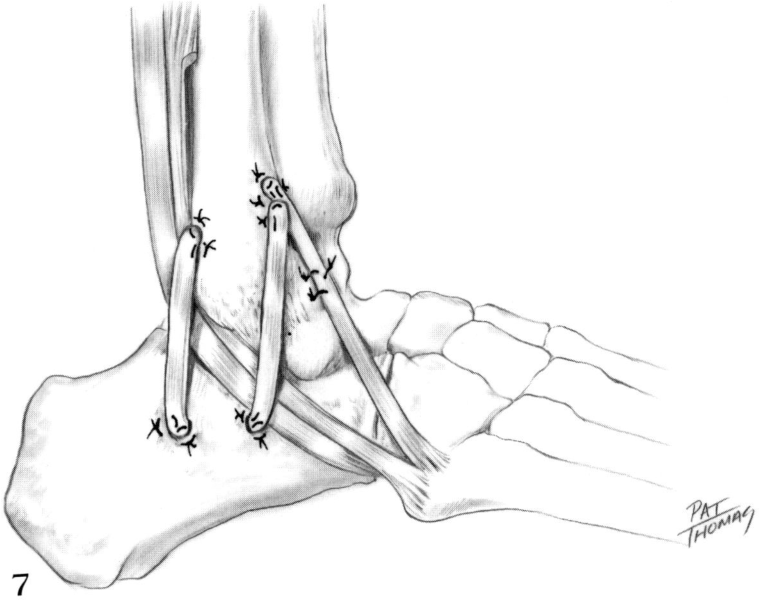

7

Postoperative Care

1. A sterile dressing is applied. A short-leg cast is applied with the foot in neutral plantarflexion-dorsiflexion and moderate eversion.
2. The sutures are removed and the cast is changed 3 weeks after surgery.
3. The patient is maintained non–weight bearing on crutches for 6 weeks after surgery.
4. After removal of the cast, the patient is allowed a slow, gradual return to weight-bearing activities in an air splint. Patients are instructed to continue non–weight bearing on crutches for 2 weeks, followed by partial weight bearing on crutches for 2 weeks, followed by full weight bearing on crutches for 2 weeks.
5. The patient may then begin ambulation with a cane.
6. A lace-up ankle brace is utilized for weight-bearing activities for up to 1 year after surgery to protect the reconstruction.

Technical Pitfalls

1. Care must be taken not to disrupt the portion of the peroneus brevis to be used as a tendon graft while splitting it longitudinally.
2. Care must be taken to avoid fracture of the cortical bone when preparing the fibular and calcaneal tunnels.
3. Excessive eversion while anchoring the graft in place may lead to residual excessive eversion and associated pain after surgery.
4. Excessive plantar flexion of the ankle during suture of the graft may result in limitation of dorsiflexion.

Complications

1. Dysesthesias in the area of the sural nerve distribution may result from swelling or scarring of the sural nerve.
2. Rerupture or attenuation of the reconstructed ligament may occur.
3. Concomitant pathologic disorders may lead to residual symptoms after ligamentous reconstruction. Ankle arthrotomy should be performed routinely during ligamentous reconstruction. Intraoperative evaluation should enable identification of intra-articular loose bodies, osteochondral fractures of the talus, impingement lesions, rupture or attenuation of the peroneal retinaculum, and injury to the peroneal tendons. If these problems are noted, appropriate surgical correction should be performed at the time of ligamentous reconstruction.
4. Loss of motion at the ankle joint may occur secondary to scarring.

BROSTRUM PROCEDURE

General Considerations

Chronic recurrent instability of the ankle is a possible sequela of a severe ankle sprain. A significant inversion injury to the ankle may result in rupture of the anterior talofibular, as well as the calcaneofibular, ligament. If the torn ligaments heal inadequately or in an elongated fashion, recurrent instability may result.

Patients describe repetitive inversion twisting injuries that may be associated with pain and swelling of the lateral ankle. Patients note a sensation of "giving way," which may occur with ambulation on uneven ground. Physical evaluation elicits tenderness over the anterior talofibular and possibly the calcaneofibular ligament. Results of an anterior drawer test may be positive. Stress radiographs taken with a local anesthetic may aid visualization of a "talar tilt" or "anterior drawer." Arthrography and magnetic resonance imaging of the ankle may help identify which ligaments are torn.

Initial treatment includes the use of a brace that prevents excessive inversion of the ankle. This device is utilized during rigorous ambulation and recreational activities. Strengthening exercises of the muscle-tendon units about the ankle, with special emphasis on the peroneal muscles, are instituted. If conservative treatment fails to prevent recurrent twisting injuries, surgical intervention may be considered.

Operative intervention consists of reconstruction of the lateral collateral ligament complex. A multitude of surgical techniques have been described in the orthopedic literature. One of the more useful surgical procedures is the modified Brostrum operation, which consists of imbrication of the remnants of the torn ligaments. Reinforcement by means of advancement of the extensor retinaculum has proved advantageous. The same inversion injury that leads to rupture of the lateral collateral ligaments may also lead to other pathologic disorders of the ankle. Physical examination and radiographic tests must be utilized to identify concomitant problems. Subluxating peroneal tendons, tears of the peroneus longus and brevis, osteochondral fractures of the talus, and impingement lesions of the ankle joint must be identified preoperatively and may be addressed surgically at the time of the ligamentous reconstruction.

Comparison of the Brostrum Procedure With Other Reconstruction Techniques

Advantages

1. This procedure allows anatomic re-creation of the lateral collateral ligament complex.
2. This technique avoids sacrifice of an adjacent tendon, which is often required in other techniques.
3. The use of autogenous soft tissue from other areas is not required.

Disadvantages

1. This technique may not be appropriate if prior inversion injuries have led to very significant attenuation or even absence of a remnant of the lateral collateral ligament complex. In this situation the available soft tissue may not be adequate to perform this procedure.
2. Patients who suffer from combined ankle and subtalar instability may be better served with a different type of reconstruction, such as the Chrisman-Snook procedure.

Patient Selection

Indications

1. Chronic recurrent twisting injuries that interfere with the patient's ability to ambulate and engage in other activities
2. Chronic recurrent instability that fails to respond to bracing and physical therapy

Contraindications

1. The procedure is contraindicated in patients with medical conditions that preclude the risks of operative intervention and general anesthesia.
2. Voluntary habitual dislocation accompanied by severe ligamentous laxity may be associated with a high recurrence rate after operative intervention.

Surgical Procedure

Operative Technique

1. A lateral longitudinal incision is made, beginning 8 cm proximal to the tip of the lateral malleolus and extending along the posterior margin of the fibula to the tip of the malleolus. The incision is then extended distally and anteriorly along the course of the peroneus brevis tendon to end just proximal to its insertion at the base of the fifth metatarsal (Fig. 1). Subcutaneous tissue is incised along the line of the skin incision. The sural nerve is identified, mobilized, and protected throughout the remainder of the procedure.
2. The skin and subcutaneous tissues are reflected anteriorly to expose the anterior talofibular ligament and the anterior ankle joint capsule. The extensor retinaculum is mobilized and tagged with a suture.
3. The peroneal tendon sheath is incised, and the peroneal tendons are mobilized (Fig. 2). The tendons are evaluated for damage, and the peroneal retinaculum is examined for possible attenuation associated with tendon subluxation. The underlying calcaneofibular ligament is identified.
4. The anterior ankle joint capsule is incised longitudinally, leaving a stump of capsule attached to the fibula for later repair. The ankle joint is explored in a systematic fashion. Loose bodies, chondral fragments, and impingement lesions are identified and treated accordingly (Fig. 3).

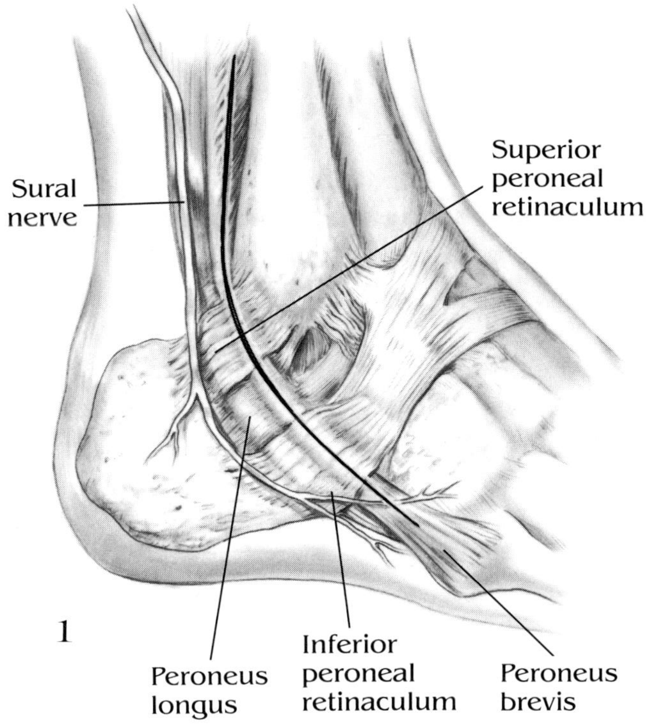
Sural nerve
Superior peroneal retinaculum
Peroneus longus
Inferior peroneal retinaculum
Peroneus brevis
1

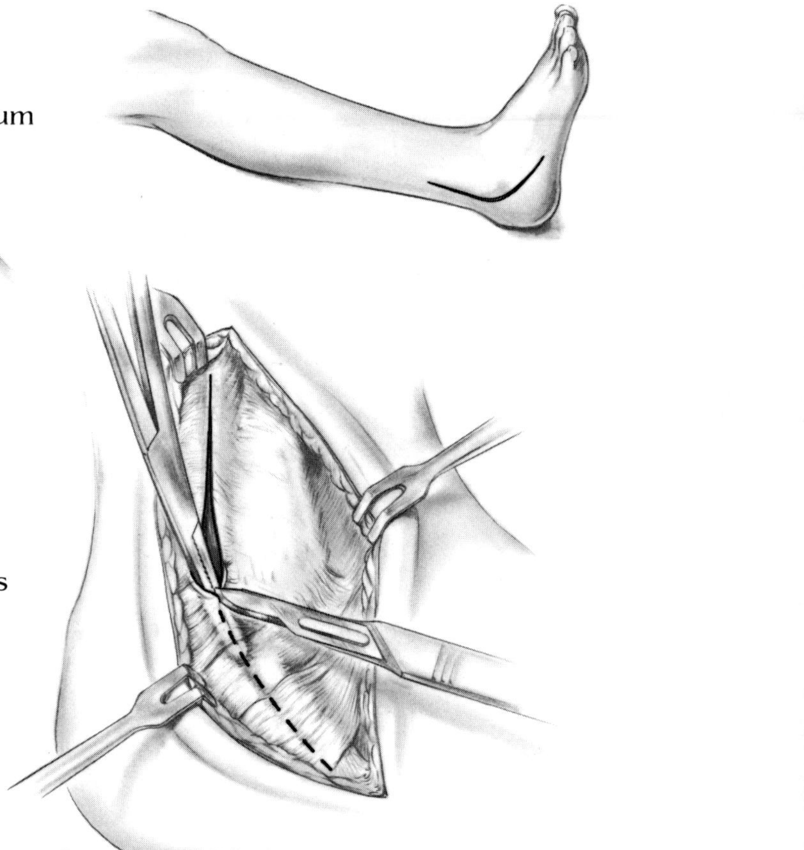
2

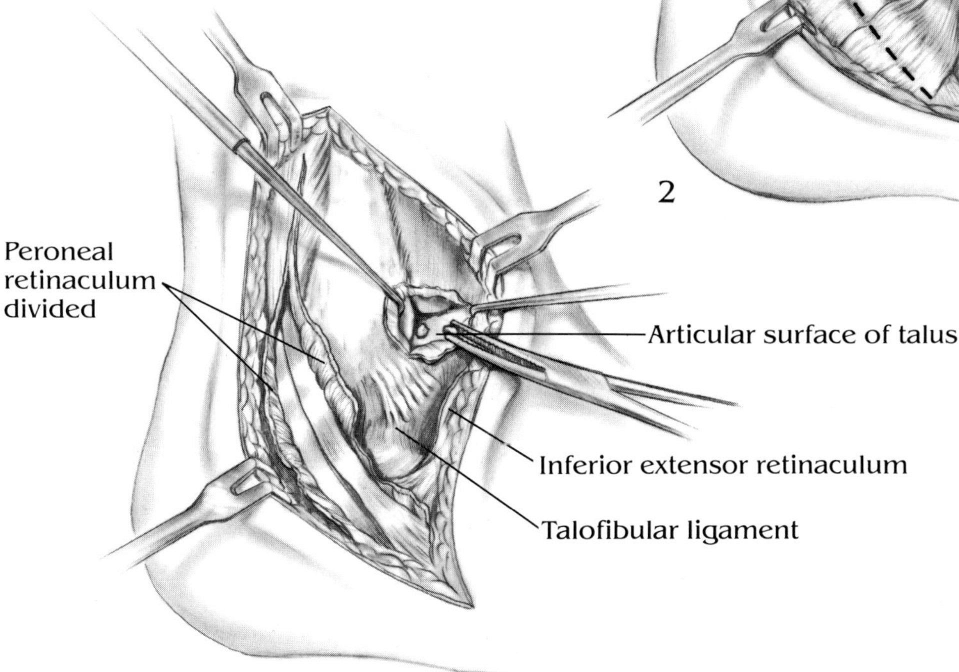
Peroneal retinaculum divided
Articular surface of talus
Inferior extensor retinaculum
Talofibular ligament
3

5. A clamp is passed under the anterior talofibular and calcaneofibular ligament. The soft tissue in this region, including the remnants of those ligaments, is divided in half over the clamp (Fig. 4).
6. Reconstruction of the calcaneofibular ligament, the anterior talofibular ligament, and the anterior ankle joint capsule is performed sequentially by means of imbrication in a vest-over-pants fashion (Fig. 5a). The distal stump is sutured to the undersurface of the base of the proximal stump with interrupted horizontal box sutures of 1-0 Dexon (Fig. 5b). The calcaneofibular ligament is repaired, followed by repair of the anterior talofibular ligament and then the anterior joint capsule. All sutures are inserted and then tied from posterior to anterior while holding the foot in neutral plantarflexion-dorsflexion and moderate eversion. The foot is held in this position throughout the remainder of the procedure.
7. The proximal stump is then sutured to the base of the distal stump with interrupted figure-of-eight sutures of 1-0 Dexon. This technique of imbrication allows tightening and doubling in thickness of the lateral collateral ligament and anterior joint capsule (Figs. 6a and 6b).

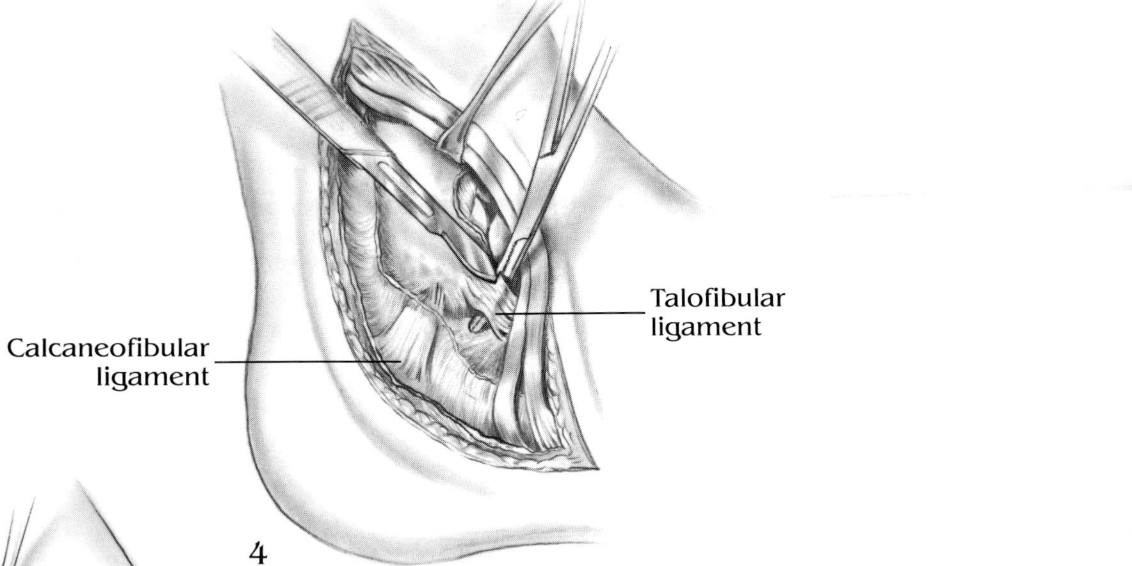

4

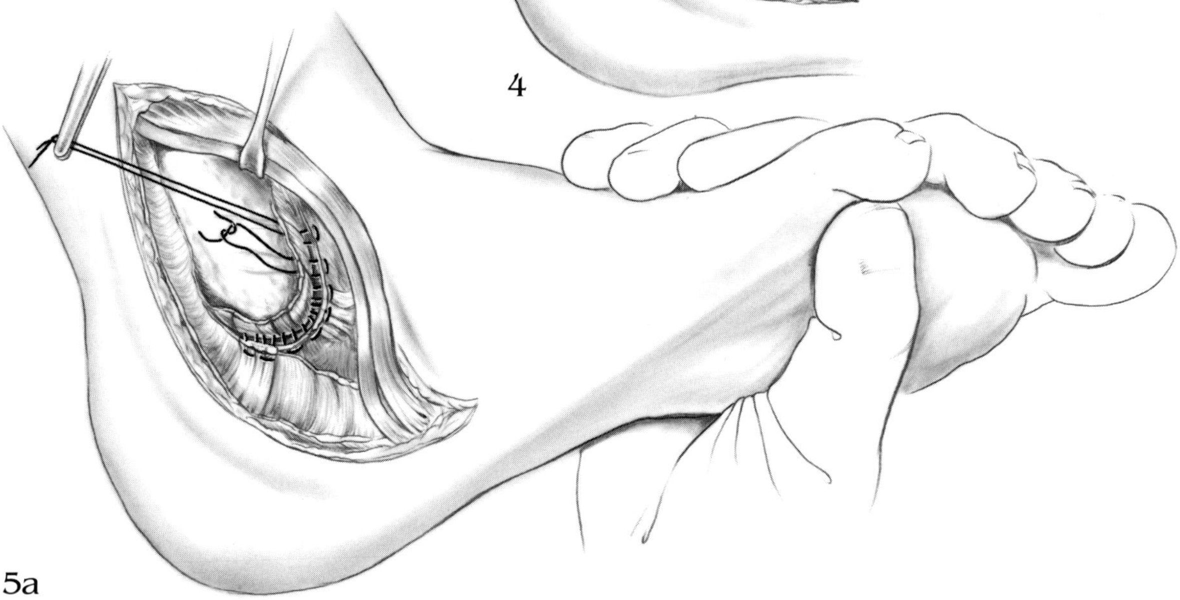

5a

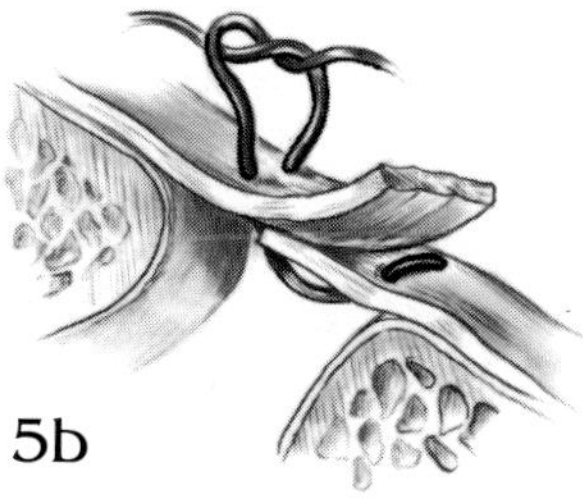

5b

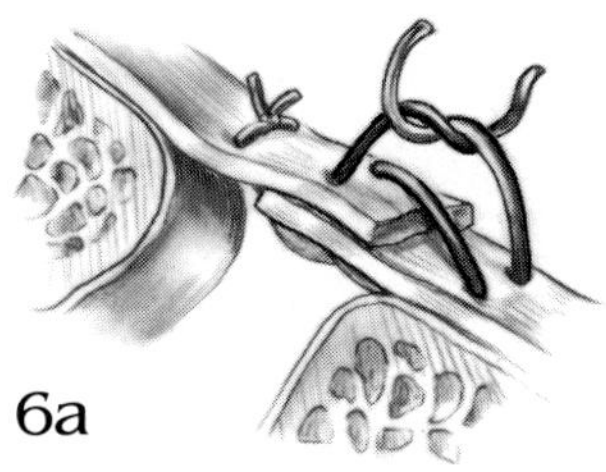

6a

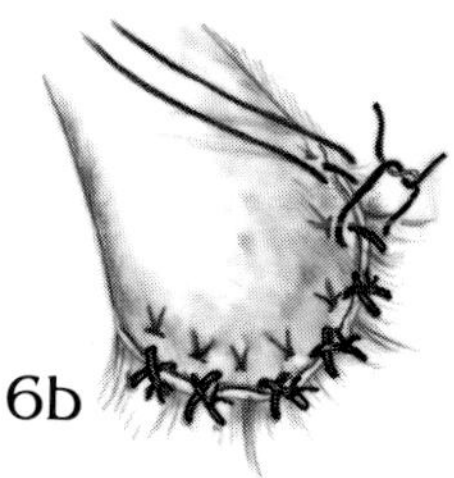

6b

8. The extensor retinaculum is mobilized and advanced. This structure is sutured to the periosteum overlying the fibula with interrupted figure-of-eight 2-0 Dexon sutures. This provides reinforcement of the ligamentous reconstruction (Fig. 7).
9. The peroneal tendons are returned to the peroneal groove behind the fibula. If intraoperative evaluation indicates attenuation of the peroneal retinaculum, this structure may be imbricated in a manner similar to that used for the lateral collateral ligament. The distal stump is sutured to the undersurface of the base of the proximal stump on the fibula with interrupted horizontal box sutures of 2-0 Dexon. The proximal stump is sutured to the distal stump with interrupted figure-of-eight 2-0 Dexon sutures (Fig. 8).
10. Subcutaneous tissue is reapproximated with interrupted simple 3-0 Vicryl sutures. The skin is closed with interrupted vertical mattress 3-0 nylon sutures (Fig. 9).

Postoperative Care

1. A sterile dressing is applied. A well-padded short-leg cast is applied with the foot in neutral dorsiflexion plantarflexion and moderate eversion.
2. The sutures are removed, and a new cast is applied 3 weeks after surgery.
3. The patient is kept non–weight bearing on crutches for 6 weeks.
4. The patient is then allowed a slow, gradual, progressive return to weight-bearing activity in an air splint.
5. Patients are instructed to wear a lace-up ankle brace during weight-bearing activities for 1 year after the surgery to protect the repair.

Technical Pitfalls

1. Care must be taken to identify, mobilize, and protect the sural nerve.
2. Adequate intraoperative examination will identify other concomitant causes of symptoms associated with inversion injuries of the ankle. These pathologic disorders must be addressed at the time of surgery, as failure to do so may lead to residual symptoms.

Complications

1. Reinjury may lead to rupture of the reconstructed ligamentous complex.
2. Attenuation of the reconstruction may occur with time. Patients are cautioned to utilize a lace-up ankle brace for recreational athletic activities to protect the repair.

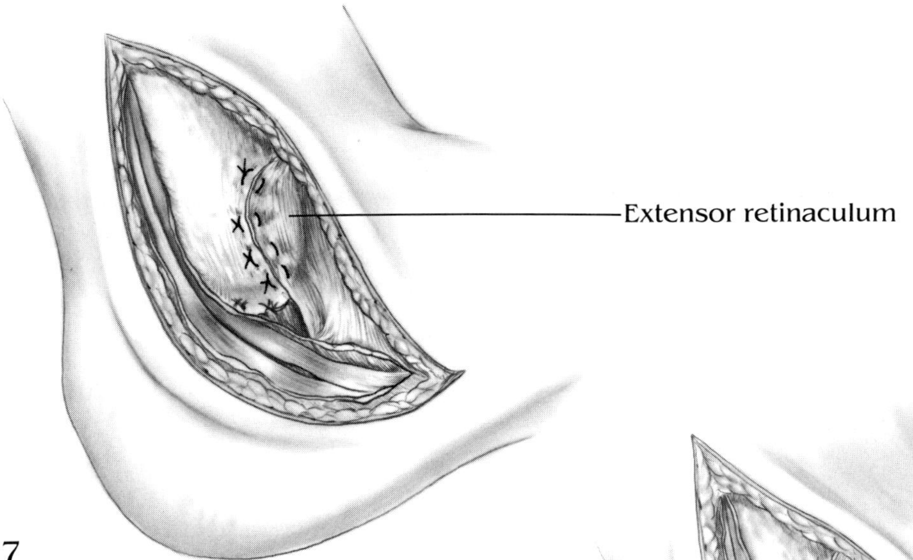

7

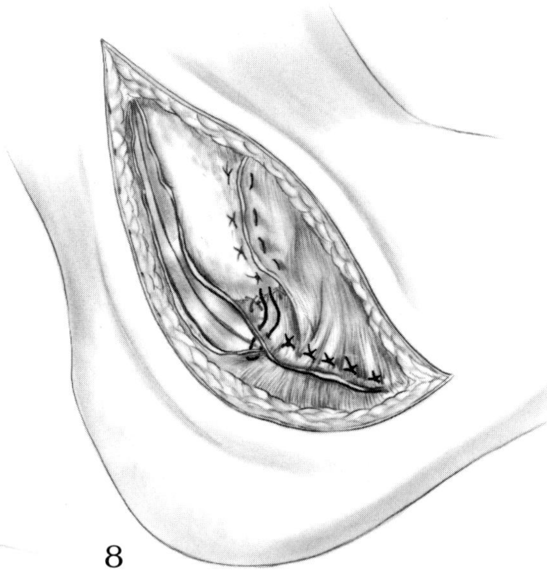

8

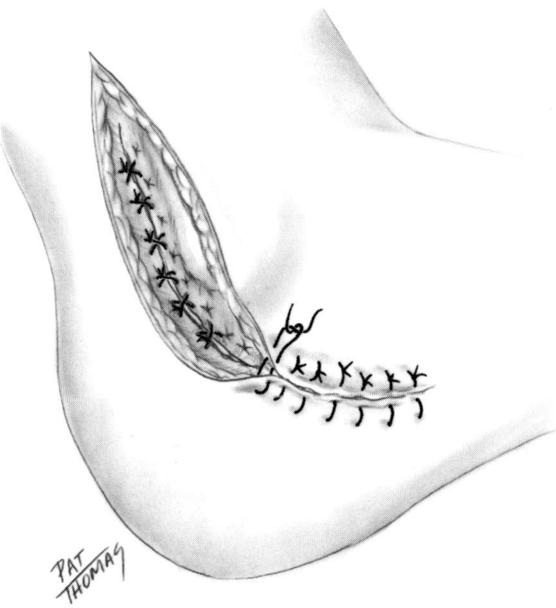

9

PART 24

Operations for Disorders of the Tendons

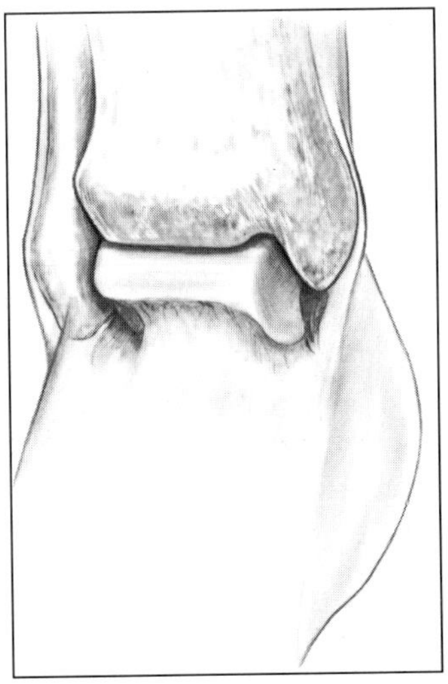

REPAIR RUPTURE ACHILLES TENDON

General Considerations

Rupture of the Achilles tendon is one of the most common tendon injuries about the ankle. This injury is typically found in a poorly conditioned middle-aged man engaged in intermittent athletic activities. It typically occurs during push-off with the knee extended or when landing from a leap with the foot in dorsiflexion. In addition, a direct blow to the tendon may cause rupture.

Clinical manifestations include pain, swelling, a palpable gap in the Achilles tendon, and weak or absent plantarflexion of the foot. The Thompson test is positive in complete ruptures, in which case the foot will not plantarflex when the calf muscle is squeezed.

There has been considerable controversy with regard to optimum treatment. Numerous authors advocate cast immobilization with the foot in plantarflexion. There has also been considerable enthusiasm for surgical repair, which is thought to provide the patient with increased strength, endurance, and power. In general, nonoperative care should be reserved for elderly patients who are not involved in strenuous activities. Surgical reapproximation with reinforcement provides optimum opportunity for return to activities in the young athletic patient. The primary technique described involves direct repair of the tendon combined with reinforcement using the plantaris tendon.

Patient Selection

Indications

1. Acute rupture of the Achilles tendon
2. Young, active patients who engage in strenuous activities

Contraindications

1. Elderly patients not involved in rigorous weight-bearing activities
2. General medical conditions that preclude operative intervention

Surgical Procedure

Positioning of the Patient

The patient is placed in the prone position on the operating room table. A bolster is placed under the leg just proximal to the ankle joint.

Operative Technique

1. A straight posterolateral longitudinal incision is made 1 cm lateral to the margin of the Achilles tendon. The incision extends from 10 cm proximal to the tendon insertion to 1 cm distal to the insertion of the tendon on the os calcis (Fig. 1).
2. Subcutaneous tissue is divided along the line of the skin incision. The sural nerve is identified, mobilized, and retracted laterally.
3. The tendon is visualized. The frayed edges are resected minimally. The tendon is repaired with a reinforcing technique using the plantaris tendon, if available. The plantaris tendon is detached as far proximally as possible. The plantaris tendon stump is placed on a large, curved needle (Fig. 2).

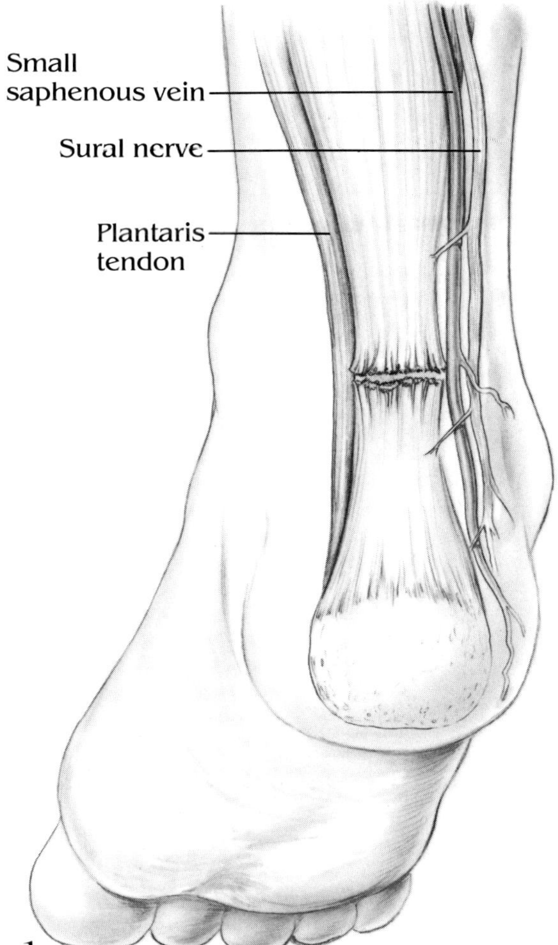

1

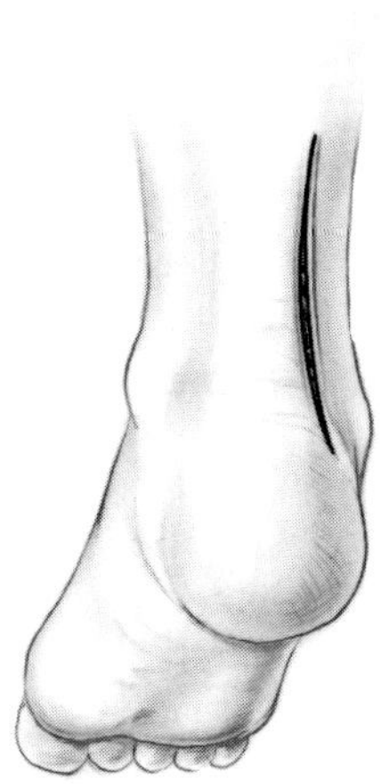

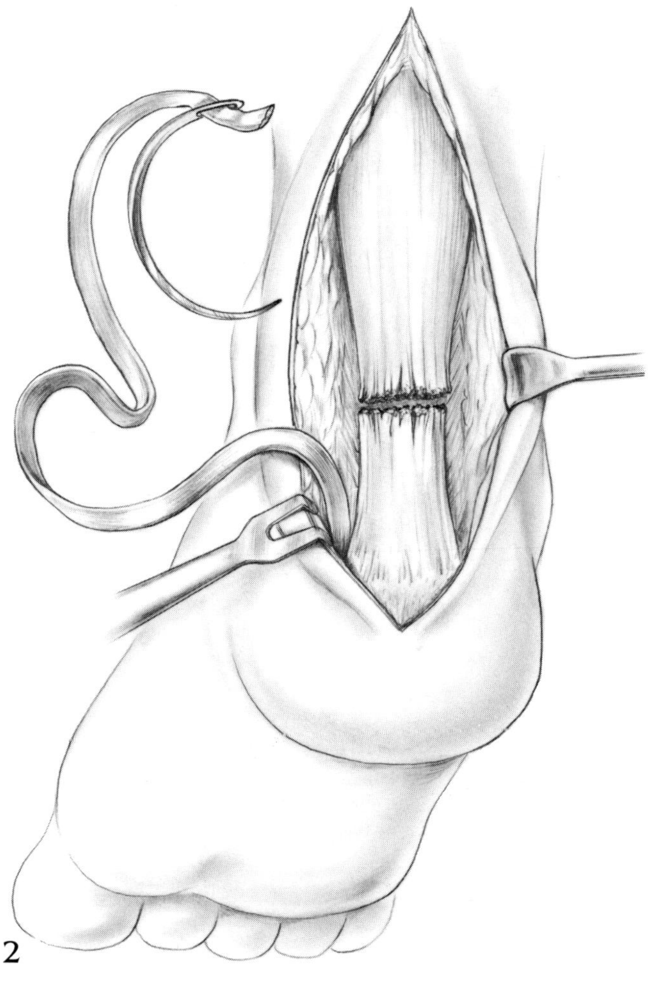

2

4. The plantaris tendon is then woven from medial to lateral through the proximal segment of the Achilles tendon and from lateral to medial through the distal segment (Fig. 3).
5. Tension is applied to approximate the tendon ends with the foot in equinus. The plantaris tendon is sutured at intervals to the Achilles tendon and then onto itself with 2-0 Dexon sutures (Fig. 4).
6. The Achilles tendon ends are reapproximated with absorbable figure-of-eight sutures to complete the repair (Fig. 4).
7. The tourniquet is deflated, hemostasis secured, and the wound closed in layers. Subcutaneous tissues are reapproximated with interrupted simple 3-0 Vicryl sutures. The skin is closed with interrupted vertical mattress 3-0 nylon sutures.

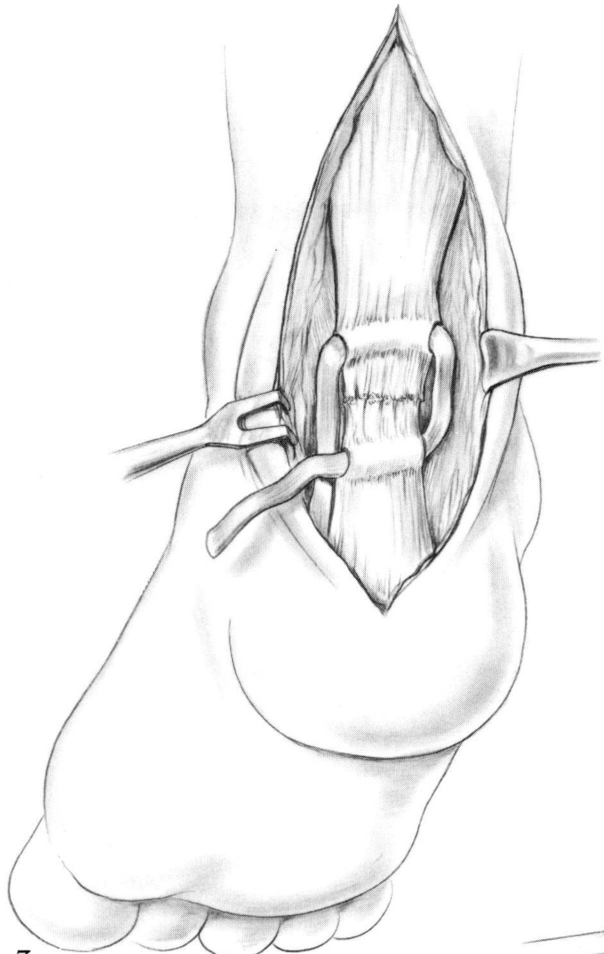

3

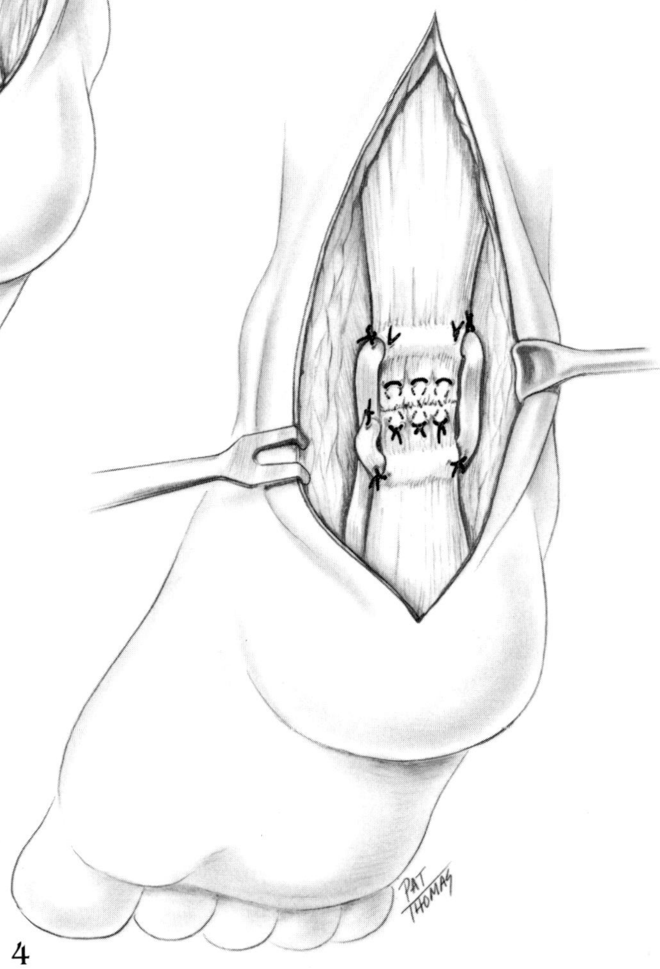

4

Alternative Surgical Repair

1. If the plantaris is not available, the tendon is repaired using a modified Kessler box suture of 1 Dexon (Fig. 5a).
2. If the tendon ends are well preserved, direct repair is then completed using absorbable figure-of-eight sutures of 1-0 Dexon to reapproximate the rupture site (Fig. 5b).
3. If the tendon ends are markedly damaged or reveal pathologic changes indicative of chronic recurrent degeneration, the repair is reinforced with a turn-down flap from the proximal aspect of the Achilles tendon. An aponeurotic flap 1.5 cm wide and long enough to cover the site of repair is created (Fig. 6a).
4. The flap is turned down and anchored in position with interrupted absorbable sutures of 2-0 Dexon. The resultant proximal defect is closed with simple interrupted absorbable sutures (Fig. 6b).

Postoperative Care

1. The patient is placed in a long-leg cast with the knee in 20 degrees of flexion and the foot in moderate plantarflexion. The patient is kept non–weight bearing on crutches.
2. The long-leg cast is removed in 6 weeks and replaced with a short-leg cast with the foot in equinus.
3. At 4 to 6 weeks the short-leg cast is removed, and the patient is allowed a slow, gradual return to weight-bearing activities.
4. The patient is instructed to wear a shoe with a 1½-inch heel. This heel height is decreased by ¼-inch increments every 2 weeks until the foot is plantigrade.

Technical Pitfalls

1. The sural nerve must be identified and protected throughout the entire operative procedure.
2. The use of absorbable sutures may help avoid the complications of wound necrosis and infection that are commonly associated with this procedure.
3. Prolonged cast immobilization and a slow, gradual return to activities may help avoid rerupture.

Potential Complications

1. Wound necrosis, superficial infection, and deep infection may occur in up to 15% of cases. Meticulous attention to operative technique may help avoid this problem. The patient should be forewarned of the possibility of wound healing problems.
2. Sural nerve injury or entrapment may occur after surgery.
3. Excessive tendon scarring may occur. Adherence of the overlying skin is possible. If the plantaris tendon is utilized for reinforcement, the remnant of the tendon may be unravelled and applied over the repair site to provide a smooth gliding surface.
4. Although more commonly seen after conservative treatment with cast immobilization, rerupture may also occur after surgical repair.

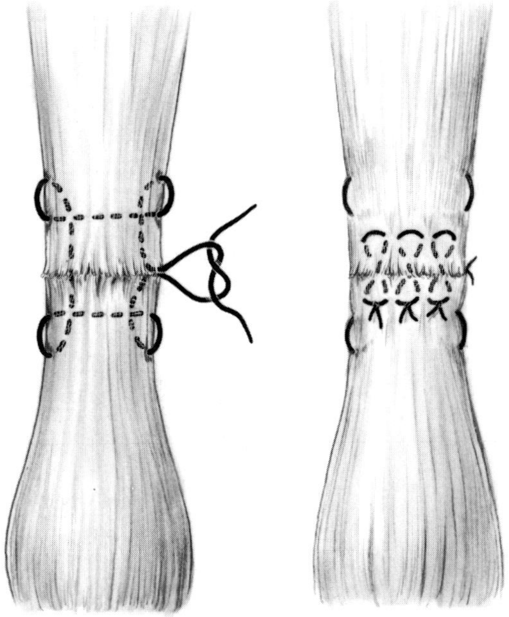

5a 5b

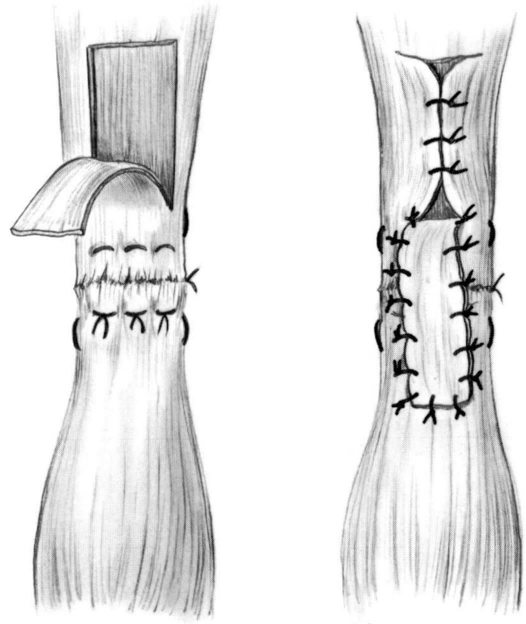

6a 6b

REPAIR RUPTURE POSTERIOR TIBIAL TENDON

General Considerations

Dysfunction of the posterior tibial tendon is thought to be one of the most common tendon disorders about the ankle. Chronic inflammation, degenerative changes, and trauma lead to synovitis, attrition, attentuation, and rupture of the tendon posterior and distal to the medial malleolus.

Women more than 40 years of age are most often affected and present with pain at the medial aspect of the ankle, swelling along the course of the tendon, progressive pronation deformity of the foot, and instability with ambulation. Physical examination reveals valgus deflection of the heel, loss in height of the medial longitudinal arch, and abduction of the forefoot at the Chopart joint. The patient has swelling and tenderness along the course of the tendon. Active inversion of the foot against resistance is weak and painful. Radiographs reveal the deformity. Tenograms and magnetic resonance imaging scans may help evaluate the tendon pathology.

A medial sole and heel wedge and an arch support may relieve stress on the tendon during the stance phase of gait. If conservative measures fail, surgical intervention may be appropriate. The specific type of repair is dependent on the specific pathology encountered at the time of surgery.

Patient Selection and Preoperative Planning

Indications for Various Procedures

1. If the synovium is hypertrophic, a synovectomy is performed.
2. The most common pathologic abnormality seen is a necrotic portion of tendon posterior and distal to the medial malleolus, evidenced by discoloration, attenuation, and longitudinal rents (see Fig. 1a). This area may be excised and the remaining tendon repaired in an end-to-end fashion. This repair is reinforced by means of a side-to-side anastomosis to the adjacent flexor digitorum longus tendon.
3. If a large gap is present, the nonviable ends are resected, and side-to-side anastomosis to the flexor digitorum longus tendon is performed.
4. If the tendon is torn off its insertion into the navicular tuberosity, nonviable tissue is resected, and the tendon is advanced and reinserted into the navicular bone by means of anchoring sutures or by passing the tendon through a drill hole and suturing it to itself.
5. Transfer of the flexor digitorum longus tendon through a drill hole in the navicular has been described and may be required if the distal aspect of the posterior tibial tendon is absent.
6. Severe deformity with hindfoot subluxation may require isolated arthrodesis of the subtalar or talonavicular joints alone or in conjunction with tendon repair.
7. Arthritis of the articulations of the hindfoot secondary to long-standing deformity may require isolated subtalar arthrodesis or triple arthrodesis with or without tendon repair.

Contraindications

1. Elderly debilitated patients may get satisfactory relief with conservative measures.
2. Surgical correction is contraindicated in patients with medical conditions that increase the risks of surgery and anesthesia.
3. Patients with peripheral neuropathy or peripheral vascular disease may have an increased risk of infection and problems with wound healing.
4. Once arthritic changes have occurred in the hindfoot, arthrodesis of the involved joints is required to eliminate symptoms.

Surgical Procedure

Operative Technique

1. A medial longitudinal incision is made, beginning 10 cm proximal to the tip of the medial malleolus and 1 cm posterior to the medial subcutaneous border of the tibia. Extend the incision distally along the medial tibial margin to the tip of the malleolus. Continue anteriorly and distally along the course of the posterior tibial tendon to end at the navicular tuberosity (Fig. 1). Incise subcutaneous tissue along the line of the skin incision and reflect to expose the tendon sheath.
2. Incise the sheath longitudinally (Fig. 2). Mobilize the tendon along its course.
3. Identify the site and extent of the rupture (Fig. 3).
4. If the synovium is hypertrophic, excise by sharp dissection with a scalpel and dissecting scissors.

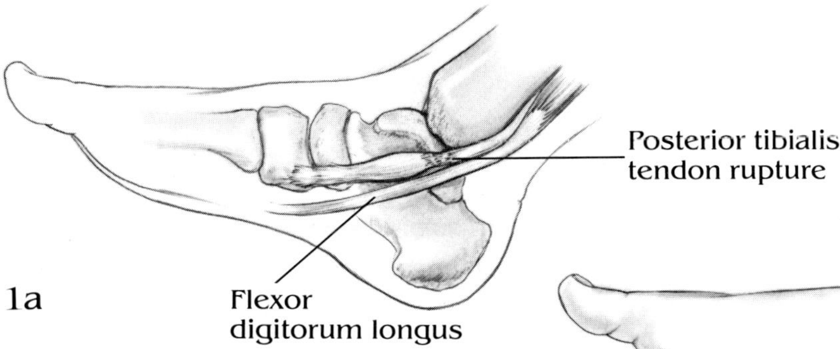
Posterior tibialis
tendon rupture
Flexor
digitorum longus

1a

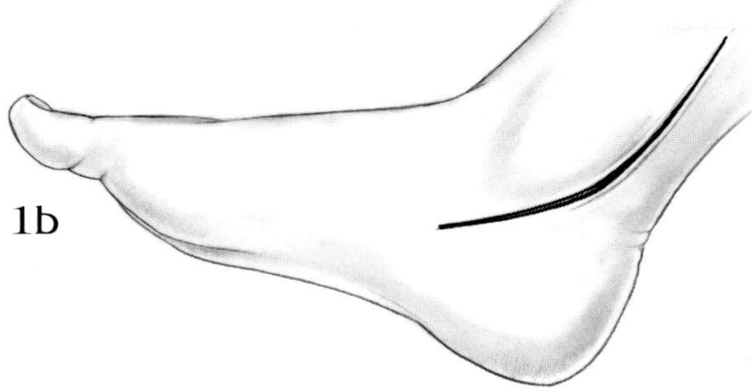

1b

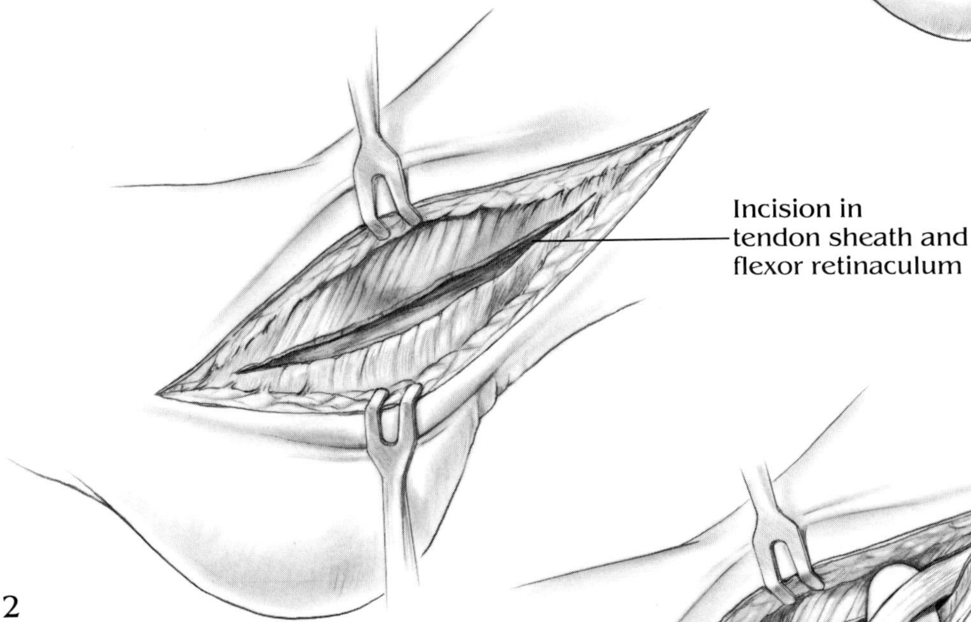
Incision in
tendon sheath and
flexor retinaculum

2

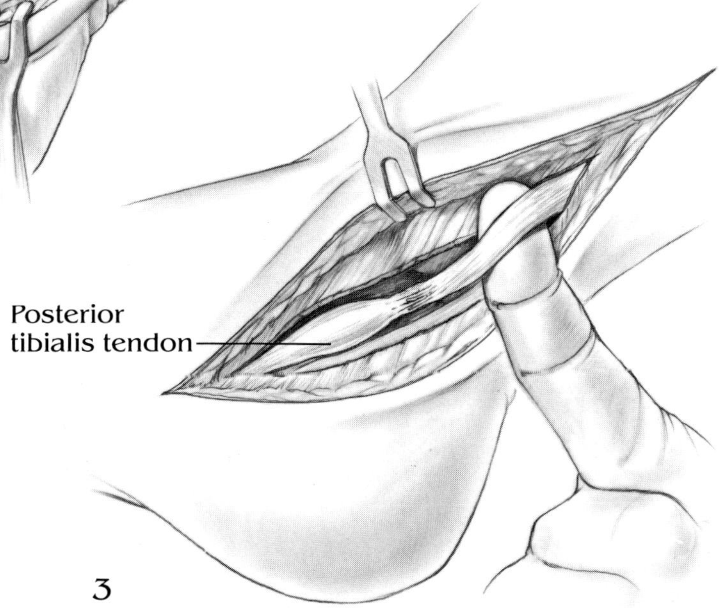
Posterior
tibialis tendon

3

5. In the most common situation, a necrotic segment of particularly discolored, attenuated, and damaged tendon is identified posterior and distal to the malleolus. This segment, or a portion of it, is excised sharply with a scalpel or razor blade (Fig. 4).
6. The proximal and distal stumps are reapproximated with a modified Kessler box suture of 1 nylon while holding the foot in plantarflexion and inversion (Figs. 5a and 5b).
7. The repair site is reinforced with interrupted buried simple sutures of 2-0 nylon (Figs. 5c and 5d).

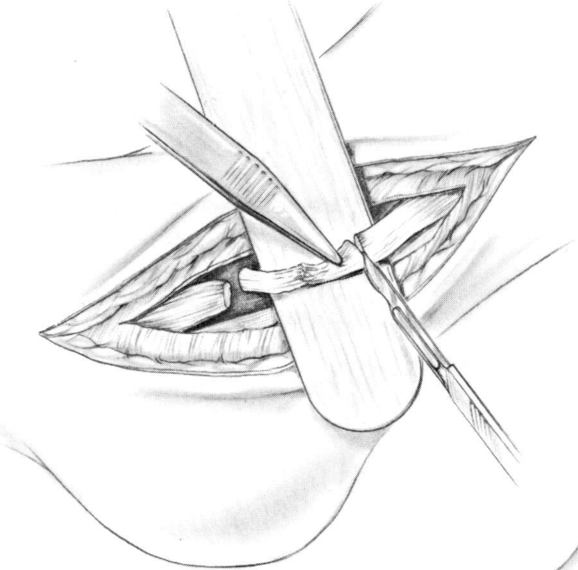

4

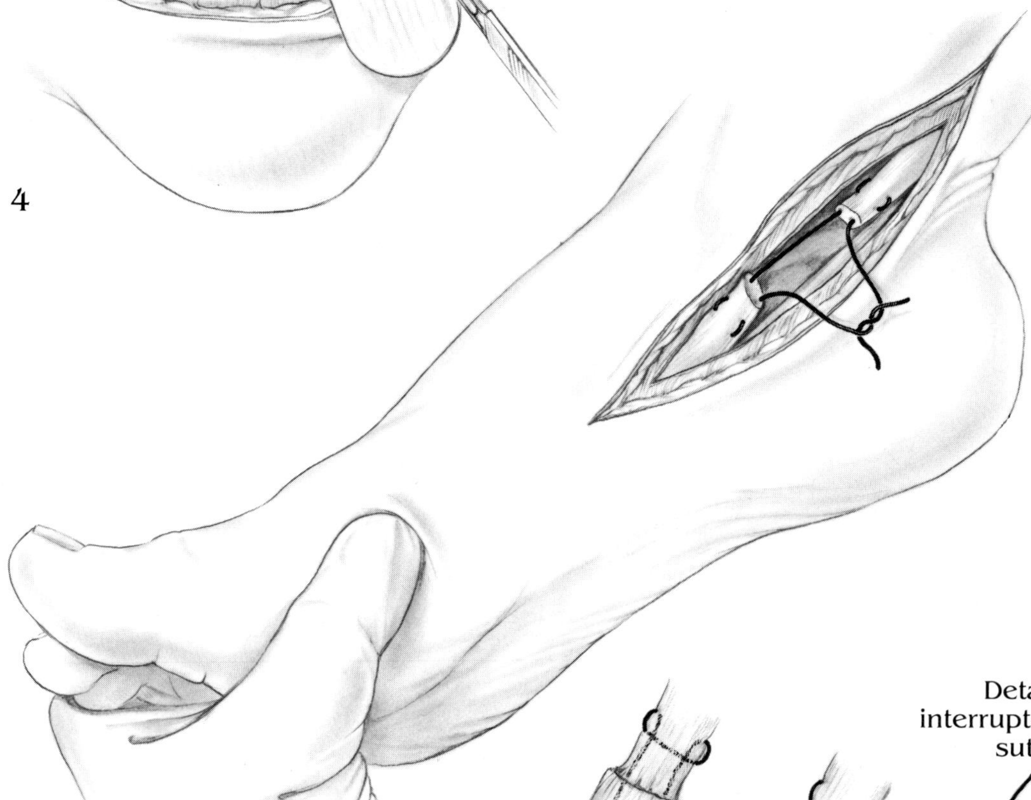

5a

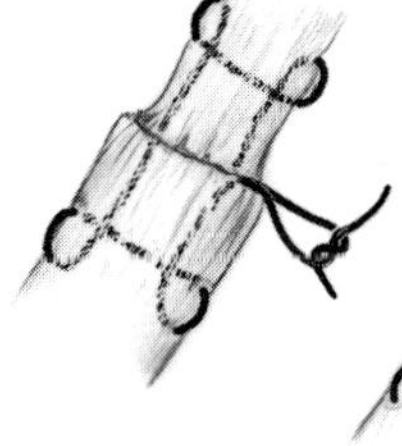

5b

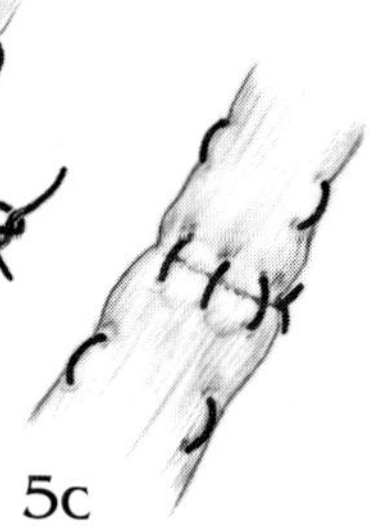

5c

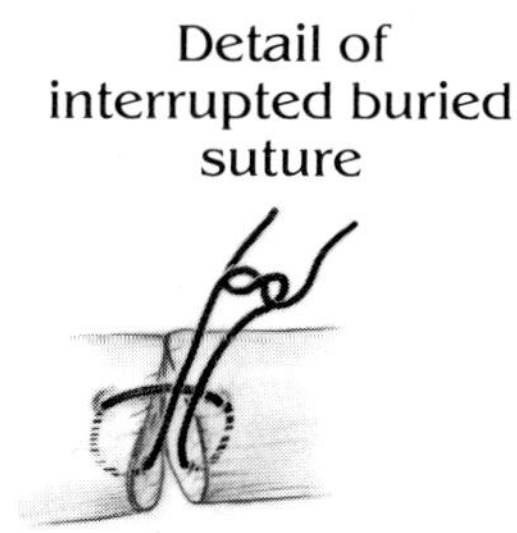

5d

8. The adjacent flexor digitorum longus tendon is identified in its sheath. Incise its sheath and mobilize the tendon (Fig. 6).
9. While holding the foot in plantarflexion and inversion with the toes hyperextended, perform a side-to-side anastomosis of the posterior tibial tendon to the flexor digitorum longus tendon with interrupted simple buried 1-0 nylon sutures (Fig. 7).
10. Re-create the pulley behind the malleolus by reapproximating the flexor retinaculum with interrupted figure-of-eight 2-0 Vicryl sutures (Fig. 8). The retinaculum is often left open for a small distance at its most distal and proximal extents to allow decompression of the tendon sheath.
11. Close subcutaneous tissue with interrupted simple 3-0 Vicryl sutures. Close the skin with interrupted vertical mattress 3-0 nylon sutures.

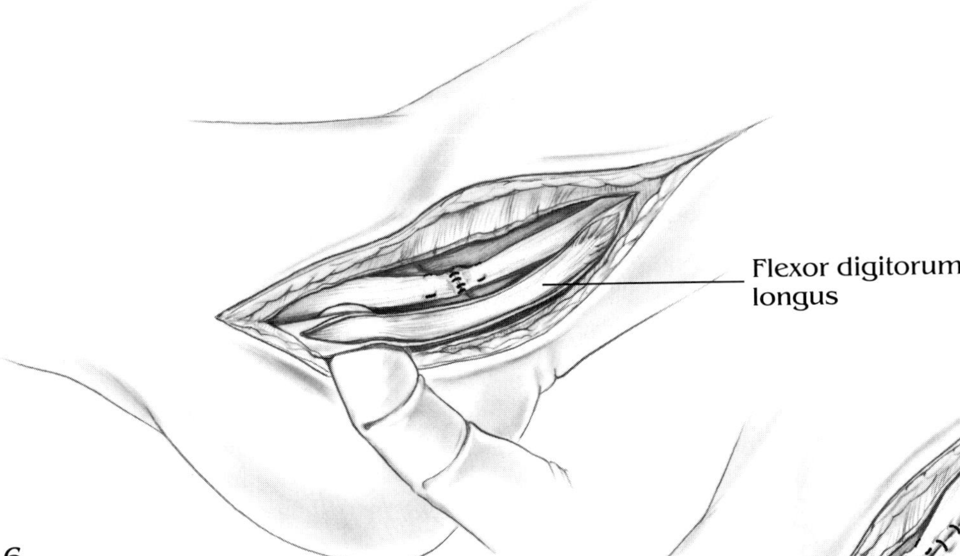

6

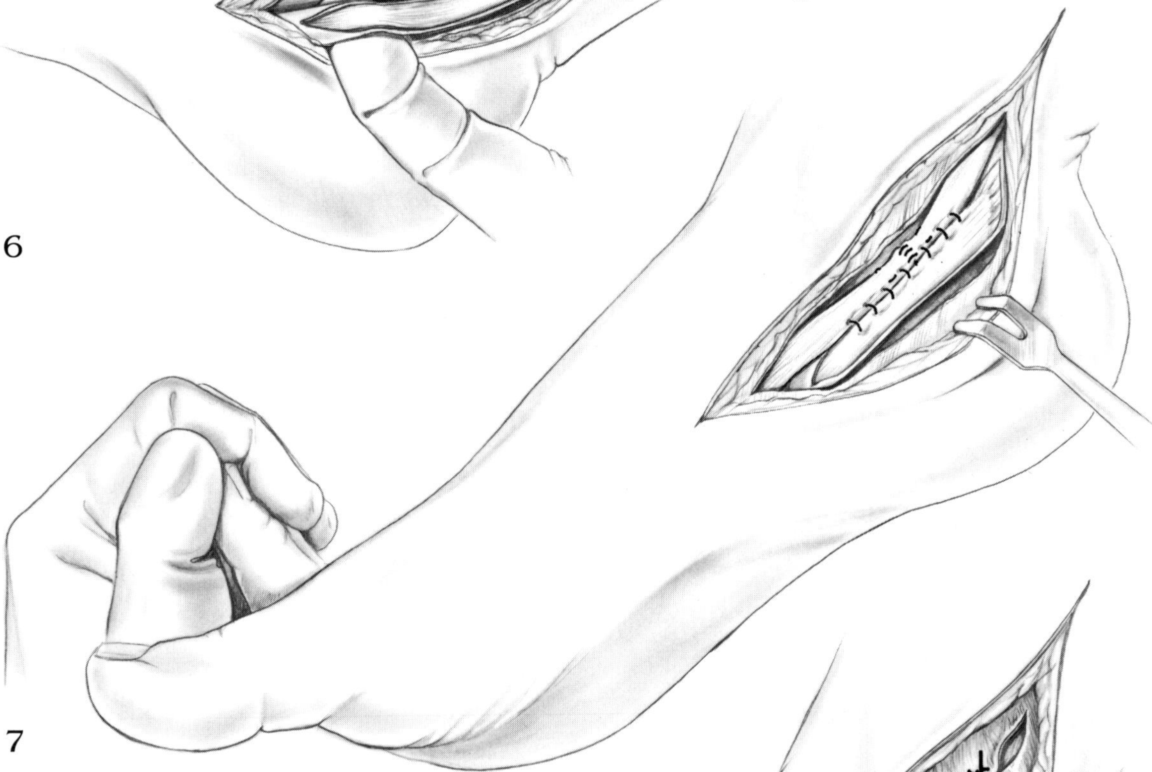

7

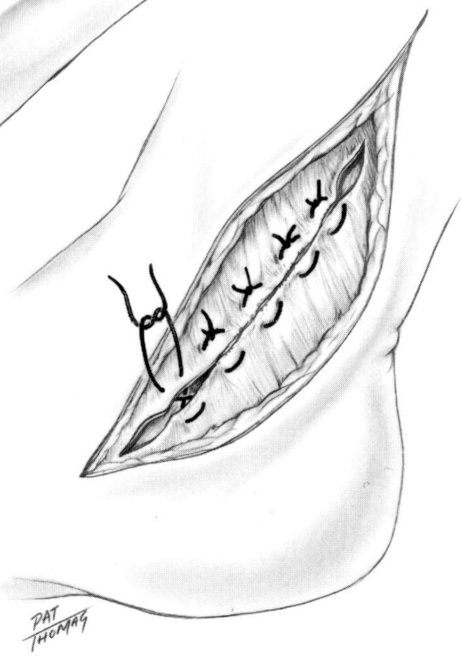

8

Postoperative Care

1. A well-padded short-leg cast is applied with the foot in plantarflexion and inversion.
2. The cast is changed and sutures removed at 3 weeks. A second cast is applied with the foot in a position somewhat closer to neutral.
3. The cast is removed 6 weeks after surgery.
4. The patient is not allowed to bear weight until the cast is removed. A slow, gradual return to weight-bearing activities is then allowed within the limits of discomfort. The patient progresses from crutch walking without weight bearing to partial weight bearing and then to full weight bearing during a 6-week period.
5. Patients are progressed to ambulation with a cane at 12 weeks after surgery.
6. A rubber-soled wedgie type shoe with a ¼-inch medial sole and heel wedge to the outer sole and a soft flexible medial arch support is recommended for the first 9 months after surgery to protect the reconstructed tendon.

Technical Variations

1. If a large gap is noted and the tendon ends cannot be reapproximated, trimming of the nonviable tendon ends and side-to-side anastomosis to the flexor digitorum longus tendon have been effective.
2. If the tendon is damaged and avulsed from the navicular tuberosity, nonviable tissue is excised, and the tendon is advanced for reinsertion into the navicular bone. This can be accomplished by means of multiple anchoring sutures into a roughened area of bone or by advancement of the tendon stump through a drill hole in the navicular tuberosity and suture of the tendon to itself.
3. Transfer of the flexor digitorum longus tendon into a drill hole in the navicular tuberosity has been described in cases in which the distal end of the tendon is absent.

Technical Considerations

1. Only enough necrotic tendon is excised to allow end-to-end repair while the foot is held in plantarflexion and inversion. This allows effective shortening of the attenuated tendon. Typically, significant abnormal tendon is retained. The incorporation of damaged tendon in the reconstruction provides good function of the repaired tendon when compared with extensive resection and reliance on the smaller flexor digitorum longus tendon.
2. The toes are held in hyperextension when performing the side-to-side anastomosis to avoid postoperative clawing deformity.
3. Buried sutures will provide increased gliding of the reconstructed tendon and will decrease postoperative tenosynovitis.
4. The use of modified shoewear with an arch support will protect the repair.

Complications

1. Correction of planovalgus deformity is inconsistent.
2. Patient expectations should include only increased stability during the stance phase of gait and possible avoidance of further progression of deformity.
3. Attenuation of the reconstructed tendon may occur with time, leading to recurrence of symptoms.
4. Rerupture may occur with an injury.
5. Arthritis of the hindfoot may progress and cause symptoms.

REPAIR SUBLUXATING PERONEAL TENDON

General Considerations

The retrofibular sulcus is a shallow groove that just accommodates the peroneus brevis tendon. The peroneus longus lies behind the peroneus brevis in a common synovial sheath. The entire complex is supported on the lateral and posterior aspects by the superior peroneal retinaculum, which is a thickened portion of the peroneal tendon sheath just proximal to the tip of the fibula. Excessive forceful dorsiflexion with eversion, combined with a violent reflex contracture of the peroneal tendons, may lead to rupture of the peroneal retinaculum and subluxation of the peroneal tendons laterally and anteriorly. This mechanism of injury is often associated with such activities as skiing, soccer, and basketball. The tendons usually reduce spontaneously.

Patients describe acute swelling and tenderness in the retromalleolar region overlying the peroneal tendons. Physical examination may enable reproduction of the subluxation by eversion of the foot. Radiographs may rarely show an avulsion fracture of the lateral ridge of the distal fibula at the insertion of the peroneal retinaculum. Initial treatment of the acute injury includes the use of a non–weight-bearing short-leg cast for 4 weeks. Unfortunately, in some patients inadequate healing of the tendon sheath and retinaculum may lead to chronic recurrent peroneal subluxation. Patients note episodic snapping and describe sensations of "giving way" as the peroneal tendons slip out of the fibular groove. Subluxations may be associated with pain and swelling posterior to the fibular malleolus overlying the peroneal tendons.

Nonoperative management of chronic recurrent subluxation may include the use of external braces, which may help hold the tendons behind the fibula. These braces may also help avoid the eversion that can induce the subluxation. If conservative measures fail, surgical intervention may be considered. Various surgical procedures have been described to hold the peroneals within the sulcus. These include a deepening of the fibular groove, bone block procedures, or soft tissue reconstruction. One technique that has proved helpful is the Ellis Jones reconstruction.

Patient Selection

Indications

1. Chronic recurrent peroneal subluxation unresponsive to conservative treatment with bracing
2. Chronic peroneal tendinitis secondary to subluxation identifiable on physical examination

Contraindications

1. Patients with a relatively limited activity level in whom peroneal subluxation is a rare event may be better treated with prophylactic bracing while engaging in rigorous athletic endeavors.
2. Surgical correction is contraindicated in patients with general medical conditions which would contraindicate general anesthesia and surgical intervention.

Surgical Procedure

Operative Technique

1. A lateral longitudinal incision 12 cm long and positioned 1 cm posterior to the fibula is made, beginning 8 cm proximal to the tip of the lateral malleolus. The incision curves around the tip of the fibula and then extends anteriorly and distally along the course of the peroneal tendons for 4 cm (Fig. 1). Subcutaneous tissue is incised along the line of the skin incision. The sural nerve is identified and protected throughout the remainder of the procedure. Skin and subcutaneous tissue are reflected to expose the peroneal tendon sheath and superior peroneal retinaculum.
2. Incise the peroneal tendon sheath and retinaculum and evaluate the peroneal tendons for damage (Fig. 2).
3. Expose the Achilles tendon and dissect a strip 6 mm wide by 6 cm long from its lateral border. The slip is freed from proximal to distal and left attached at its insertion on the os calcis (Fig. 3).

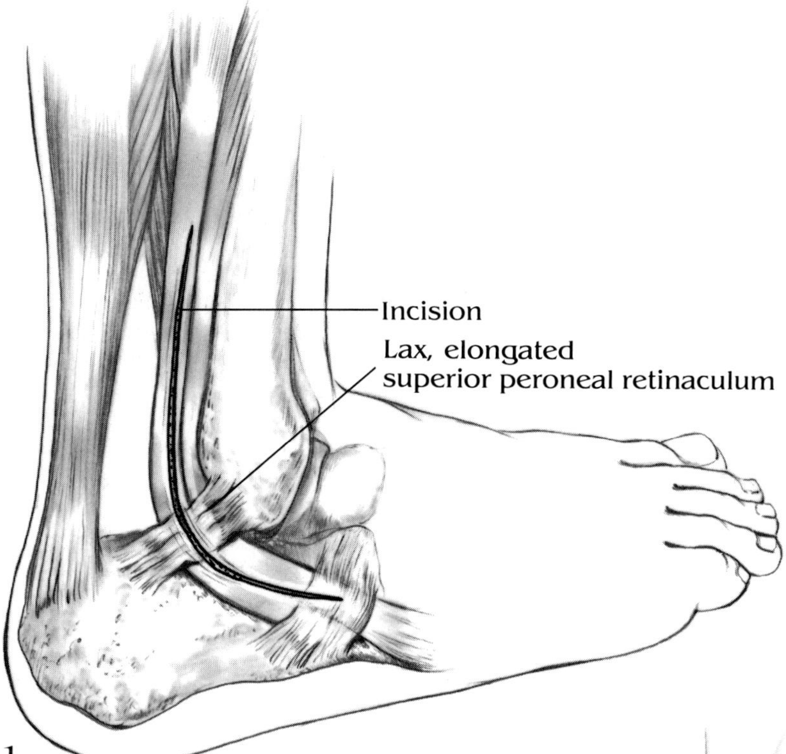
Incision
Lax, elongated
superior peroneal retinaculum

1

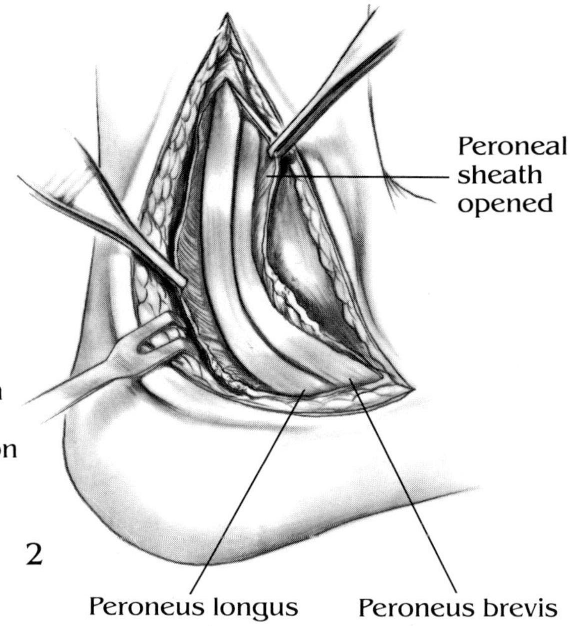
Peroneal
sheath
opened
Peroneus longus
Peroneus brevis

2

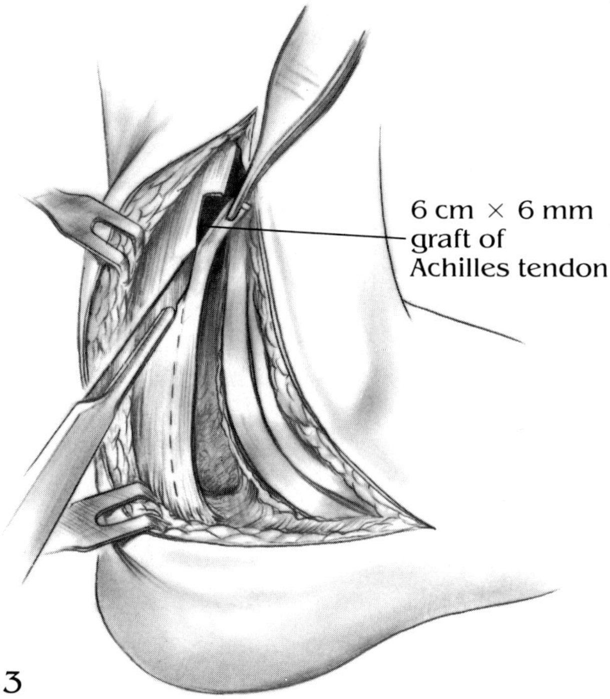
6 cm × 6 mm
graft of
Achilles tendon

3

4. Expose the lateral malleolus and drill a hole transversely through the fibula. The hole is placed approximately 2 cm proximal to the tip of the malleolus from anterior to posterior through the lateral cortex of the fibula (Fig. 4).
5. The tendon slip is passed from posterior to anterior through the drill hole. While holding the foot in neutral position at the ankle and with the graft held taut, the tendon graft is sutured to itself with interrupted buried 1-0 Dexon sutures (Fig. 5).
6. Reinforcement of the anchor of the tendon graft is achieved by suturing the graft to the periosteum overlying the fibula with interrupted figure-of-eight 2-0 Dexon sutures (Fig. 6).
7. The peroneal sheath and retinaculum is reapproximated with interrupted figure-of-eight 2-0 Dexon sutures (Fig. 7).
8. The subcutaneous tissue is closed with interrupted simple 3-0 Vicryl sutures. The skin is closed with interrupted vertical mattress 3-0 nylon sutures.

Postoperative Care

1. A sterile dressing is applied. A short-leg cast is applied with the foot in neutral position at the ankle.
2. The patient is maintained non–weight bearing on crutches for 6 weeks.
3. The cast is changed and sutures removed 3 weeks after surgery.
4. Once the cast is removed, the patient is allowed to begin a slow, gradual return to weight-bearing activity.
5. An air splint is used to protect the repair for 6 weeks after cast removal.
6. The patient is advised to utilize immobilization in the form of an air splint or lace-up brace for rigorous walking and other recreational activities for up to 9 months to 1 year after surgery.

Technical Pitfalls

1. Care must be taken to avoid cracking through the fibula when preparing the drill holes.
2. The drill hole must be placed in such a way as to be certain that the tendon graft lies at the lateral ridge of the fibular groove. This position ensures that the peroneal tendons will remain in the peroneal groove.
3. The sural nerve should be identified in the subcutaneous tissue during the approach. The nerve is identified, mobilized, and protected throughout the remainder of the case.

Potential Complications

1. Attenuation of the tendon graft may occur with time. This may lead to recurrent peroneal subluxations.
2. Rerupture of the tendon graft may occur with a new injury.
3. Injury to the sural nerve may lead to neurogenic symptoms.

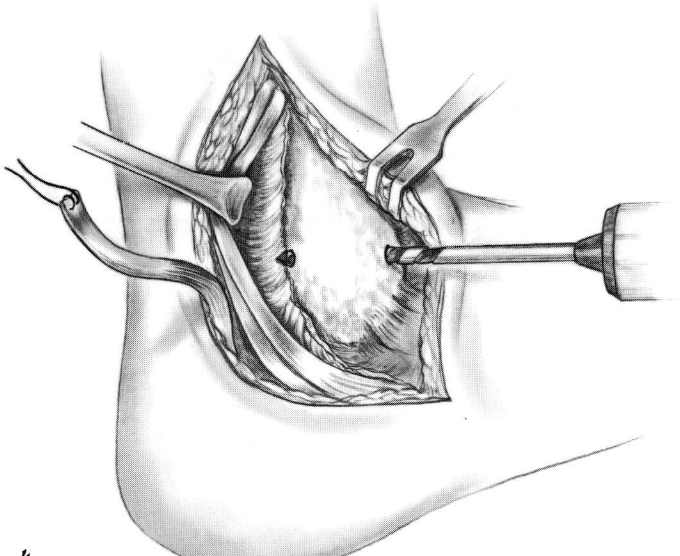

4

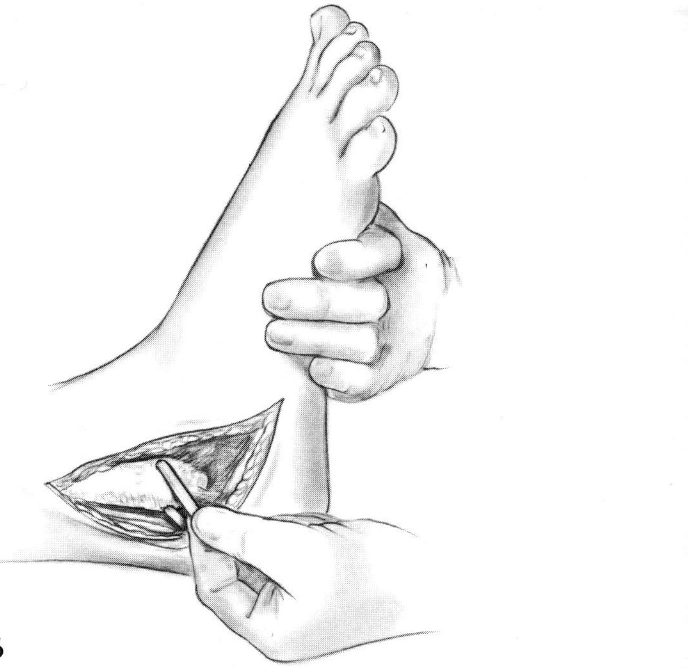

5

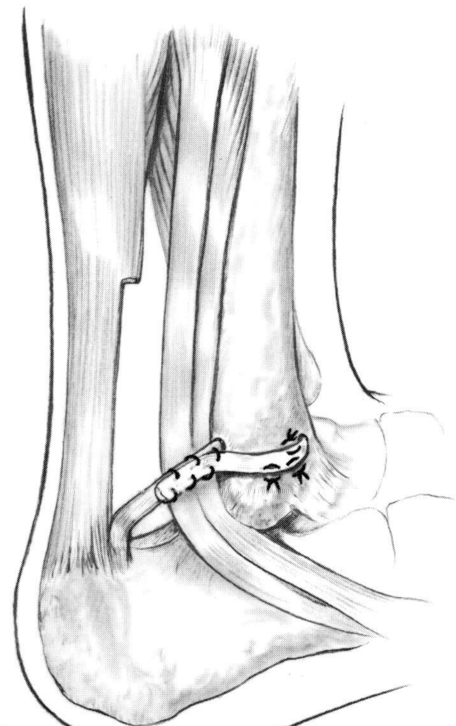

6

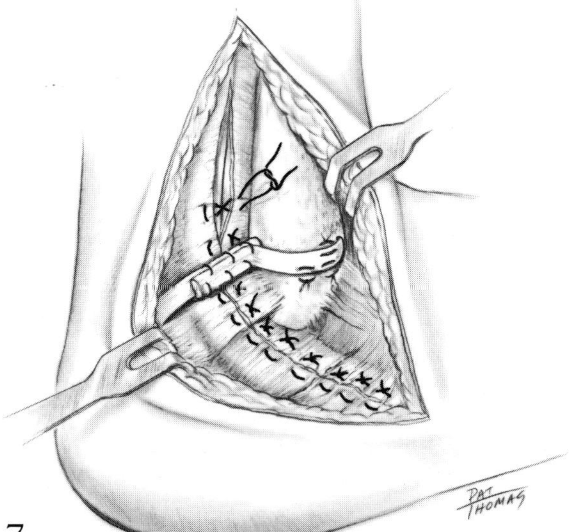

7

PART 25

Ankle Arthrodesis

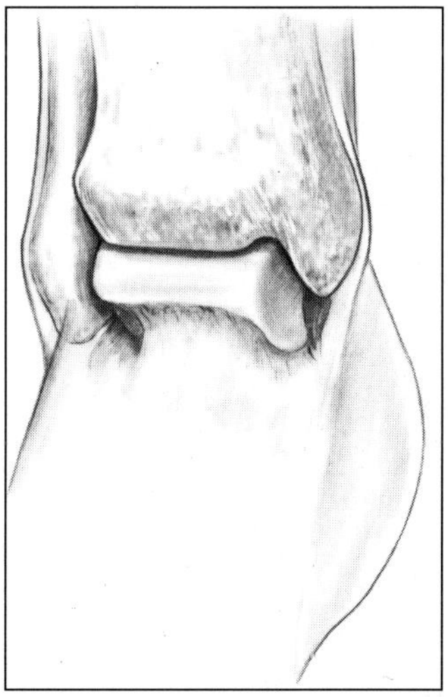

ARTHRODESIS OF THE ANKLE JOINT

General Considerations

Arthritis of the ankle joint may lead to localized pain and swelling as the incongruous articular surfaces grind against each other during activities that require motion or weight bearing. Symptoms may be controlled with bracing, anti-inflammatory medications, and other conservative measures. If these modalities fail to provide relief, surgical stabilization of the ankle may be appropriate. The technique described in this chapter uses internal fixation with compression screws. Inlaid iliac bone graft may help ensure osseous union.

Patient Selection

Indications

1. Degenerative arthritis of the ankle joint
2. Traumatic arthritis secondary to fractures of the distal tibia, malleoli, or talus
3. Rheumatoid arthritis and other seronegative arthropathies of the tibiotalar joint
4. Metabolic disorders such as gout that may lead to loss of articular cartilage and narrowing of the joint space
5. Infectious arthritis
6. Neoplastic disorders resulting in articular damage
7. Malposition of the foot at the tibiotalar joint, including varus, valgus, equinus, or calcaneus deformities caused by congenital abnormalities, neuromuscular disorders, traumatic injuries, or other acquired disorders.

Contraindications

1. Elderly debilitated patients whose general medical condition increases the risks of general anesthesia and surgery
2. Diabetes mellitus
3. Neuropathic disorders
4. Circulatory disorders that increase the risk of vascular compromise or delayed wound healing
5. Active infection
6. The presence of arthritis at the subtalar and/or Chopart joint, which may require inclusion of these joints in the form of a pantalar arthrodesis.

Comparison of This Technique With Other Forms of Arthrodesis

Advantages

1. The bimalleolar approach allows for excellent visualization of articular surfaces, as well as decompression of the typical bulbous distention of the ankle secondary to chronic recurrent inflammation and arthritis.
2. Exposure of the distal tibia medially and laterally allows for meticulous intraoperative evaluation of the accuracy of the cuts and the overall alignment of the distal peripheral extremity.
3. Internal fixation avoids pin tract infection and other problems often associated with external fixators.
4. Compression screw fixation allows excellent approximation of cut surfaces and rapid osseous union.
5. Inlaid iliac bone graft may decrease the risk of pseudarthrosis.

Disadvantages

1. Two incisions are required.
2. Osteotomy and removal of the medial and lateral malleolus may mean that less surface area is available for fusion.
3. If fixation is inadequate, a third screw (posterior or anterior) or an external fixation device may be required.

Surgical Procedure

Operative Technique

1. A longitudinal incision 10 cm long and centered over the fibula is made. This incision extends from 1 cm distal to the tip of the malleolus to 9 cm proximal to the malleolus (Fig. 1). The deep fascia and periosteum are incised along the line of the skin incision. The fibula is exposed subperiosteally. Osteotomize the fibula 6 cm proximal to the tip of the malleolus with a power saw. The osteotomy is oriented from proximolateral to distomedial (Fig. 2). Rotate the fragment externally and remove by sharp dissection with a scalpel and periosteal elevator.
2. Incise the periosteum and ankle capsule posterior to the insertion of the interosseous membrane. Expose the distal tibia subperiosteally. Incise the capsule over the talus and expose the body and neck of the talus subperiosteally (Fig. 3).
3. A longitudinal incision 8 cm long and centered over the medial malleolus is made (Fig. 4). Incise the periosteum along the incision and expose the malleolus subperiosteally. Osteotomize the malleolus at the level of its junction with the shaft of the tibia. The osteotomy is oriented from proximomedial to distolateral (Fig. 2). Remove the malleolar fragment by incising the deltoid ligament (Fig. 5).

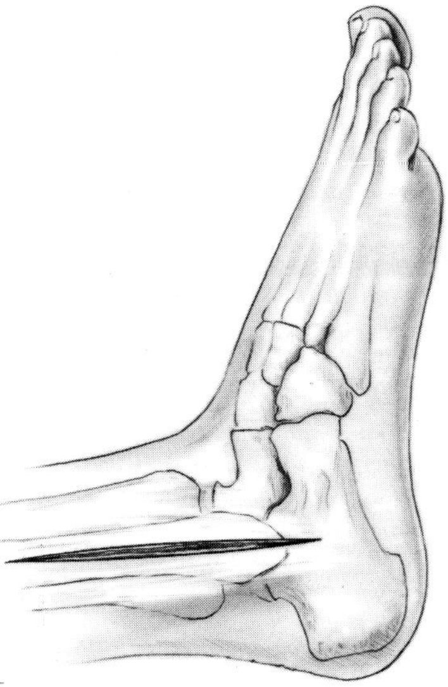

1

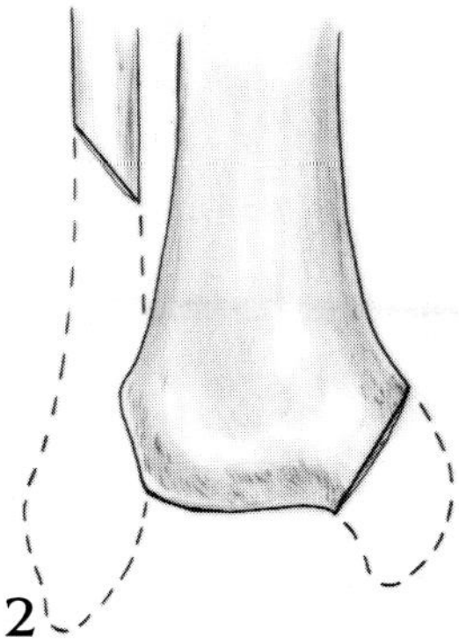

2

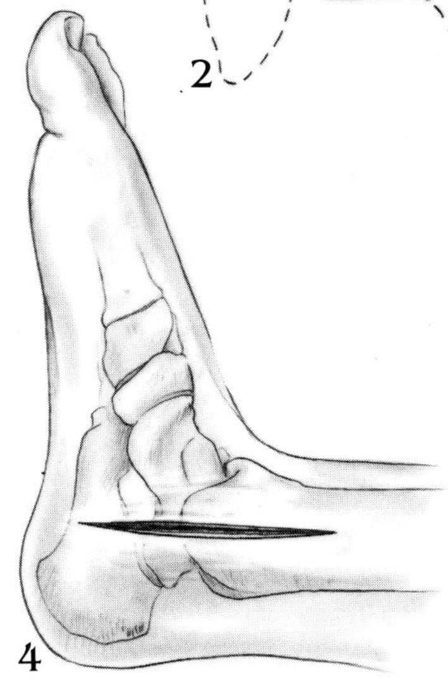

4

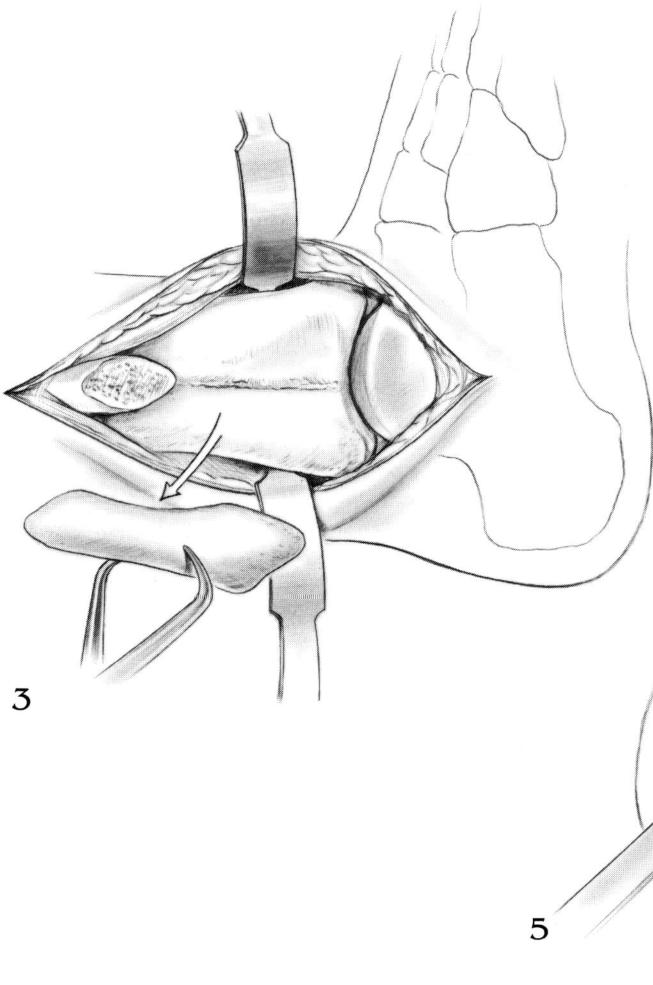

3

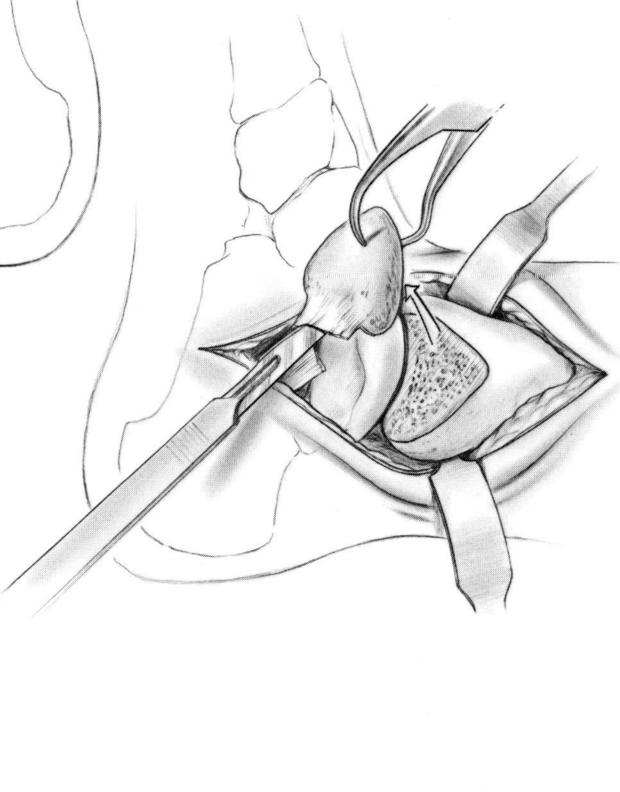

5

4. Excise the articular surface of the tibia from the lateral side. The tibia is cut transversely with the power saw perpendicular to its longitudinal axis (Fig. 6).
5. An axial pin is inserted from the heel into the tibia while holding the foot in neutral plantarflexion-dorsiflexion and varus-valgus (Fig. 7).
6. Excise the articular surface of the dome of the talus with the power saw to the pin. Remove the pin, complete the cut, and reinsert the pin into the tibia.
7. Fixation is accomplished by means of a lateral screw inserted from the lateral tibial metaphysis and a medial screw inserted from the medial tibial metaphysis and extending into the body of the talus (Fig. 8). The lateral screw is oriented 20 degrees anteriorly, and the medial screw is oriented 20 degrees posteriorly. A 6.5-mm cancellous screw or a 7.0-mm cannulated cancellous screw is inserted in the usual fashion.
8. Create a trough 4 cm long and 1 cm wide across the fusion site with a microsagittal saw and osteotome. One trough is made medially and one laterally. Pack with corticocancellous iliac bone graft (Fig. 9).
9. Hemostasis is obtained. Subcutaneous tissue is reapproximated with interrupted simple 3-0 Vicryl sutures. The skin is closed with interrupted vertical mattress 3-0 nylon sutures. A Robert Jones compression dressing is applied.

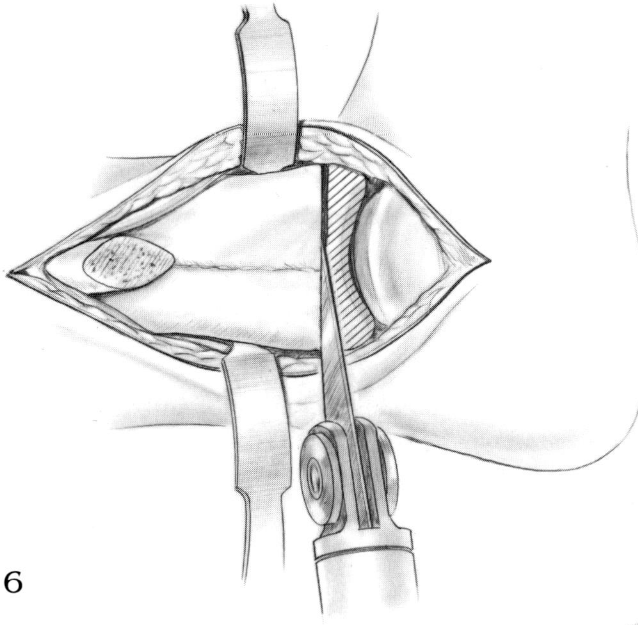

6

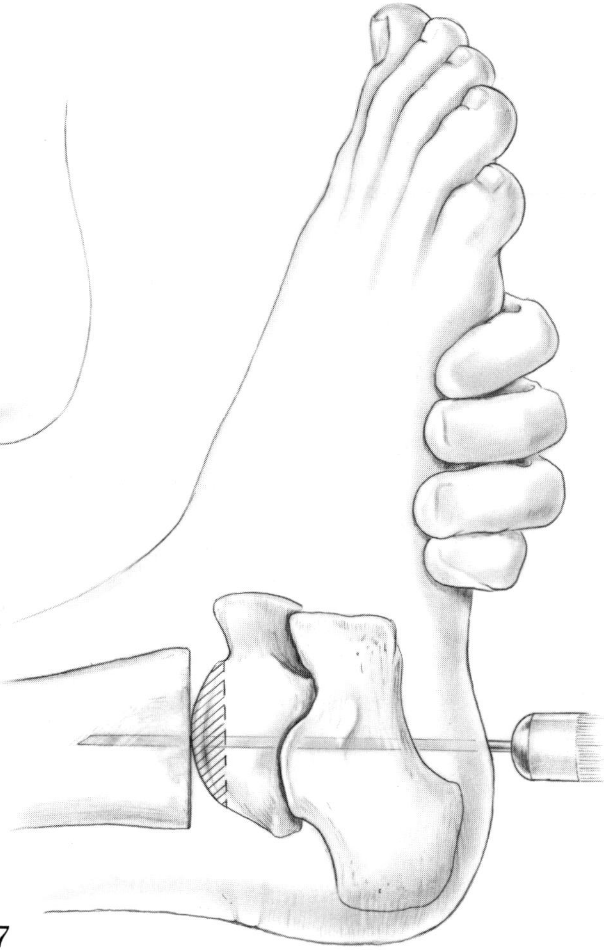

7

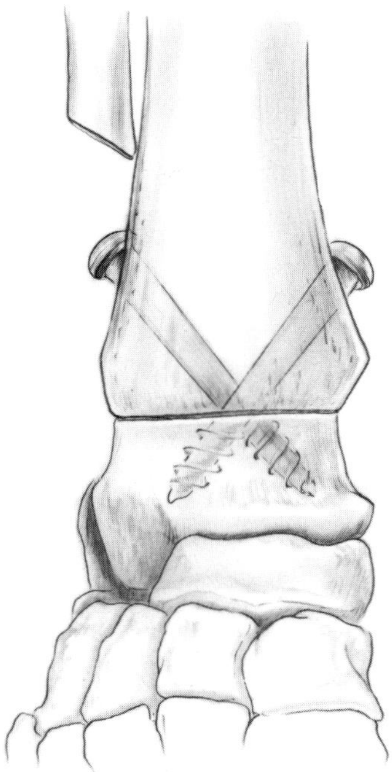

8

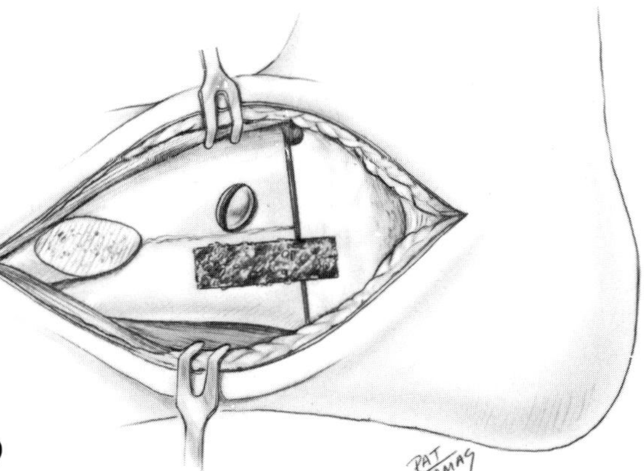

9

Postoperative Care

1. A soft compression dressing is maintained for 48 hours.
2. A short-leg cast is applied.
3. The cast is changed and sutures removed 3 weeks after surgery.
4. The patient is maintained non–weight bearing on crutches for 6 weeks.
5. A short-leg walking cast is applied 6 weeks after surgery. Partial weight bearing is allowed.
6. The cast is removed at 12 weeks after surgery or maintained until radiographs reveal osseous union.

Technical Pitfalls

1. Osteotomy of the medial malleolus performed too obliquely may result in the removal of a portion of the tibial plafond. This error will decrease the contact area available for fusion.
2. Excessive removal of bone will result in shortening of the lower extremity.
3. Inaccurate positioning of the foot on the tibia may result in deformity. The optimum position for fusion is neutral varus-valgus and neutral plantarflexion-dorsiflexion or up to 5 degrees of plantarflexion.
4. Inadequate fixation may require the addition of a third screw anteriorly or posteriorly. If screw fixation is inappropriate, external fixation may be considered. The Calandruccio triangular compression device has proved to be most effective for ankle arthrodesis.

Potential Complications

1. Delayed union
2. Nonunion
3. Malunion resulting in a nonplantigrade foot producing abnormal weight-bearing pressures during the stance phase of gait
4. Infection
5. Excessive shortening requiring external lifts to equalize leg length discrepancies

APPENDIX: Radiographic Supplement

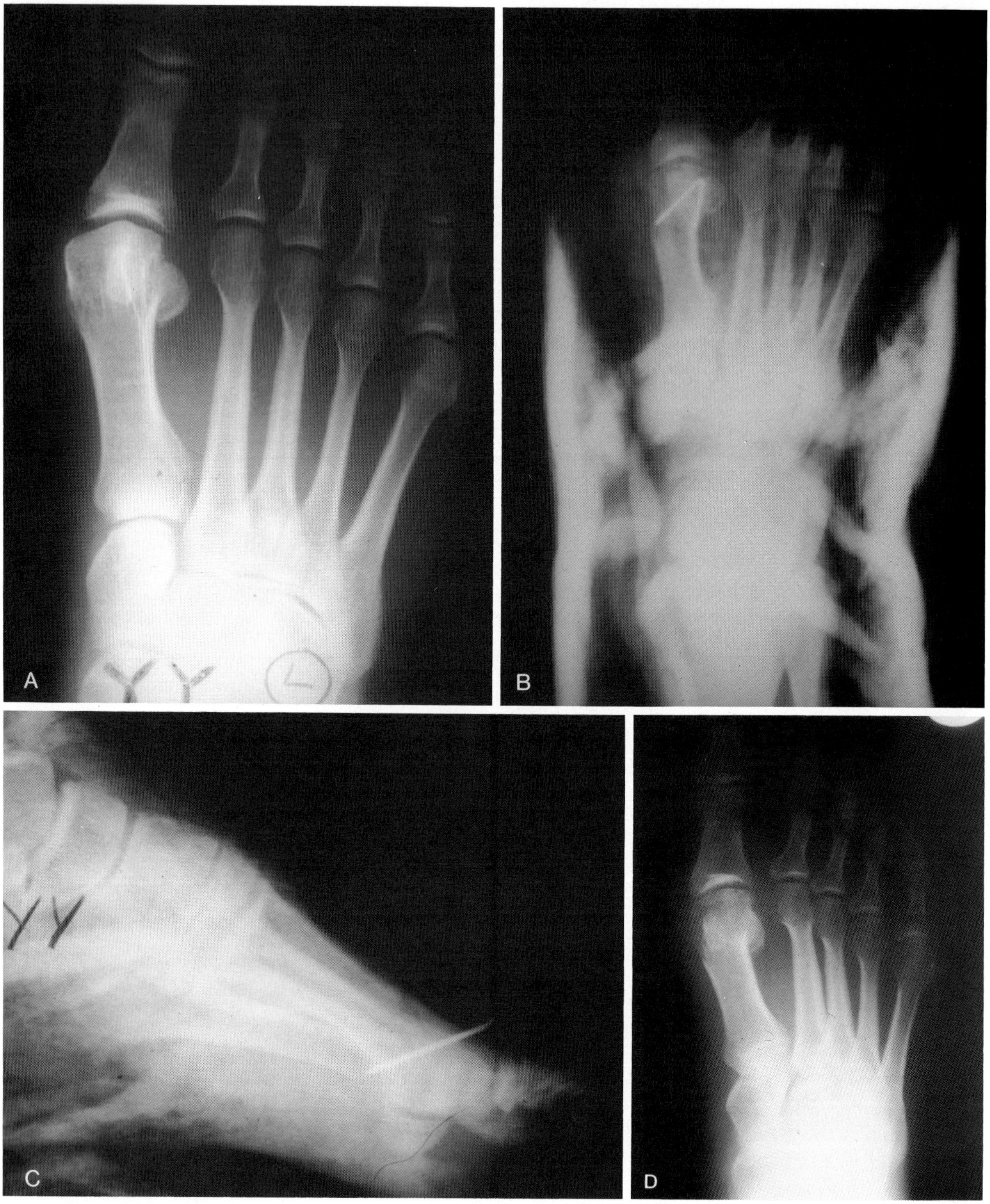

FIGURE 1. Chevron osteotomy. The chevron osteotomy may be utilized to correct a mild to moderate hallux valgus deformity. This procedure provides for reduction of the metatarsus primus varus, narrowing of the forefoot, resection of the prominent medial eminence, and correction of the valgus deviation of the hallux.

1A. Preoperative anteroposterior radiograph: Note the moderate deformity including hallux valgus, metatarsus primus varus, and prominent medial eminence of the first metatarsal head.

1B. Postoperative anteroposterior radiograph: Note the resection of the prominent medial eminence and the lateral translocation of the distal fragment.

1C. Postoperative lateral radiograph: Note the pin placement.

1D. Postoperative anteroposterior radiograph: After pin removal.

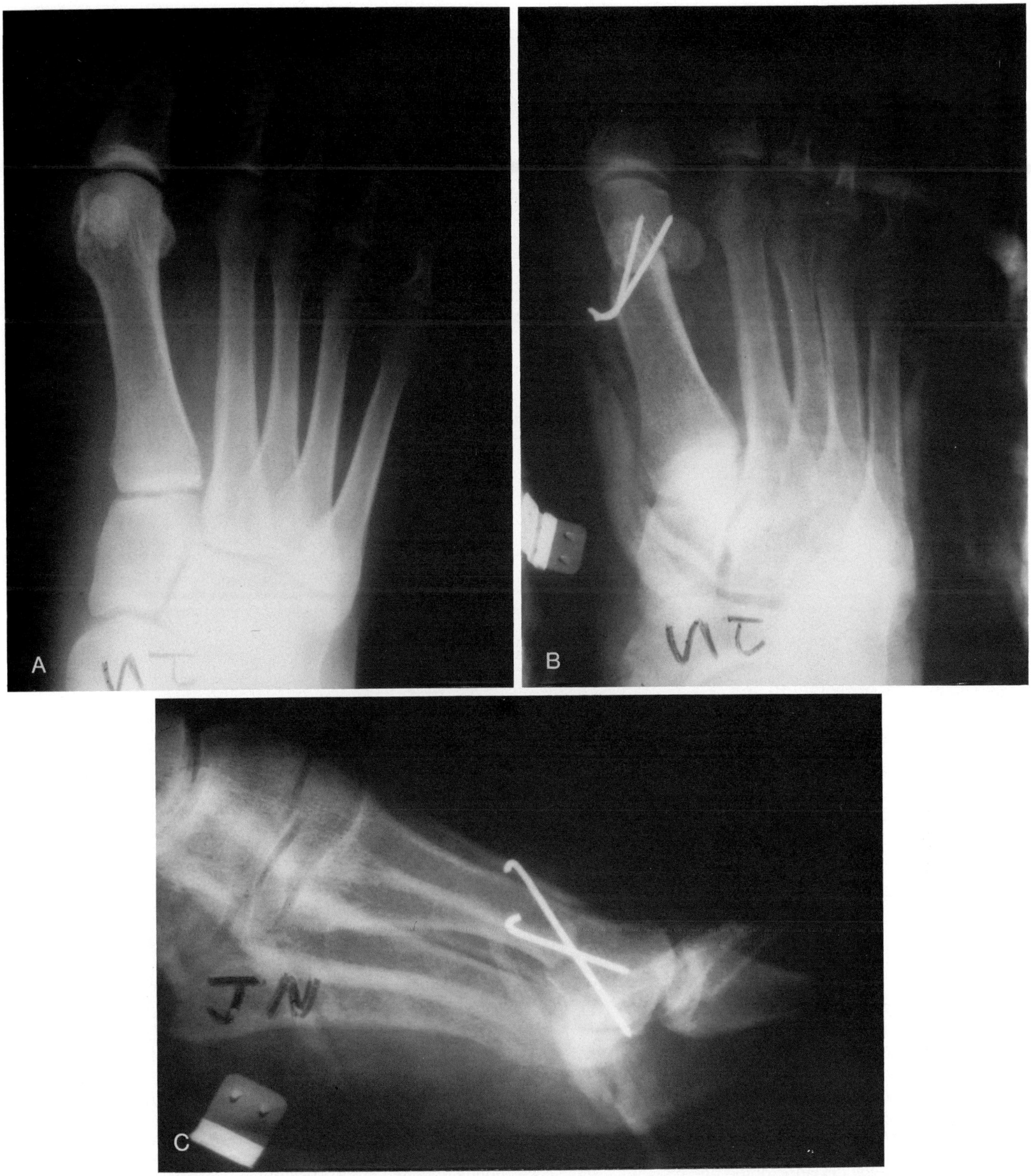

FIGURE 2. Modified Mitchell osteotomy. This operation utilizes a transverse osteotomy made perpendicular to the longitudinal axis of the first metatarsal at its neck. The metatarsal head is shifted laterally to correct the metatarsus primus varus. Plantar displacement of the distal fragment allows for increased weight bearing at the first metatarsal head. Fixation is best accomplished with two cross Kirschner wires as shown here.

2A. Preoperative anteroposterior radiograph: Note the moderate hallux valgus deformity.

2B. Postoperative anteroposterior radiograph: Note the lateral translocation of the distal fragment.

2C. Postoperative lateral radiograph: Note the plantarward displacement of the distal fragment and the crossed K-wire fixation.

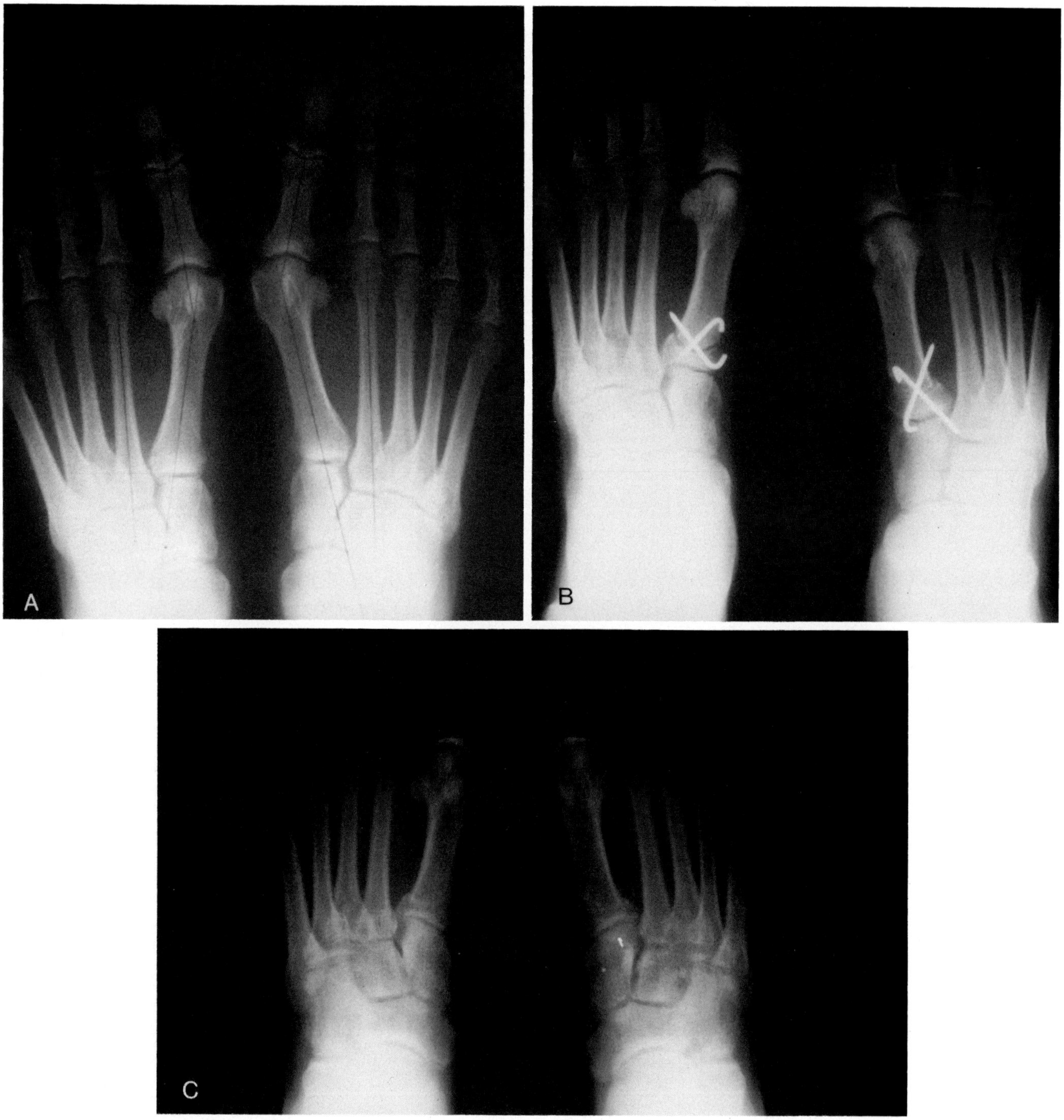

FIGURE 3. Basilar crescentic osteotomy and web space release for hallux valgus. Patients with moderate to severe hallux valgus deformity often require more extensive reconstructive procedures to gain correction of the various components of the deformity. Reconstructive surgery requires release of contracted lateral soft tissue structures, medial capsulorrhaphy, excision of the prominent medial eminence, and osteotomy at the proximal aspect of the first metatarsal. Basilar osteotomy provides greater improvement of more severe medial deviation of the first metatarsal since correction is obtained at the apex of the deformity.

3A. Preoperative anteroposterior radiograph: Note the marked deformity with metatarsus primus varus, hallux valgus, and prominent medial eminence of the first metatarsal head.

3B. Postoperative anteroposterior radiograph: Note the significant correction of the metatarsus primus varus and the hallux valgus deformity. Note also the crossed K-wire fixation.

3C. Postoperative anteroposterior radiograph: After pin removal.

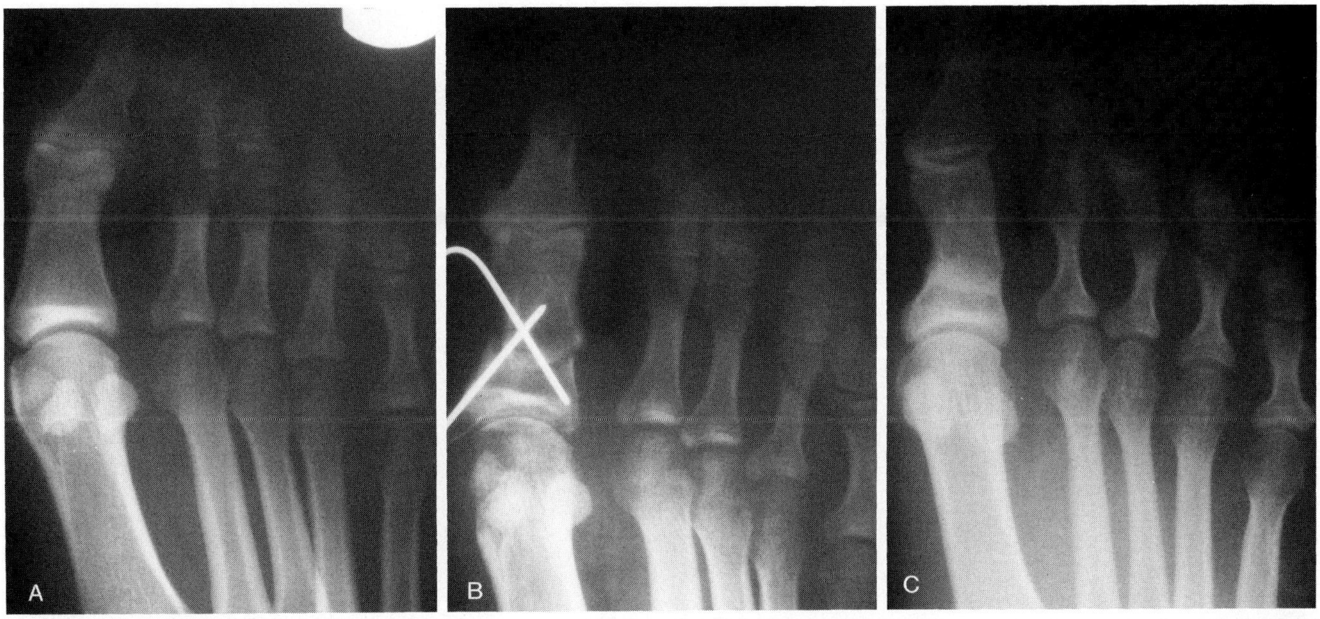

FIGURE 4. Proximal phalangeal osteotomy for hallux valgus. This procedure is useful for correction of hallux valgus interphalangeal, in which lateral deviation of the great toe occurs at the interphalangeal joint. It may also provide adequate correction for patients with hallux valgus with minimal or no metatarsus primus varus. The arcuate configuration of the osteotomy avoids shortening and allows for intraoperative correction of alignment of the great toe if intraoperative radiographs reveal the correction to be inadequate or overzealous.

4A. Preoperative anteroposterior radiograph: Note the significant hallux valgus interphalangeal deformity.

4B. Postoperative anteroposterior radiograph: Note the arcuate configuration of the osteotomy. Note the fixation technique utilizing two crossed K-wires.

4C. Postoperative anteroposterior radiograph: After pin removal.

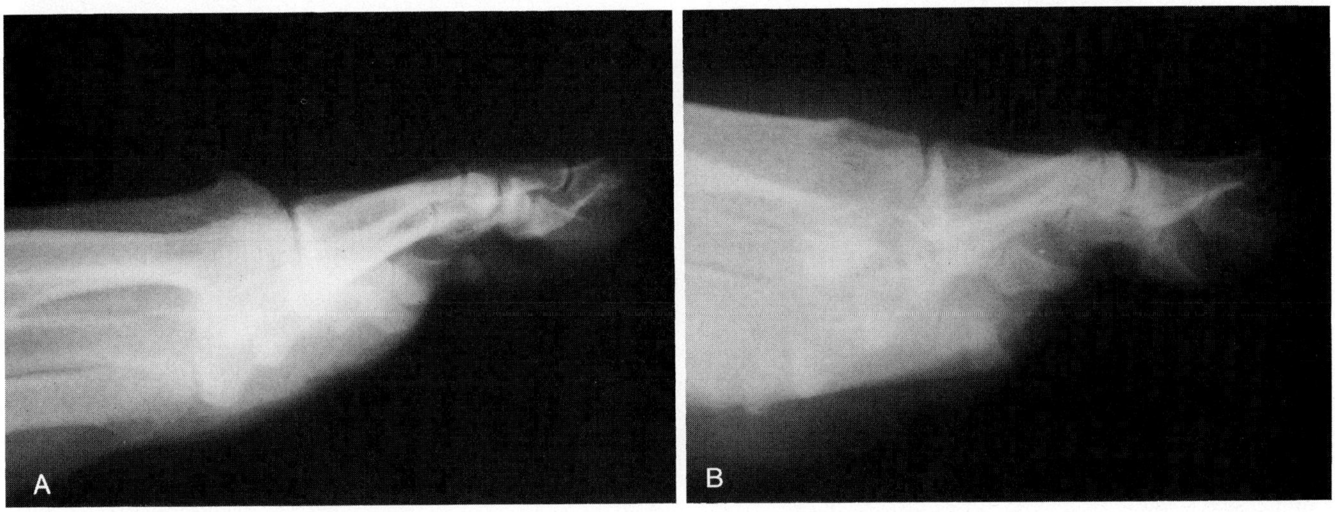

FIGURE 5. Cheilectomy for hallux rigidus. In this procedure the dorsal exostosis at the first metatarsal head, as well as any concomitant osteophyte at the base of the proximal phalanx, is resected. Cheilectomy alleviates the mechanical block to dorsiflexion caused by impingement of osteophytes at the dorsal aspect of the first metatarsophalangeal joint.

5A. Preoperative lateral radiograph: Note the hallux rigidus deformity consisting of a dorsal exostosis of the metatarsal head.

5B. Postoperative lateral radiograph: Note the resection of the incongruous articular surface and the osteophyte at the dorsal aspect of the joint.

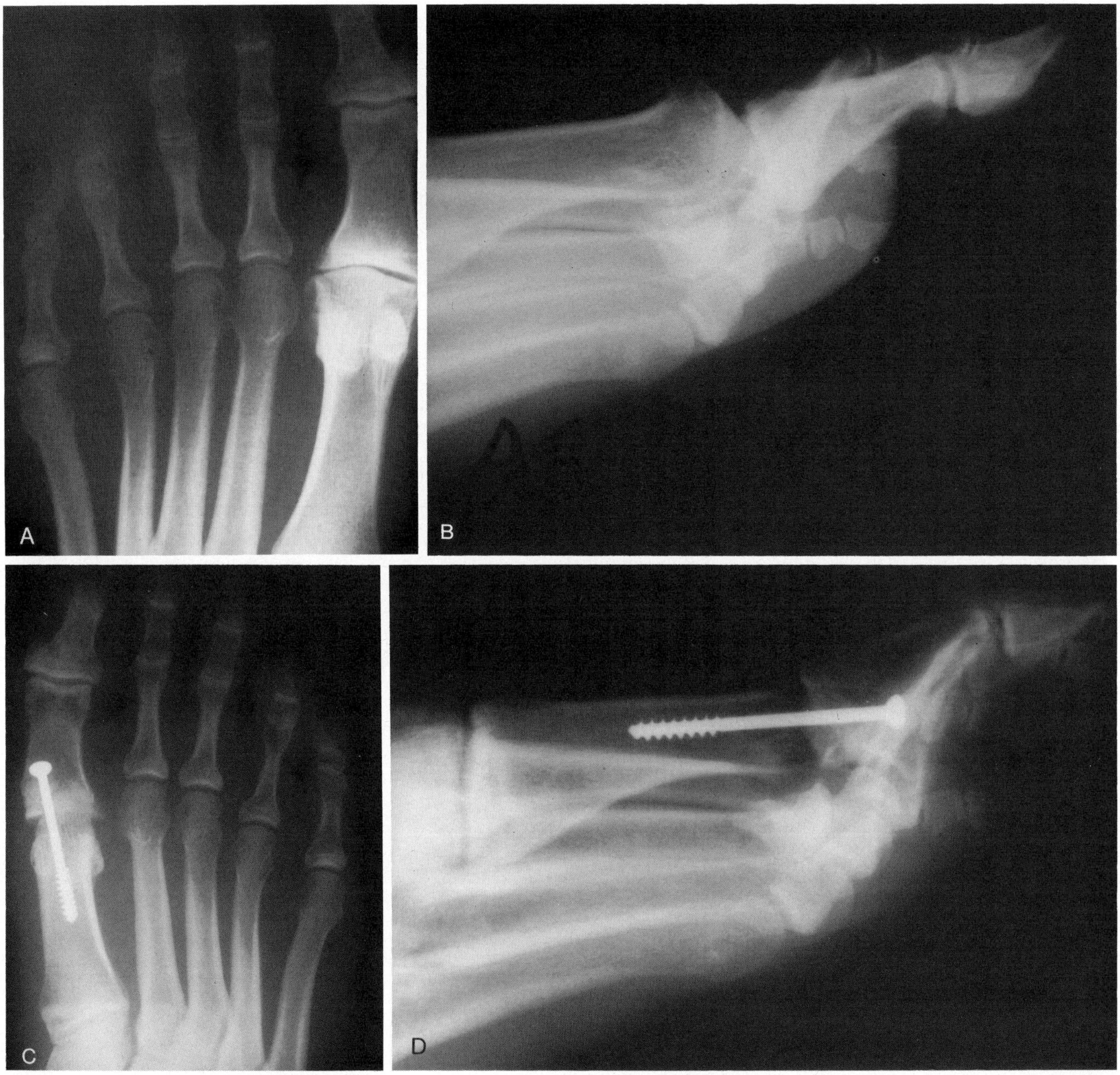

FIGURE 6. Arthrodesis of the first metatarsophalangeal joint. Arthrodesis of this joint eliminates painful motion associated with intra-articular arthritis. Note the cup-and-cone configuration of the bones and fixation with a 4-mm AO compression screw.

6A. Preoperative anteroposterior radiograph: Note the extensive intra-articular arthritis present diffusely throughout the joint.

6B. Preoperative lateral radiograph: Note the articular incongruity present from the dorsal to the plantar aspect of the joint.

6C. Postoperative anteroposterior radiograph: Note the alignment of the great toe. Note the internal fixation with the AO compression screw.

6D. Postoperative lateral radiograph: Note the dorsiflexed position of the great toe and internal fixation.

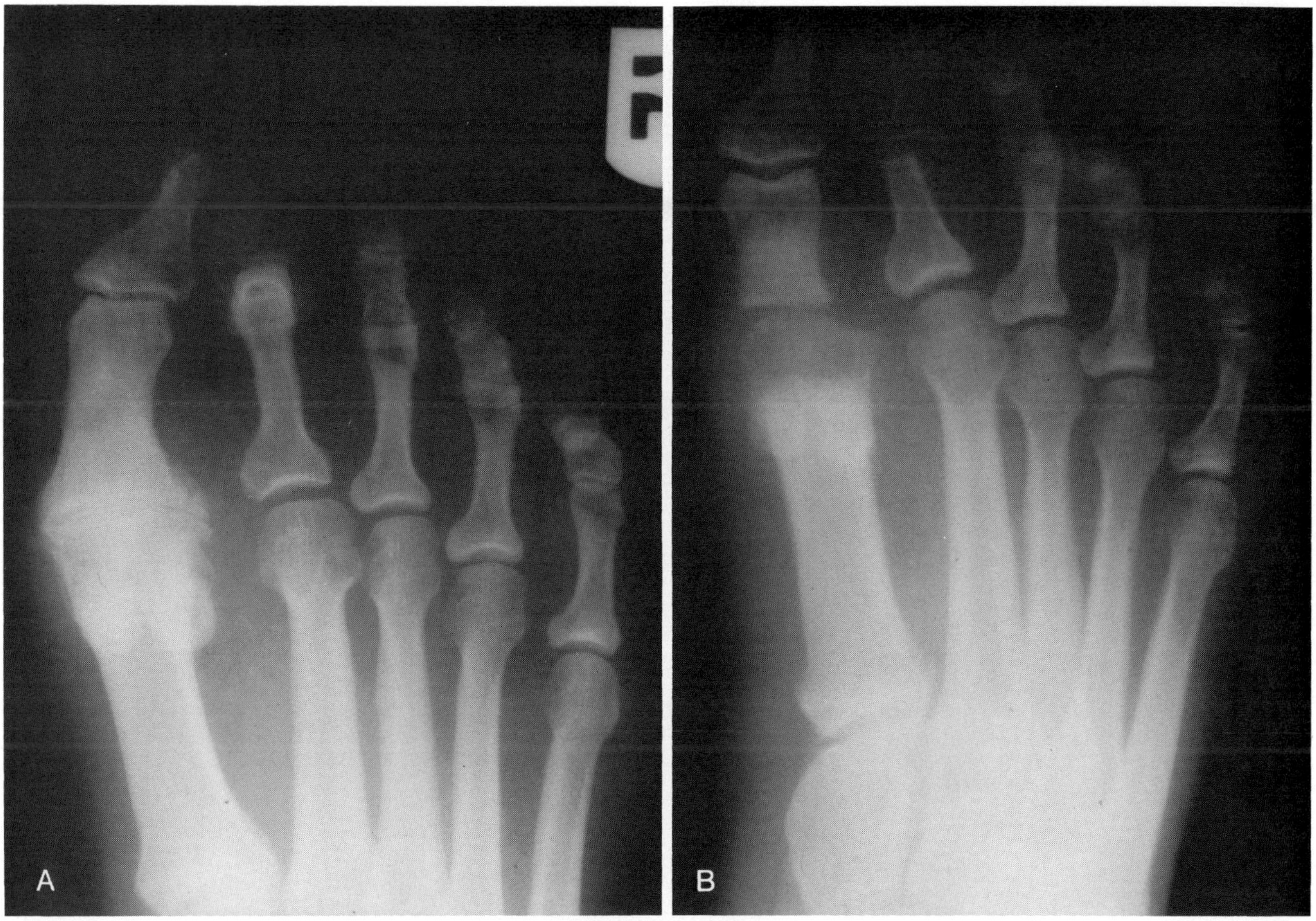

FIGURE 7. Keller resection arthroplasty. This procedure is utilized for correction of severe hallux rigidus and hallux valgus associated with arthrosis of the metatarsophalangeal articulation. It is generally reserved for elderly individuals with limited weight-bearing or ambulatory status.

7A. Preoperative anteroposterior radiograph: Note the severe arthrosis of the metatarsophalangeal articulation.

7B. Postoperative anteroposterior radiograph: Note the resection of the proximal portion of the proximal phalanx. Note correction of the claw toe deformity of the second toe by means of resection of the distal portion of the proximal phalanx.

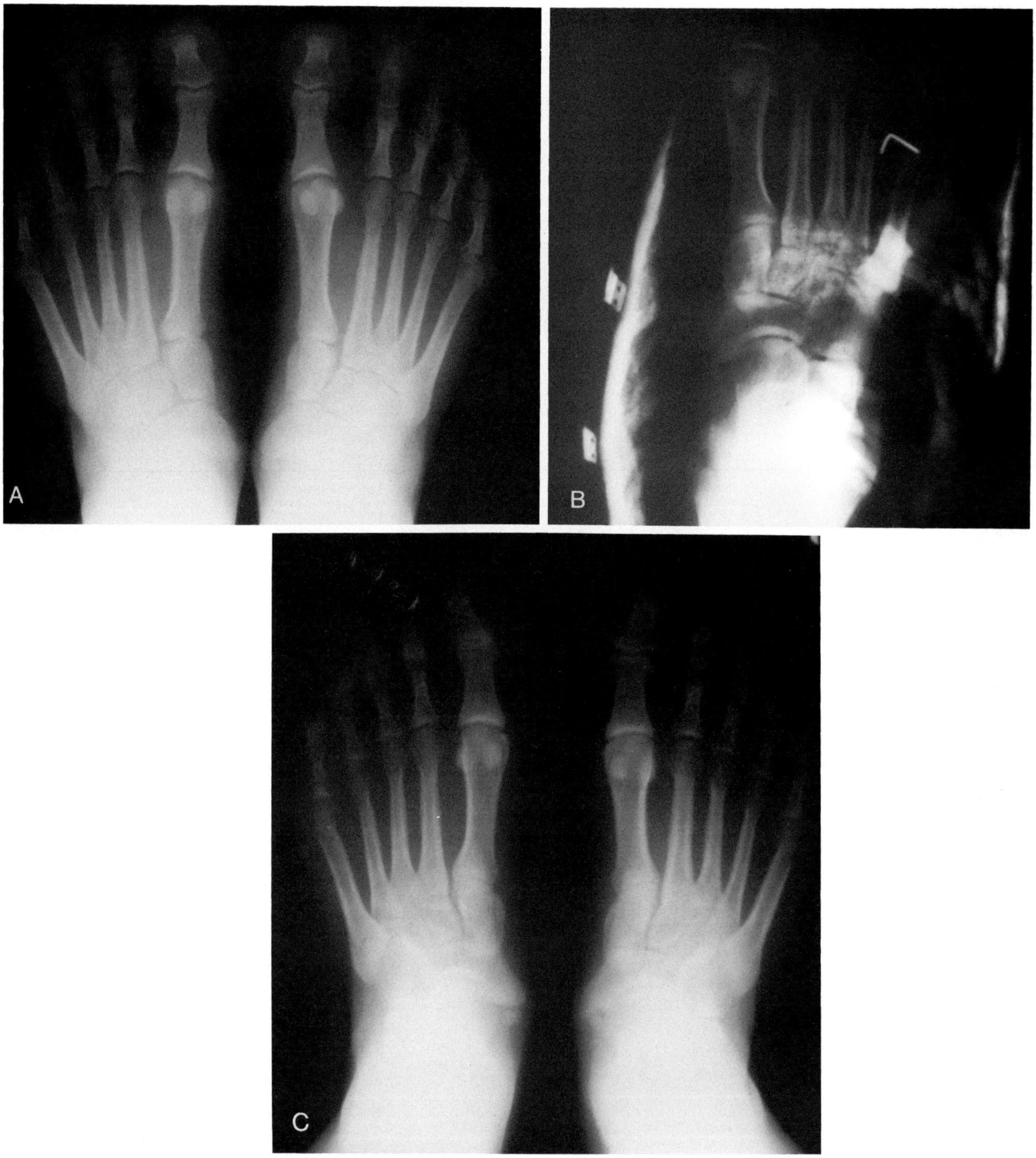

FIGURE 8. Chevron osteotomy fifth metatarsal. The chevron osteotomy may be utilized to correct a "bunionette" deformity. This procedure provides narrowing of the forefoot width, excision of the prominent lateral eminence, and correction of the metatarsus quintus valgus, as well as the medial deviation of the fifth toe.

8A. Preoperative anteroposterior radiograph: Note the bunionette deformity with metatarsus quintus valgus and the medial deviation of the fifth toe.

8B. Postoperative anteroposterior radiograph: Note the correction of the metatarsus quintus valgus and the single pin fixation.

8C. Postoperative anteroposterior radiograph: After pin removal.

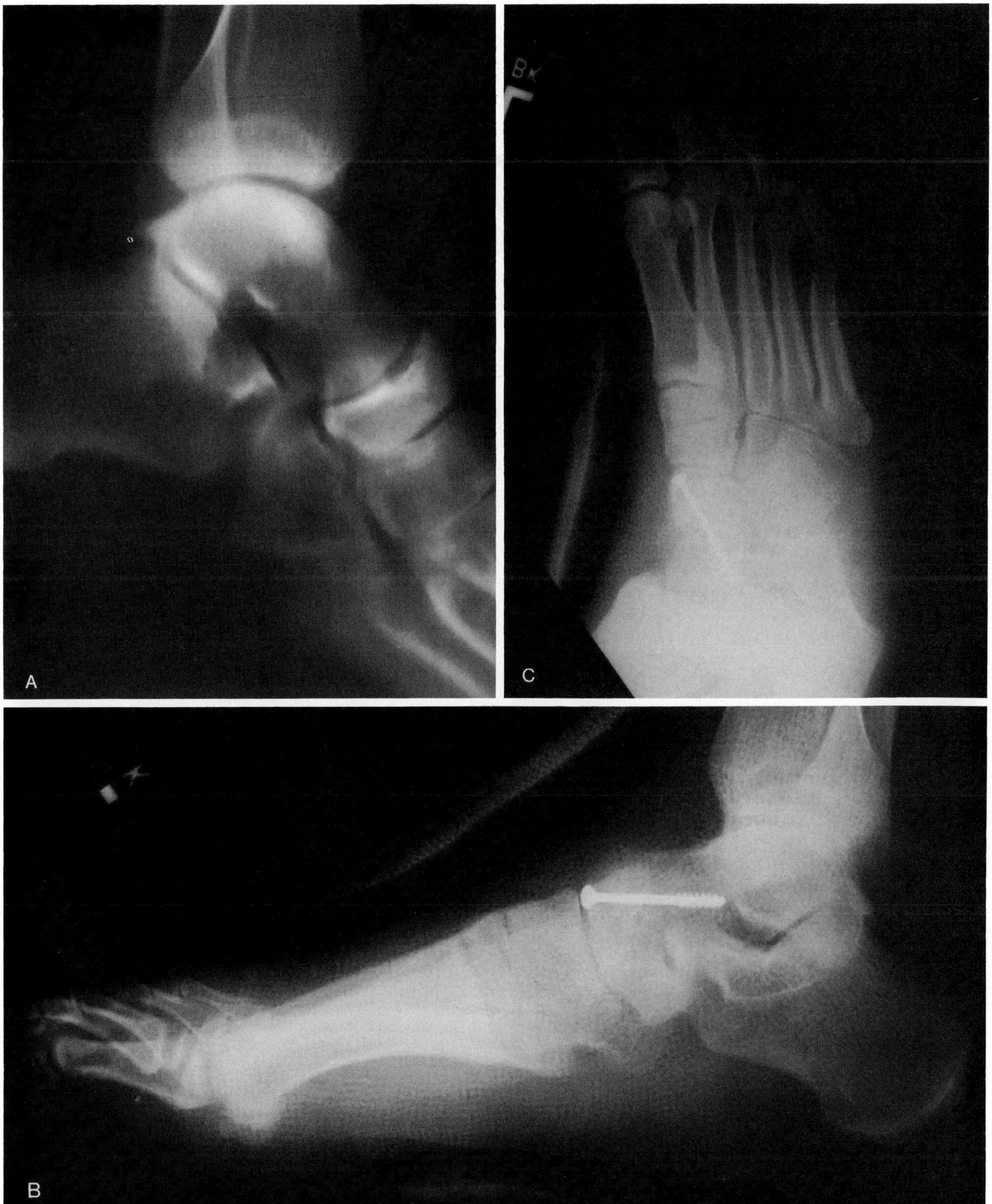

FIGURE 9. Isolated talonavicular arthrodesis. Fusion of the talonavicular joint eliminates pain due to degenerative, traumatic, or inflammatory arthritis of this articulation. The technique decribed utilizes compression screw fixation with an inlaid iliac bone graft.

9A. Preoperative lateral tomogram: Note the incongruous collapsed articular surface in this patient with avascular necrosis of the tarsal navicular.

9B. Postoperative lateral radiograph: Note the cancellous AO screw utilized to obtain fixation and compression.

9C. Postoperative anteroposterior radiograph: Iliac bone graft is utilized to hasten osseous union.

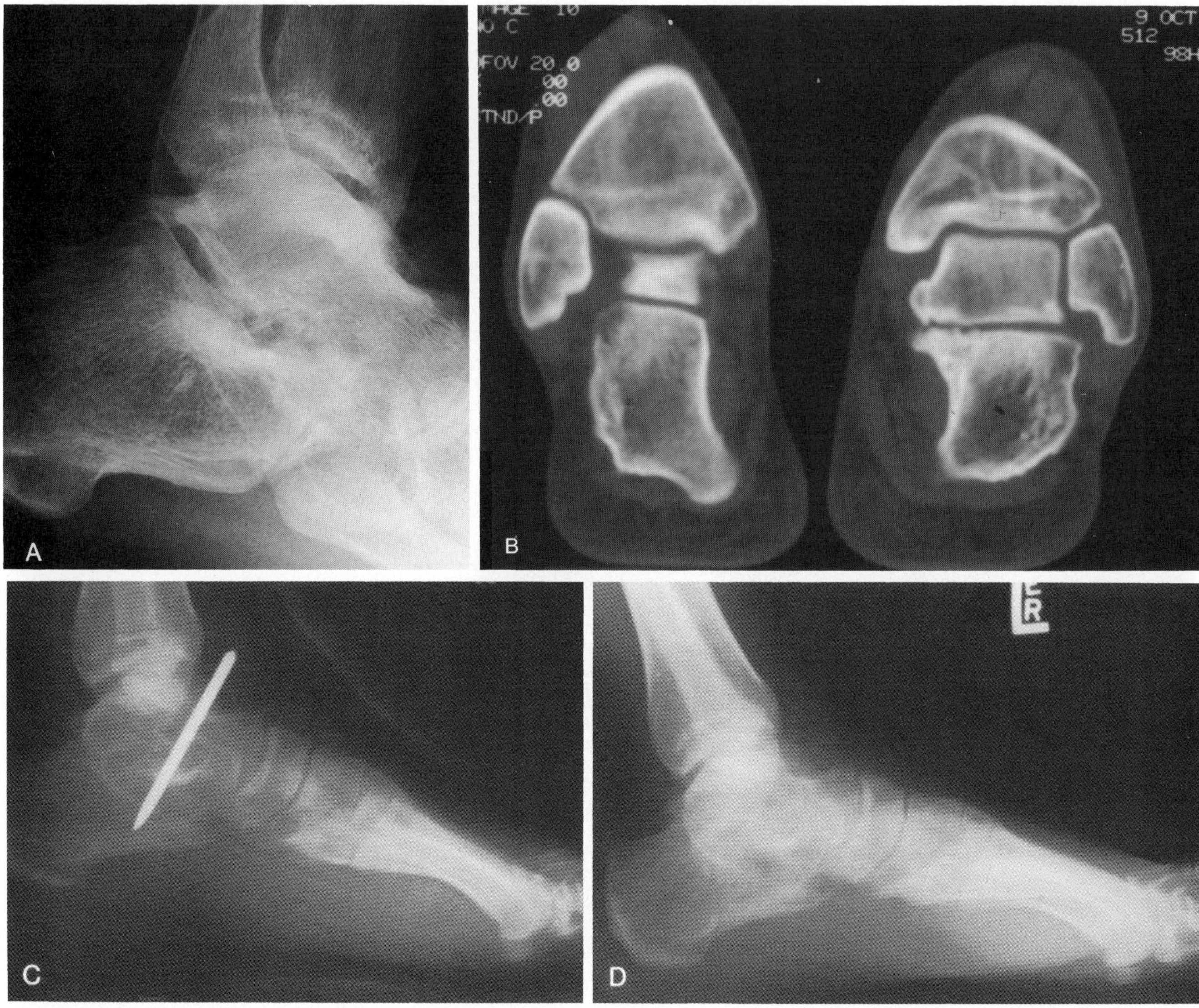

FIGURE 10. Isolated subtalar arthrodesis. This operation provides for surgical stabilization of a deformed or arthritic hindfoot. Note the localized arthrosis in the subtalar joint as evidenced on the lateral and axial radiographs. Note the single pin fixation utilized to maintain alignment while osseous union progresses.

10A. Preoperative lateral radiograph: Note the incongruous articular surface most visible at the middle subtalar joint.

10B. Preoperative tomogram of the calcaneus: Note the articular arthrosis at the middle and posterior facets.

10C. Postoperative lateral radiograph: Note the fixation with a single oblique Steinmann pin inserted from the dorsum of the neck of the talus into the calcaneus.

10D. Postoperative lateral radiograph after pin removal: Note the osseous union at the arthrodesis site.

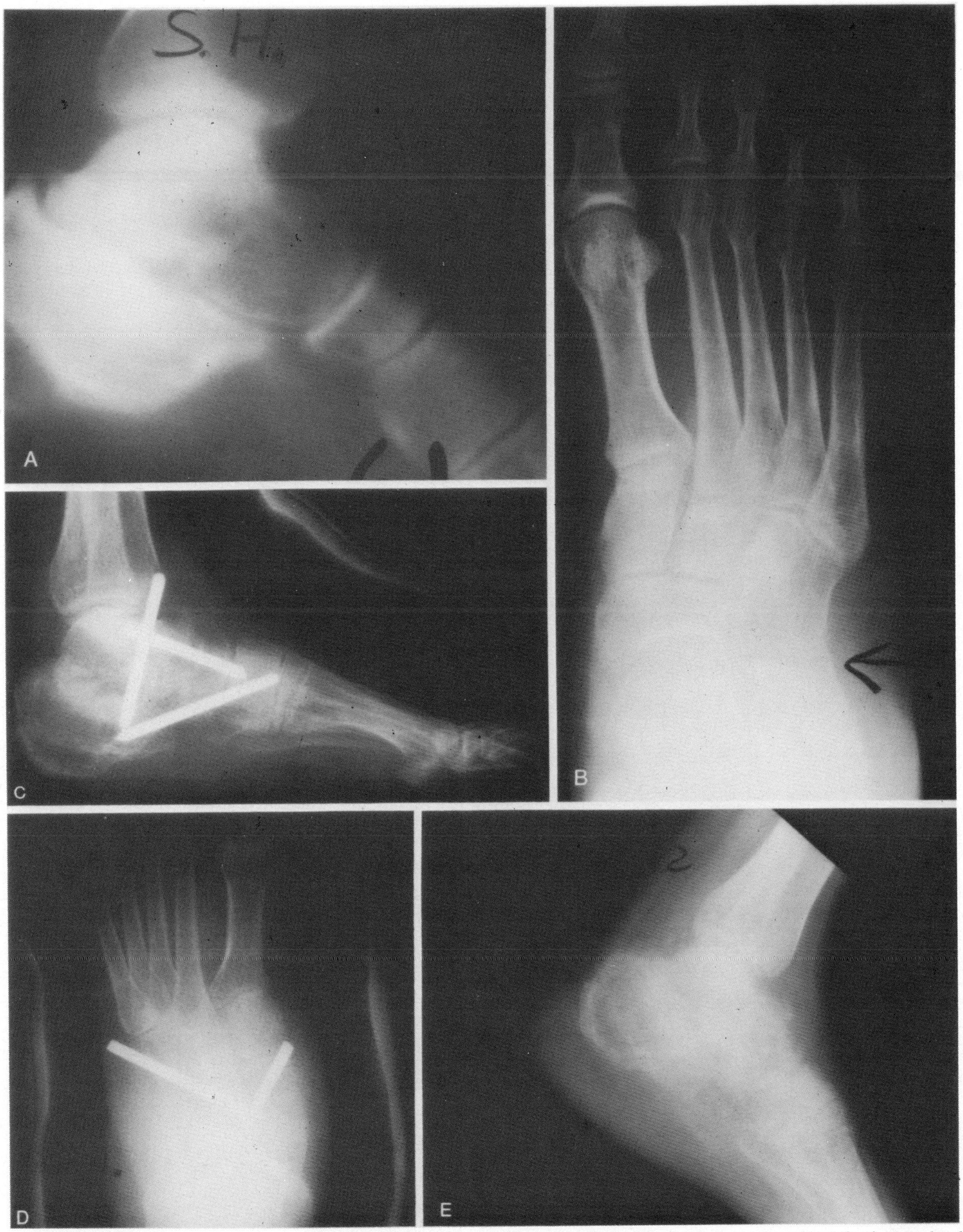

FIGURE 11. Quadruple arthrodesis. This surgical procedure is a further extension of the technique described for isolated subtalar arthrodesis. This operation enables correction of deformity at Chopart's joints as well as the talocalcaneal joints. Note the pin fixation of the talocalcaneal joints, talonavicular joints, and calcaneocuboid joints. The addition of cancellous iliac bone graft optimizes osseous union.

11A. Preoperative lateral tomogram: Note the diffuse articular arthritis at the posterior, middle, and anterior facets of the subtalar joint.

11B. Preoperative anteroposterior radiograph: Note articular incongruity at the calcaneocuboid joint.

11C. Postoperative lateral radiograph: A single smooth Steinmann pin is utilized to fix each of the joints fused.

11D. Postoperative anteroposterior radiograph: Note the pins fixing the talonavicular and calcaneocuboid joints.

11E. Postoperative lateral radiograph: After pin removal: Note the successful osseous union of all articulations in the hindfoot.

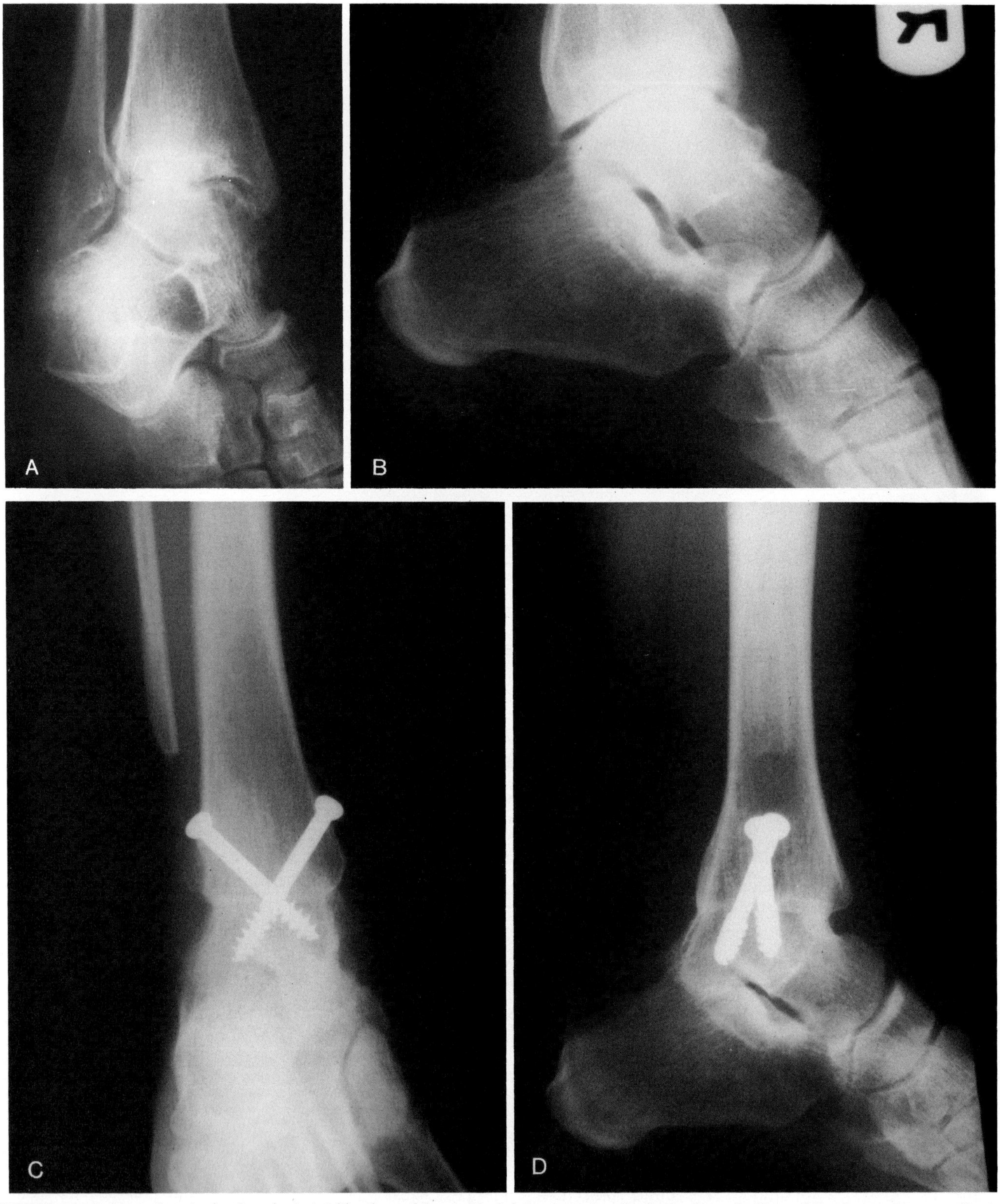

FIGURE 12. Ankle arthrodesis. Surgical stabilization of the ankle joint serves to eliminate the grinding of the incongruous articular surfaces associated with arthritis of the joint. The technique described in this book utilizes internal fixation with compression screws. Inlaid iliac bone grafts may help ensure osseous union.

12A. Preoperative anteroposterior radiograph of the ankle: Note the severe arthrosis present diffusely throughout the entire articulation.

12B. Preoperative lateral radiograph: Note the articular incongruity visualized in this view.

12C. Postoperative anteroposterior radiograph: The technique described in this textbook utilizes a bimalleolar approach and internal fixation with compression screws.

12D. Postoperative lateral radiograph: Note the compression achieved at the fusion site.

REFERENCES

Banks, S.W., Laufman, H. An Atlas of Surgical Exposures of the Extremities. Philadelphia: W.B. Saunders, 1953, pp. 347–349.

Bordelon, R.L. A Surgical and Conservative Foot Care: A Unified Approach to Principles and Practice. Thorofare, New Jersey: Slack, Inc., 1988.

Chapman, M.W. Operative Orthopaedics. Vol. 3. Part XIII. The Foot. Philadelphia: J.B. Lippincott, 1988, pp. 1717–1859.

Evarts, C.M. Surgery of the Musculoskeletal System. Vol. 3, section 8, chaps. 4–6. Vol. 4, section 9, chaps. 1–24. New York: Churchill Livingstone, 1983, pp. 8:115–8:205, 9:3–9:255.

Giannestras, N.J. Foot Disorders: Medical and Surgical Management. 2nd ed. Philadelphia: Lea and Febiger, 1976.

Gould, J.S. The Foot Book. Baltimore: Williams & Wilkins, 1988.

Gould, J.S. Operative Foot Surgery. Philadelphia: W.B. Saunders, in press.

Guhl, J.F. Ankle Arthroscopy: Pathology and Surgical Techniques. Thorofare, New Jersey: Slack, Inc., 1988.

Hamilton, W.C. Traumatic Disorders of the Ankle. New York: Springer-Verlag, 1984.

Heim, U., Pfeiffer, K.M. Internal Fixation of Small Fractures: Technique Recommended by the AO-ASIF Group—Small Fragment Set Manual. 3rd ed. New York: Springer-Verlag, 1987.

Hoppenfeld, S., deBoer, P. Surgical Exposures in Orthopaedics: The Anatomic Approach. Philadelphia: J.B. Lippincott, 1984.

Jahss, M.H. Disorders of the Foot and Ankle: Medical and Surgical Management. 3rd ed. Philadelphia: W.B. Saunders, 1991.

Johnson, K.A. Surgery of the Foot and Ankle. New York: Raven Press, 1989.

Kelikian, H., Kelikian, A.S. Disorders of the Ankle. Philadelphia: W.B. Saunders, 1985.

Levin, M.E., O'Neill, L.W. The Diabetic Foot. 3rd ed. St. Louis: C.V. Mosby, 1983.

Mann, R.A. Surgery of the Foot. 5th ed. St. Louis: C.V. Mosby, 1986.

Mueller, M.E., Allgower, M., Schneider, R., Willenegger, H. Manual of Internal Fixation: Techniques Recommended by the A-O Group. 2nd ed. New York: Springer-Verlag, 1979.

Parisien, J.S. Arthroscopic surgery of the ankle. In: Parisien, J.S. (ed.). Arthroscopic Surgery. New York: McGraw-Hill, 1988, pp. 259–281.

Richardson, E.G. The foot in adolescents and adults. In: Crenshaw, A.H. (ed.). Campbell's Operative Orthopaedics. 7th ed. St. Louis: C.V. Mosby, 1987, pp. 829–988.

Sammarco, G.J. Foot and Ankle Manual. Philadelphia: Lea and Febiger, 1991.

Sammarco, G.J. The Foot in Diabetes. Philadelphia: Lea and Febiger, 1991.

Sarrafian, S.K. Anatomy of the Foot and Ankle: Descriptive, Topographic, Functional. Philadelphia: J.B. Lippincott, 1983.

Tillmann, K. The Rheumatoid Foot: Diagnosis, Pathomechanics and Treatment. Stuttgart, Germany: Georg Thieme, 1979.

Yablon, I.G., Segal, D., Leach, R.E. Ankle Injuries. New York: Churchill Livingstone, 1983.

INDEX

Note: Page numbers in *italic* indicate figures